5624 25/3/88

31.95

WU230 GRO

ENDODONTIC PRACTICE

Endodontics is that branch of dentistry that deals with the etiology, diagnosis, prevention, and treatment of diseases of the pulp and periapical tissues compatible with good health. Its scope encompasses those disturbances or diseases of the pulp requiring pulpotomy or pulp extirpation; treatment and filling of infected root canals by conservative means; surgical removal of pathologic periapical tissue when indicated; restoration of the natural appearance of the crown when discolored; replantation of teeth when avulsed or luxated; intentional replantation of teeth; transplantation of teeth; hemisection or radisectomy; and endodontic implants.

"Never must the physician say the disease is incurable. By that admission he denies God, our Creator; he doubts Nature with her profuseness of hidden powers and mysteries."

—PARACELSUS

ENDODONTIC PRACTICE

LOUIS I. GROSSMAN, D.D.S., Dr. med. dent., Sc.D. (hon.)

Emeritus Professor of Endodontics
School of Dental Medicine, University of Pennsylvania;
Honorary Lecturer, Tokyo Dental College

SEYMOUR OLIET, D.D.S.

Professor of Endodontics
School of Dental Medicine, University of Pennsylvania
Philadelphia, Pennsylvania

CARLOS E. DEL RÍO, D.D.S.

Chairman and Professor of Endodontics
University of Texas Health Science Center Dental School
San Antonio, Texas

ELEVENTH EDITION

 LEA & FEBIGER
Philadelphia   1988

Lea & Febiger
600 Washington Square
Philadelphia, PA   19106-4198
U.S.A.
(215) 922-1330

1st Edition, 1940
2nd Edition, 1946
3rd Edition, 1950
4th Edition, 1955
5th Edition, 1960
6th Edition, 1965
7th Edition, 1970
8th Edition, 1974
9th Edition, 1978
10th Edition, 1981

In Chinese translation
    by Dr. C. C. Dien, 1951

In Portuguese translation
    by Dr. Sylvio Bevilacqua
from the Third edition, 1954
from the Fourth edition, 1956
from the Fifth edition, 1963
from the Seventh edition, 1973
from the Eighth edition, 1978
from the Tenth edition, 1983

In Spanish translation
    by Dra. Margarita Muruzabal
from the Fourth edition, 1957
from the Fifth edition, 1963
from the Seventh edition, 1973
from the Ninth edition 1981

In Persian translation
    by Bahram Nowparast, 1962

In Italian translation
    by Dr. Umberto Bar
from the Sixth edition, 1968
from the Ninth edition, 1980

In German translation
    by Dr. Dieter Schlegel
from the Sixth edition, 1968

In Japanese translation
    by Dr. Kensaku Suzuki
from the Eighth edition, 1977
from the Ninth edition, 1980
from the Tenth edition, 1983

Library of Congress Cataloging-in-Publication Data

Grossman, Louis Irwin.
  Endodontic practice.

  Includes bibliographies and index.
  1. Endodontics. I. Oliet, Seymour. II. Del Rio,
Carlos E. [DNLM: 1. Endodontics. WU 230 G878r]
RK351.G78 1987   617.6'342   87-3272
ISBN 0-8121-1070-6

PRINTED IN THE UNITED STATES OF AMERICA

Print No.   4   3   2   1

Affectionately Dedicated

to my wife
   Emma May
our children
   Clara Ruth and Richard Alan
our grandchildren
   David and Bryan

L.I.G.

to my wife
   Sherry
our children
   Eric, Mary, Amy, and David
our grandchildren
   Jennifer, Daniel, Stephanie, Lauren, Amanda, and Katie

S.O.

to my wife
   Colette Marie
our children
   Carlos Miguel, Denise Marie, Roxanne Marie, and Michael George
our grandchildren
   Christopher Clayton, Colette Jeanine, and Lauren Nicole

C.E. del R.

Preface

In this eleventh edition of *Endodontic Practice,* the reader will encounter two collaborators, Drs. Seymour Oliet and Carlos E. del Río. Both are seasoned practitioners and teachers of endodontics, yet young enough to be aware of the progress made during the last decade in the various disciplines that make up the scope of endodontics.

In a previous edition, I stated, "It is expected that the next great advance in endodontics will be in obturation of the root canal." During the last decade there has been a proliferation of both filling materials and methods of filling the root canal. This has given dentists a greater choice of materials and methods for obturating root canals. Their success in sealing the canal will depend upon their intelligent use of the materials and the care and time taken to obturate the canal. They must be concerned, however, that endodontics does not become more technologic than biologic, and the individual is still the key to good endodontic practice.

I want to thank Lea & Febiger for their excellent cooperation in publishing this and former editions of *Endodontic Practice;* particularly Thomas J. Colaiezzi, Samuel A. Rondinelli, Raymond R. Kersey, Holly Campbell Lukens, and Tanya Lazar.

Finally, I wish to express my gratitude to Drs. Oliet and del Río for relieving me of the burden of revising many of the chapters in the book and contributing new material.

Philadelphia   *Louis I. Grossman*

Acknowledgments

I wish to thank Drs. Joel B. Alexander and Maria L. Canales for their valuable editorial contribution during the preparation of the manuscript. My special thanks to Lynn A. Higginbotham for proofreading and typing the manuscript.

C.E. del R.

My thanks to Hazel Dean, Janice Meier, and Sylvia Cohen, who assisted in the preparation of this manuscript.

S.O.

Contents

1 Clinical Diagnostic Methods

Correct treatment begins with a correct diagnosis. Arriving at a correct diagnosis requires knowledge, skill, and art: knowledge of the diseases and their symptoms, skill to apply proper test procedures, and the art of synthesizing impressions, facts, and experience into understanding.

Symptoms are the units of information sought in clinical diagnosis. They are defined as phenomena or signs of a departure from the normal and indicative of illness. Symptoms can be classified accordingly: subjective symptoms are those experienced and reported to the clinician by the patient; objective symptoms are those ascertained by the clinician through various tests. Understanding of both is essential to the correct identification of disease and thereby to a diagnosis of the problem that brought the patient to the clinician.

Because many diseases have similar symptoms, the clinician must be astute in determining the correct diagnosis. Differential diagnosis is the most common procedure. This technique distinguishes one disease from several other similar disorders by identifying their differences. Diagnosis by exclusion, on the other hand, eliminates all possible diseases under consideration until one remaining disease correctly explains the patient's symptoms. Although proper clinical diagnosis may appear to be simple, it can tax the most experienced clinician.

The process begins with the initial telephone call requesting an appointment for some specific reason, usually a complaint of pain. Subjective information is supplied by the written history or questionnaire that each patient completes and signs. Further information is obtained by the clinician, who reviews the questionnaire and asks specific questions regarding the patient's chief complaint, past medical history, past dental history, and current medical and dental status. The clinician should not hesitate to consult the patient's physician whenever the patient appears to be medically compromised or "brittle," or when the gleaned information is inadequate or unclear. More often than not, a patient's medical problem affects the course of treatment, especially concerning the use of anesthetics, antibiotics, and analgesics. On occasion, however, the patient's medical status bears a direct relation to the clinical diagnosis. For example, diffuse pain in the mandibular left molars may be referred pain caused by angina pectoris, or bizarre symptoms may be the result of psychogenic or neurologic disorders (Fig. 1–1).

HISTORY AND RECORD

To avoid irrelevant information and to prevent errors of omission in clinical tests, the clinician must establish a routine for examination. The sequence of examination should be printed on the patient's chart and should act as a guide to proper diagnostic habits (Fig. 1–2).

Questions concerning the patient's chief complaint, past medical history, and past dental history are reviewed. If more information is needed, further questions should be directed to the patient and should be recorded carefully.

Subjective Symptoms

The completed medical form concerning the patient's past medical and dental history consists of subjective symptoms. Included in this category is the patient's reason for seeing the dentist, or chief complaint. Generally, a chief complaint relates to pain, swelling, lack of function, or esthetics. It may be simply "something on the x ray," which the patient has brought with him. Whatever the reason, the patient's chief complaint is the best starting point for a correct diagnosis.

Pain

The most common complaint that leads to dental treatment is pain. Judicious questioning about the pain can aid the diagnostician in developing a tentative diagnosis quickly.

Seymour Oliet, D.D.S. Associates

Seymour Oliet, D.D.S. • *Alan M. Barnett, B.D.S.* • *Andrew D. Greenstein, D.M.D.*

ENDODONTICS

HEALTH QUESTIONNAIRE   (PLEASE PRINT)

Name ――――――――――――――――――――――――― Spouse's Name ―――――――――――――
            Last   First   M.I.

Address   H: ――――――――――――――――――――――― Home Phone ――――――――――――――

            City   State   Zip Code

            W: ――――――――――――――――――――――― Work Phone ――――――――――――――

            City   State   Zip Code

Birthdate ――――――――――― Sex ――――――― Height ――――――― Weight ――――――――

Occupation ――――――――――――――――――――――――――

PLEASE ANSWER EACH QUESTION   CIRCLE

1. Are you in good health?   Yes   No

2. Name & Address of your physician ――――――――――――――――――――――――
    ――
    ――

3. Have you been a patient in a hospital during the past 2 years? Yes   No

4. Have you been under the care of a physician during
        the past 2 years?   Yes   No

5. Have you taken any kind of medicine or drugs during
        the past year?   Yes   No

6. Are you taking any medication now? If so, name them. ――――――――――――
    ――
    ――

7. Are you allergic to penicillin, local anaesthetics, pain killers, or any drugs?
    If so, which drugs: ――――――――――――――――――――――――――――――
    ――

8. Circle any of the following which you have had:

heart trouble	high blood pressure	sinus trouble	OTHER:
— angina/coronary	abnormal bleeding	asthma	―――――
— heart murmur	anemia	tuberculosis	―――――
— congenital heart lesions	jaundice	stroke	―――――
— rheumatic fever	hepatitis/AIDS	epilepsy	―――――
diabetes	arthritis	psychiatric treatment	―――――

9.   Do you have a pacemaker?   Yes   No

10. Are you pregnant now?   Yes   No

Date: ――――――――― Signature of Patient ――――――――――――――――――

Fig. 1–1. Medical history form, completed and signed by patient.

One should ask the patient about the kind of pain, its location, its duration, what causes it, what alleviates it, and whether or not it has been referred to another site.

Generally, pulpal pain is described by a patient in one of two ways; sharp, piercing, and lancinating; or dull, boring, gnawing, and excruciating. The first group of painful responses is consistent with those usually associated with excitation of the "A delta" nerve fibers in the pulp, whereas the second group of painful responses is consistent with those resulting from excitation and slower rate of transmission of the "C" nerve fibers

DR.

MR.

MS. _____ FEE _____ RECALL _____

ADDRESS _____ CITY _____

PARENT OR GUARDIAN _____ PHONE: HOME _____

DATE OF BIRTH _____ OCCUPATION _____ BUS. _____

REFERRED BY _____ PHYSICIAN _____

| R | 1 | 2 | 3 | 4 | 5 | 6 | 7 | 8 | 9 | 10 | 11 | 12 | 13 | 14 | 15 | 16 | L |
| | 32 | 31 | 30 | 29 | 28 | 27 | 26 | 25 | 24 | 23 | 22 | 21 | 20 | 19 | 18 | 17 | |

DATE	SERVICE RENDERED	Credit	Balance

BACTERIOLOGIC RECORD   LABORATORY RECORD

DATE				
CULTURE				

DENTAL HISTORY

Chief complaint (c.c.): _____

History of involved tooth: _____

Subjective Symptoms:

Pain: Present ☐ or absent ☐; sharp ☐ or dull ☐; localized ☐ or diffuse ☐; throbbing ☐, intermittent ☐, or continuous ☐; lasting seconds ☐, minutes ☐, or hours ☐; increased by cold ☐, heat ☐, pressure ☐, mastication ☐, lying down ☐, sweet ☐, sour ☐, or other _____

Objective Symptoms:

Extraoral swelling ☐; intraoral swelling ☐; sinus tract (fistula) ☐

Lymph nodes involved: Submaxillary ☐; submental ☐; other _____

Tooth discolored ☐; painful on percussion ☐; mobile ☐

Tissue tender on palpation ☐

Electric test: Control tooth respond at no. ___ test tooth at no. ___

Thermal test: Normal ☐; abnormal response to cold ☐ or heat ☐; no response ☐

Radiograph: Periapical radiolucency present ☐ or absent ☐; thickened periodontal ligament ☐; internal resorption ☐; external resorption ☐; calcification ☐; crown or root fracture ☐; periodontal disease ☐; caries ☐; atypical anatomy _____

Pulp exposure by _____ Pulp affected by _____

Clinical Diagnosis

Pulpitis: Acute reversible (hyperemia) ☐; acute irreversible, responsive to heat ☐ or to cold ☐; chronic irreversible ☐

Degenerative changes: Calcification ☐; resorption ☐; necrosis ☐

Periapical lesion: Abscess/pericementitis: acute ☐; subacute ☐; chronic ☐

Intentional extirpation ☐; retreatment ☐

Prognosis of tooth: Favorable ☐; questionable ☐; unfavorable ☐

MEDICAL HISTORY

_____

_____

REMARKS

_____

_____

_____

Fig. 1–2. Record.

in the pulp. Determining the category of the pain is important in suggesting the next group of questions to be asked.

The ability to localize the pain is obviously important. Pain is localized when the patient can point to a specific tooth or site with assurance and speed when asked to do so. Sharp, piercing, lancinating pain in a tooth usually responds promptly to cold and is easy to localize. Symptoms from such teeth are rarely referred to other sites.

When the pain is diffuse, however, the patient describes an area of discomfort rather than a specific site. When the patient is asked to point to the most painful spot, the patient's finger moves along the dental arch or between the maxilla and the mandible. This diffuseness is diagnostic because the inability to localize the pain frequently relates to dental pain that is dull, boring, and gnawing, from a tooth that responds abnormally to heat more than to cold and with symptoms that can be referred to other sites.

The duration of the pain is also diagnostic. At times, pulpal pain lasts only as long as an irritant is present. At other times, it lasts for minutes to hours. The pain may either be intermittent or constant. Clinical experience has shown that a tooth with fleeting pulpal pain that disappears on removal of the irritant has an excellent chance of recovery without the need for endodontic treatment.

This condition, acute reversible pulpitis (hyperemia), is characterized by pain of short duration, caused by a specific irritant, that disappears as soon as the irritant is removed. The pain is usually localized and is more responsive to cold than to heat. If the pain persists, or if it occurs without any apparent cause, the pulpitis will usually be irreversible, and the patient will require endodontic therapy.

Abnormal dental pain caused by heat usually requires endodontic treatment. Pain that occurs on changing the position of the head, awakens the patient from sleep, or occurs during mastication of food in a cariously exposed tooth usually indicates a need for endodontic treatment. Spontaneous pain and pain of long duration are symptoms of irreversible pulpitis.

Objective Symptoms

Objective symptoms are determined by tests and observations performed by the clinician. These tests are as follows: (1) visual and tactile inspection; (2) percussion; (3) pal-pation; (4) mobility and depressibility; (5) radiograph; (6) electric pulp test; (7) thermal tests (hot and cold); (8) anesthetic test; and (9) test cavity.

Although it may not be necessary to perform all these tests at any one time, a combination of corroborating tests is desirable to ensure a correct diagnosis. One should not rely on the results of any single test.

Visual and Tactile Inspection

The simplest clinical test is visual examination. Too often, it is done only casually during examination, and as a result, much essential information is lost inadvertently. A thorough visual, tactile examination of hard and soft tissue relies on checking the "three Cs": color, contour, and consistency. In soft tissue, such as gingiva, deviation from the healthy, pink color is readily recognized when inflammation is present. A change in contour occurs with swelling, and the consistency of soft, fluctuant, or spongy tissue differs from that of normal, healthy, firm tissue and is indicative of a pathologic condition (Fig. 1–3).

Similarly, teeth should be visually examined using the "three Cs." A normal-appearing crown has a lifelike translucency and sparkle that is missing in pulpless teeth. Teeth that are discolored, opaque, and less lifelike in appearance should be carefully evaluated because the pulp may already be inflamed, degenerated, or necrotic. Not all discolored teeth need endodontic treatment; staining may be caused by old amalgam restorations, root canal filling materials and medicaments, or systemic medication, such as tetracycline staining. Many discolorations, however, are the result of diseases commonly associated with necrotic, gangrenous pulps, internal or external resorption, and carious exposure.

Crown contours should be examined. Because fractures, wear facets, and restorations change the crown's contour, the clinician should be prepared to evaluate the possible effects of such changes on the pulp.

Ravn observed enamel cracks in 1300 teeth over a 2-year period following traumatic injury.[25] Of this number, 3.5% resulted in death of the pulp. Abou-Rass recommends endodontic treatment and crown restoration once a cracked tooth develops symptoms because tooth cracks can become tooth fractures.[1]

Consistency of the hard tissue relates to the

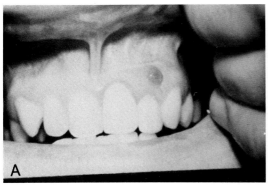

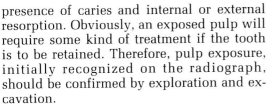

Fig. 1–3. *A*, Visual examination: sinus tract foramen (stoma) between lateral incisor and cuspid, scar tissue present from healed incision from previous endodontic surgical procedure. *B*, Sinus tract, gingival recession and root exposure of maxillary right cuspid.

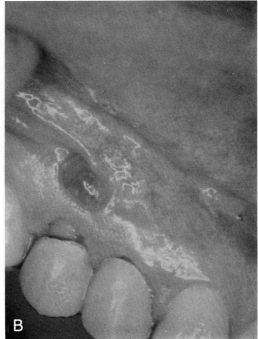

presence of caries and internal or external resorption. Obviously, an exposed pulp will require some kind of treatment if the tooth is to be retained. Therefore, pulp exposure, initially recognized on the radiograph, should be confirmed by exploration and excavation.

The technique of visual and tactile examination is simple. One uses one's eyes, fingers, an explorer, and the periodontal probe. The patient's teeth and periodontium should be examined in good light under dry conditions. For example, a sinus tract (fistula) might escape detection if it is covered by saliva, or an interproximal cavity may escape notice if it is filled with food. Loss of translucency, slight color changes, and cracks may not be apparent in poor light. In fact, a transilluminator may aid in detecting enamel cracks or crown fractures.

Visual examination should include the soft tissue adjacent to the involved tooth, for detection of swelling. The periodontal probe should be used routinely to determine the periodontal status of the suspected tooth and adjacent teeth. Sinus tracts opening into the gingival crevice or deep infrabony pockets may go undetected because of failure to use the periodontal probe. The crown of the tooth should be carefully evaluated, to determine whether it can be restored properly after completion of endodontic treatment. Finally, a rapid survey of the entire mouth should be made, to ascertain whether the tooth requiring treatment is a strategic tooth.

Percussion

This test enables one to evaluate the status of the periodontium surrounding a tooth. The tooth is struck a quick, moderate blow, initially with low intensity by the finger, then with increasing intensity by using the handle of an instrument, to determine whether the tooth is tender. A sensitive response, differing from that of the adjacent teeth, usually indicates the presence of pericementitis (periodontitis). Although percussion is a simple method of testing, it may be misleading if used alone. To eliminate bias on the part of the patient, one must change the sequence of the teeth percussed on successive tests. Moreover, one should change the direction of the blow from the vertical-occlusal to the buccal or lingual surface of the crown and strike separate cusps in a differing order (Fig. 1–4). Finally, while the clinician questions the patient about tenderness of a tooth, a more valid response can be obtained if at the same time, the patient's body movement, reflex pain reaction, or even an unspoken response is observed. One must not percuss a sensitive tooth beyond the patient's tolerance. This problem can be avoided by lightly pressing several teeth prior to percussing them.

Percussion is used in conjunction with

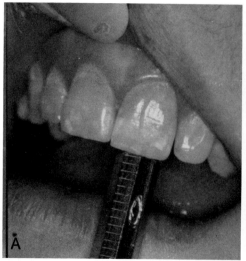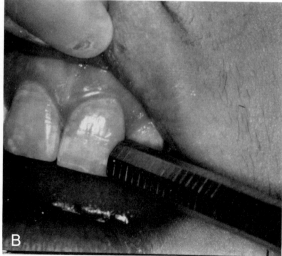

Fig. 1—4. *A,* Vertical percussion using the handle of an operative instrument. *B,* Horizontal percussion; before percussing a tooth with a metal handle, initially test the patient's response by lightly tapping the suspected tooth with your finger.

other periodontal tests, namely, palpation, mobility, and depressibility. These tests help to corroborate the presence of periodontitis. The presence of this disorder is not a true indication of irreversible pulpitis or pulp necrosis, however. Although periodontitis may be a response to pulp necrosis, it can also occur around a tooth with a vital, clinically normal pulp, as in acute periodontal abscess. When periodontitis occurs unrelated to a periodontal cause, it is usually the result of, and a sequela to, pulp necrosis. One infrequent exception occurs in the late stages of irreversible pulpitis, when the tooth is abnormally responsive to heat. The pulp still has some vitality, but the tooth is sensitive to percussion.

Palpation

This simple test is done with the fingertip, using light pressure to examine tissue consistency and pain response. Although simple, it is an important test. Its value lies in locating the swelling over an involved tooth and determining the following: (1) whether the tissue is fluctuant and enlarged sufficiently for incision and drainage; (2) the presence, intensity, and location of pain; (3) the presence and location of adenopathy (Fig. 1—5); and (4) the presence of bone crepitus.

When palpation is used to determine adenopathy, it is advisable to exercise caution when palpating lymph nodes in the presence of an acute infection, to avoid the possible spread of infection through the lymphatic vessels. Diagnostically, when the posterior teeth are infected, the submaxillary lymph nodes become involved. Infection of the lower anterior teeth may cause swelling of the submental lymph nodes. When the infection is confined to the pulp and has not progressed into the periodontium, palpation is not diagnostic. Palpation, percussion, mobility, and depressibility test the integrity of the attachment apparatus, that is, periodontal ligament and bone, and are not diagnostic when the disease is confined within the pulp cavity of a tooth. In short, percussion, palpation, mobility, and depressibility are tests of the periodontium rather than of the pulp.

Mobility-Depressibility Testing

The mobility test is used to evaluate the integrity of the attachment apparatus surrounding the tooth. The test consists of moving a tooth laterally in its socket by using the fingers or, preferably, the handles of two instruments (Fig. 1—6). The objective of this test is to determine whether the tooth is firmly or loosely attached to its alveolus. The amount of movement is indicative of the condition of the periodontium; the greater the movement, the poorer the periodontal status.

Similarly, the test for depressibility consists of moving a tooth vertically in its socket. This test may be done with the fingers or with an instrument. When depressibility exists, the chance for retaining the tooth ranges from poor to hopeless.

One classification for mobility defines

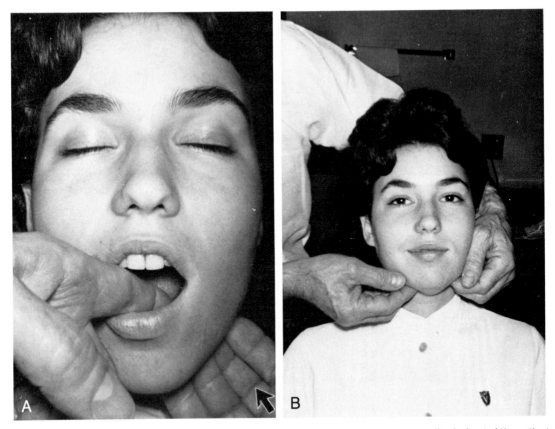

Fig. 1–5. *A*, Palpation of submaxillary lymph nodes (arrow) bimanually with the operator standing in front of the patient. *B*, Bimanual palpation of submaxillary lymph nodes with the operator standing behind the patient.

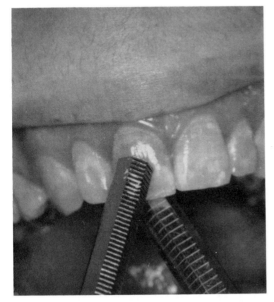

Fig. 1–6. Mobility is determined by moving a tooth laterally using the handles of two operative instruments.

first-degree mobility as a noticeable movement of the tooth in its socket; second-degree mobility as movement of a tooth within a range of 1 mm; and third-degree mobility as movement greater than 1 mm or when the tooth can be depressed. Endodontic treatment should not be carried out on teeth with third-degree mobility unless mobility is reduced when pressure in the periodontium has been relieved. For example, this situation could occur in the case of an acute apical abscess if sufficient drainage was established and pus escaped after the root canal was opened, sufficiently enlarged, and left patent.

Radiography

The radiograph is one of the most important clinical tools in making a diagnosis. It permits visual examination of the oral structures that would otherwise be unseen by the naked eye. Without it, diagnosis, case selection, treatment, and evaluation of healing would be impossible. The practice of dentistry would be impossible without radiographs.

To use radiographs properly, the clinician must have the knowledge and skill necessary to interpret them correctly. Required is a thorough understanding of the underlying normal or anomalous anatomy and the changes that can occur due to aging, trauma, disease, and healing. Only then will these two-dimensional black-and-white shadows on processed film have meaning (Figs. 1–7 and 1–8).

Because the information contained within a radiograph is so essential to dental practice, it is important that radiographs be of excellent quality. An excellent radiograph may be difficult to interpret, but a poor radiograph is impossible to "read." To produce an excellent radiograph, one must master the necessary skills: proper placement of the film in the patient's mouth; correct angulation of the cone in relation to the film and oral structures to prevent distortion of the anatomic images; correct exposure time, so the images are recorded with identifiable contrasts, and proper developing technique to ensure a clear, permanent record that can be retained and stored for future use. Minor deviation

from any of the foregoing will result in a poor radiograph with little or no value.

Radiographs can contain information on the presence of caries that may involve or may threaten to involve the pulp. Radiographs may show the number, course, shape, length, and width of root canals, the presence of calcified material in the pulp chamber or root canal, the resorption of dentin originating within the root canal (internal resorption) or from the root surface (external resorption), calcification or obliteration of the pulp cavity, thickening of the periodontal ligament, resorption of cementum, and nature and extent of periapical and alveolar bone destruction.

Thus, radiographs provide pertinent information concerning diagnosis, prognosis, case selection, instrumentation, obturation, and repair of bone and cementum. They can be used to alert the clinician to impending difficulties caused by calcifications, periodontal problems, perforations, blockages, and fractures (Figs. 1–9 to 1–11). Nevertheless, radiographs can be misleading and must be viewed with caution. The interpretation of radiographs is not an exact science. For example, a radiograph cannot be used to differentiate reliably among a chronic abscess,

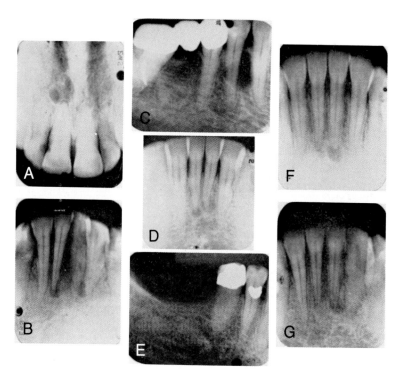

Fig. 1–7. Radiolucent areas associated with vital teeth. A, Incisive foramen; B, periapical osteofibrosis; C, periodontal cyst; D, periapical osteofibrosis; E, mental foramen; F and G, periapical osteofibrosis.

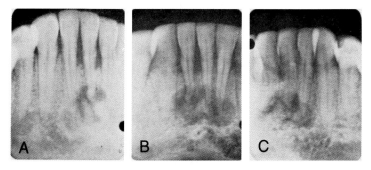

Fig. 1–8. *A* to *C,* Periapical osteofibrosis.

a granuloma, or a cyst. To be accurate, such differentiation requires histopathologic evidence.

Concomitantly, the presence of periapical radiolucency on a tooth does not automatically indicate a diseased tooth. In many instances, an area of rarefaction that appears to be on the root apex of a tooth in a radiograph is actually a superimposition of an image on the root apex (Fig. 1–12). This phenomenon may occur where the anatomy is normal, such as in the maxillary sinus, incisive foramen, mental foramen, medullary spaces, or where a disorder is present but not pulpally related, such as a traumatic bone cyst, ameloblastoma, periodontal cyst, and malignant tumors (Fig. 1–13).

Periapical osteofibrosis (ossifying periapical fibroma, periapical rarefying osteitis, ossifying fibroma, cementoma, cementoblastoma, osseous dysplasia), as described by Stafne,[29] is another entity that can lead to radiographic misinterpretation. Periapical osteofibrosis is recognizable by a radiolucent area surrounding the apex of a tooth whose pulp is normal and tests accordingly. Gen-

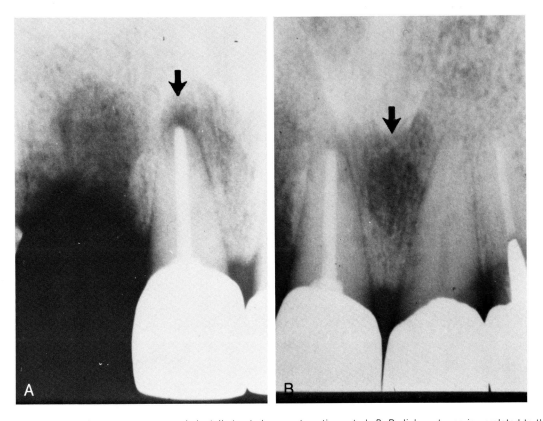

Fig. 1–9. *A,* Radiolucent area over endodontally treated, asymptomatic central. *B,* Radiolucent area is unrelated to the tooth and is the incisive foramen.

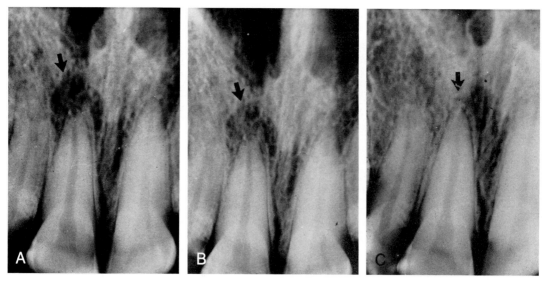

Fig. 1–10.   Patient had been in an automobile accident several months previously. *A,* Area of rarefaction (arrow) present over central, but all tests were negative and the tooth was asymptomatic. *B,* Another radiograph taken of the same area (arrow) also showed a radiolucent area. *C,* Radiograph taken at a greater angle shows normal bone structure and lamina dura (arrow). Radiolucent area is the incisive foramen.

erally, one sees evidence of bone trabeculae in the area, and at times, cementum. The radiolucent area is often delineated at the periphery by sclerotic bone. Nevertheless, periapical osteofibrosis may be misdiagnosed as a granuloma, chronic abscess, or cyst. Because the affected teeth require no treatment, it is essential to differentiate periapical osteofibrosis from those diseases that require endodontic therapy or extraction.

The conclusion of a study by Bender and Seltzer,[3] confirmed in a later study by Schwartz and Foster,[28] stated that a lesion in cancellous bone is not discernible on a radiograph until the cortical bone has been reached or penetrated. Bender later reconfirmed that loss of cancellous bone is undetectable until at least 6.6% of the mineral content of the cortical bone in the direct path of the x-ray beam has been lost.[2] In other words, a periapical lesion is usually larger than its image on a radiograph. A pathologic area therefore can be present, yet be obscured by a plate of cortical bone, and an acute abscess in a tooth can have a normal radiographic appearance with no apparent radiolucency.

Radiographs have other limitations. Goldman and co-workers found that when 5 dentists examined the same endodontic radiographs, their interpretations concurred in only 67% of cases.[14] Nielsen's study of radiographic interpretation showed that the

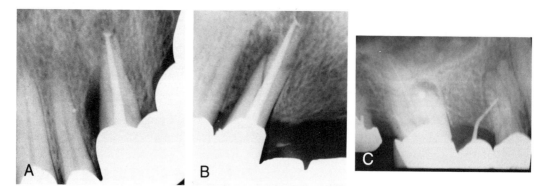

Fig. 1–11.   *A,* Apparent periodontal involvement of an upper cuspid tooth, with swelling, which could also be mistaken for periapical involvement because of endodontally treated tooth. *B,* Radiograph taken at a marked change in horizontal angulation shows evidence of a fractured root, which is the cause of the swelling. *C,* Radiographic aid to diagnosis: trace the origin of a sinus tract by insinuating a gutta-percha cone into the tract.

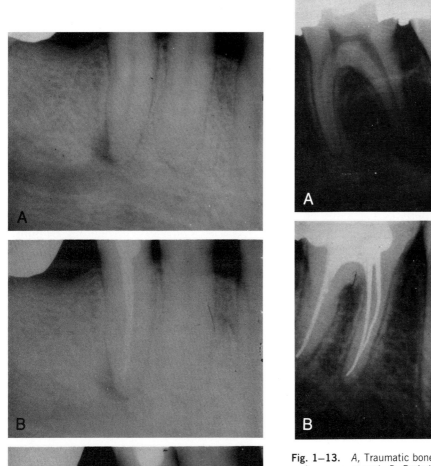

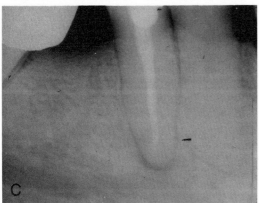

Fig. 1–12. *A*, Area of rarefaction: Is this periapical rarefaction the result of a chronic periapical lesion or the mental foramen superimposed over the root apex? *B*, Area of rarefaction is both a chronic periapical lesion (pulp tested nonvital to electric pulp testing, cold application, and test cavity) and the mental foramen. Endodontic treatment completed without anesthesia. *C*, Recall radiograph at 6 months.

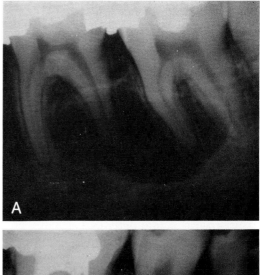

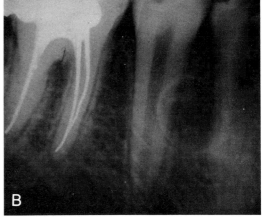

Fig. 1–13. *A*, Traumatic bone cyst; vitality tests for both molars were normal. *B*, Periodontal cyst; vitality tests for both premolars were normal.

examiners agreed on 65 to 75% of cases, but the percentage increased when the same examiner re-examined the same radiographs.[21] Gelfand and associates showed that visual interpretation of radiographs varies among general dentists and endodontists.[13] In addition, the examiners disagreed with themselves 21.8% of the time when they viewed the same radiograph a second time. Pitfalls of radiographic interpretation have also been demonstrated by Roit and Gröndahl.[27]

Priebe and colleagues questioned the value of a radiograph for differentiating different types of periapical lesions.[24] Brynolf reported that an accurate interpretation is possible 74% of the time using a single radiograph and 90% of the time when using 3 radiographs taken at different angles of the same area.[4] Brynolf also found that a "histologically correct diagnosis of changes in the periapical area can be made in 82 to 95% of cases."[5] Suzuki reported that histologic examination confirmed that the radiograph was reliable in 83% of cases when endodontic treatment led to a reduction in size of the periapical radiolucency and an increase in trabeculation.[30] Pitt Ford found no dependable relationship between radiographic and histologic findings of periapical tissue in dogs.[23]

Several published reports have described a newly developed dental radiograph called the xeroradiograph. This radiograph can be exposed by a conventional x-ray machine using less-than-usual radiation, automatically processed, and delivered as a dry, laminated permanent film in 25 sec. In addition, it can be viewed as a black-and-white photograph or as a traditional radiograph using transilluminated lighting. Leff and associates compared the diagnostic value of images produced by conventional radiography and with that of images produced by xeroradiography.[18] These workers reported that the images were of equal diagnostic value, but xeroradiography produced images of sharper clarity and finer detail.

The paradox of the radiograph is that it does not always lend itself to correct interpretation, yet it has contributed more than any other diagnostic test toward the scientific practice of dentistry. Without it, we could not properly diagnose dental structures with any reasonable degree of accuracy. Nevertheless, other tests must be used in conjunction with the radiograph to corroborate the interpretation.

Electric Pulp Testing

The electric pulp test is more accurate than some of the tests used to determine pulp vitality. Although pulp vitality is dependent on intrapulpal blood circulation, no practical, clinical test has been devised to test circulation. The electric tester, when testing for pulp vitality, uses nerve stimulation instead. The objective is to stimulate a pulpal response by subjecting the tooth to an increasing degree of electric current. A positive response is an indication of vitality and helps in determining the normality or abnormality of that pulp. No response to the electrical stimulus can be an indication of pulp necrosis (Fig. 1–14).

A simple technique for electrical pulp testing is as follows:

1. Describe the test to the patient in a way that will reduce anxiety and will eliminate a biased response.
2. Isolate the area of teeth to be tested with cotton rolls and a saliva ejector, and air dry all the teeth.
3. Check the electric pulp tester for function, and determine that current is passing through the electrode.
4. Apply an electrolyte (toothpaste) on the tooth electrode, and place it against the dried enamel of the crown's occlusobuccal or incisolabial surface (Fig. 1–15). It is important to avoid contacting any restorations in the tooth or the adjacent gingival tissue with the electrolyte or the electrode; this would cause a false and misleading response.
5. Retract the patient's cheek away from the tooth electrode with the free hand. This hand contact with the patient's cheek completes the electrical circuit.
6. Turn the rheostat slowly to introduce minimal current into the tooth, and increase the current slowly. Ask the patient to indicate when sensation occurs by using such words as "tingling" or "warmth." Record the result according to the numeric scale on the pulp tester.
7. Repeat the foregoing for each tooth to be tested.

Because errors in technique or in response can occur easily, it is wise to recheck all results for accuracy whenever in doubt about the validity of the test. Testing the accuracy of the patient's response with the unit off or changing the sequence of the teeth being tested prevents the accuracy of the results from being affected by the patient's reaction because of bias or anxiety. A radiograph of all teeth being tested should be visible for reference during the test. Finally, one should not rely on the results of any one test or reaction to any one tooth without similarly testing and comparing the response to a control tooth.

The electric pulp test cannot be solely depended on for testing pulp vitality, and results should be corroborated with those of other tests, such as the cold test or test cavity. At times, the results of the electric pulp test are misleading. For example, a false-positive response can occur when moist gangrenous pulp is present in a root canal. This situation is uncommon and requires the passage of maximum current through the tooth to elicit

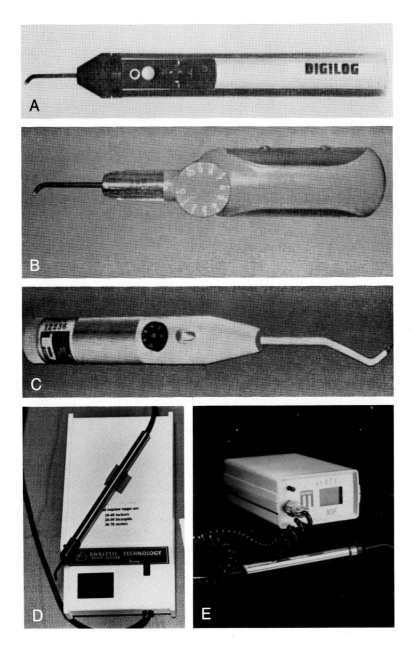

Fig. 1—14. Electric Pulp Testers. *A*, Digilog pulp tester, battery operated. *B*, Pelton-Crane compact, transistorized battery-operated electric pulp tester. *C*, Battery-operated Parkell pulp tester. *D*, Analytic Technology pulp tester. *E*, Neotest ADP (automatic digital pulp tester).

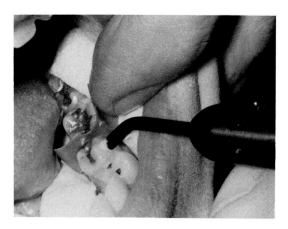

Fig. 1–15. Electric pulp testing: the electrode is placed against the occlusobuccal enamel surface of the isolated and dried tooth crown using toothpaste as an electrolyte; the current is slowly increased until the patient feels "tingling" or "heat."

a response. Another cause for confusion can occur in multirooted teeth in which the pulp is partially necrotic, with some nerve fibers still vital in one or more of the root canals.

A false-negative result with no apparent response to electrical stimulation is misleading more often than a false-positive response. A negative response can occur when calcification in the pulp tissue or dentin has been extensive. More current is needed to elicit a response in a tooth with increased reparative dentin and a diminishing pulp cavity, or in fibrotic pulp. Other factors that may affect response are: (1) teeth with extensive restorations and a pulp-protecting base; (2) recently traumatized teeth; (3) recently erupted teeth with incomplete root formation; (4) sedative medication taken by patient; and (5) patients with an unusually high pain threshold.

Electric pulp testing is not done on teeth with full-coverage restorations because an electrical stimulus cannot pass undistorted through acrylic, ceramic, or metallic portions of a crown. These teeth can be tested for vitality using a test cavity, but such a test should be done only under limited circumstances because it requires cavity preparation in the occlusal surface of the crown. Application of carbon dioxide snow ($-78°C$) or Frigident spray ($-50°C$) is the test of choice under such circumstances.

Problems encountered in electric pulp testing have been discussed by Mumford and Bjorn.[20] Degering found that an electrical stimulus was the most reliable method of testing.[7] Mumford stated that the electric pulp test was superior to thermal tests, for both accuracy and reproducibility.[19] Harris also confirmed the diagnostic value of electric pulp testing.[15] In comparative tests, Teitler and associates found a better correlation between the clinical status of the tooth and the electric pulp test than with the ethyl chloride cold test.[31]

Other studies have explained why the results of electric pulp testing are difficult to interpret quantitatively. Klein found that 16 to 36% of anterior teeth of children, ages 6 to 11, did not respond to the electric pulp test.[17] Dummer and colleagues, who correlated the patients' history, thermal tests, and electric pulp tests of 98 painful teeth with histologic examination, found a higher reading in 10% of teeth with uninflamed pulps and in 38% of teeth with inflamed pulps and a lower reading in 5% of teeth with uninflamed and in 23% of teeth with inflamed pulps.[9]

Thermal Testing

These tests involve the application of cold and heat to a tooth, to determine sensitivity to thermal changes. Although both are tests of sensitivity, they are dissimilar and are conducted for different diagnostic reasons. A response to cold indicates a vital pulp, regardless of whether that pulp is normal or abnormal. A heat test is not a test of pulp vitality. An abnormal response to heat usually indicates the presence of a pulpal or periapical disorder requiring endodontic treatment.

Other diagnostic differences exist between heat and cold tests. When a reaction to cold occurs, the patient can quickly point to the painful tooth. The heat response, when described by the patient, can be localized or diffuse, and, at times, referred to a different site. A positive response to the application of heat on a single tooth during the examination, however, results in a localized, painful, and momentarily delayed reaction. The results of the thermal test should be correlated with the results of other tests, to ensure validity.

Heat Testing. The heat test can be performed using different techniques that deliver different degrees of temperature (Fig. 1–16). The area to be tested is isolated and dried, warm air is directed to the exposed surface of the tooth and the patient's response is noted. If a higher temperature is

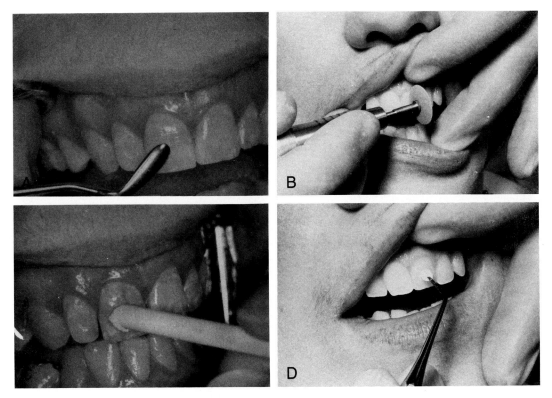

Fig. 1–16. Heat testing. *A,* Applying hot blade of plastic instrument against buccal surface of crown enamel. *B,* Frictional heat created by rotating polishing disc. *C* and *D,* Applying hot gutta-percha to tooth surface.

needed to elicit a response, one should use hot water, a hot burnisher, hot gutta-percha, or hot compound, or any instrument that can deliver a controlled temperature to the tooth. When using a solid substance, such as hot gutta-percha, the heat is applied to the occluso-buccal third of the exposed crown. If no response occurs, the host substance can be moved to the central portion of the crown or closer to the tooth cervix. When a response occurs, the heat should be removed immediately. Care should be taken to avoid using excessive heat or prolonged application of heat to the tooth.

A different technique is required for the application of hot water. The tooth to be tested is isolated under a rubber dam. The tooth is then immersed in "coffee-hot" water delivered from a syringe, and the patient's reaction is noted. Because the hot water is contained in the rubber dam, the response is limited to the tooth tested.

Cold Testing. Cold can be applied in several different ways (Fig. 1–17). A stream of cold air can be directed against the crown of the previously dried tooth and also at the gingival margin. If no reaction occurs, the

tooth can be isolated under a rubber dam and sprayed with ethyl chloride, which evaporates so rapidly that it absorbs heat and thereby cools the tooth. A more common method is to apply a cotton pellet saturated with ethyl chloride to the tooth being tested. Although the temperature is not as cold as with an ethyl chloride spray, it is generally cold enough to elicit a valid response.

A simple means of applying cold to a tooth is to wrap a sliver of ice in wet gauze, to place it against the facial surface of the tooth, and to compare the reaction to a control tooth. Pencils of ice can be made by filling discarded anesthetic carpules with water and freezing them in an upright position in a refrigerator. The rubber stopper should be at the base of the carpule, to enable one to force the ice out of the carpule and thereby to obtain a pencil of ice. Dachi and associates recommended that a quarter-inch-diameter cone of ice be placed against a tooth for 5 sec to quantify cold testing.[6]

Carbon dioxide (dry ice) snow has also been used for application of cold to teeth. The use of dry ice has been described by Ehrmann.[10] Because the temperature of dry

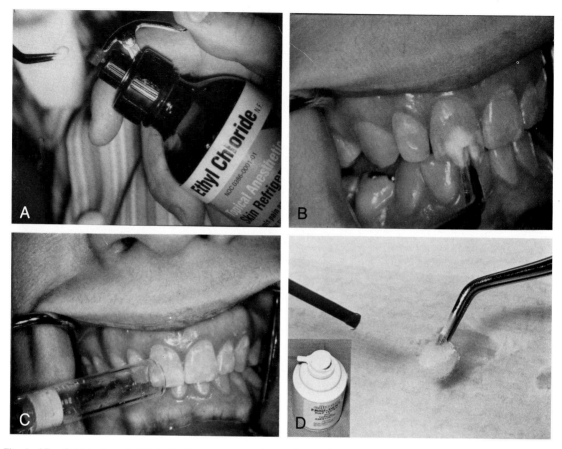

Fig. 1–17. Cold testing. *A,* Ethyl chloride spray on a cotton pellet; rapid evaporation creates cold sensation. *B,* Sprayed cotton pellet applied to tooth crown; a positive response indicates pulp vitality in a tooth whose pulp is normal or abnormal. *C,* Water frozen inside an empty anesthetic carpule creates an ice stick for cold testing. *D,* Cotton pellet sprayed with Frigident (inset), to be applied to crown surface; Frigident, at approximately − 50°C, when sprayed on enamel or restored surface of tooth crown is the most accurate test for pulp vitality.

ice is − 78°C, one is able to penetrate full-coverage restorations and to elicit a reaction from the underlying tooth to the cold. The reaction of the pulp to the dry-ice method of thermal testing has been studied by Dowden and co-workers, who applied a temperature of − 80°C for 1 to 3 min to the teeth of monkeys.[8] Pulpal injury resulted, but recovery occurred when the teeth were re-examined 47 to 63 days later. Ingram and Peters have shown that carbon dioxide snow did not cause any permanent deleterious effect on enamel or pulp when it was applied to the teeth of dogs.[16] Rickoff and colleagues have studied the effect of carbon dioxide snow and hot gutta-percha on human teeth and have reported no significant injury to the pulp.[26] That carbon dioxide snow is a reliable means of testing pulp sensitivity has been shown by Fulling and Andreasen.[11] Fuss and associates, in an in vivo study comparing tooth

vitality, produced a positive vitality response of 98.7% with dichloro-difluoro methane (DDM), 97.4% with carbon dioxide snow, 94.8% with the electric pulp tester, 53.2% with ethyl chloride, and 32.5% with ice.[12] Mumford claimed that the electric pulp test was easily reproduced and more reliable than the thermal tests,[19] but his study did not compare EPT to the application of DDM or carbon dioxide snow.

Anesthetic Testing

This test is restricted to patients who are in pain at the time of the test, when the usual tests have failed to enable one to identify the tooth. The objective is to anesthetize a single tooth at a time until the pain disappears and is localized to a specific tooth (Fig. 1–18).

The technique is as follows: Using either infiltration or the intraligament injection, inject the most posterior tooth in the area suspected of being the cause of pain. If pain

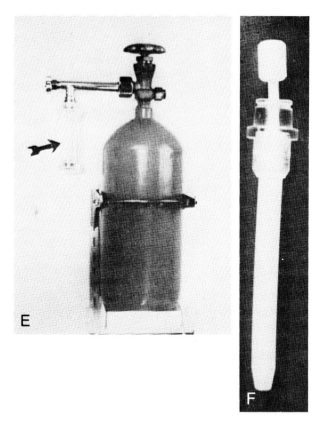

Fig. 1–17 (continued). *E,* Apparatus for producing carbon dioxide snow, attached to wall. Arrow points to pencil-type applicator in plastic receptacle. *F,* Applicator for applying carbon dioxide snow to tooth.

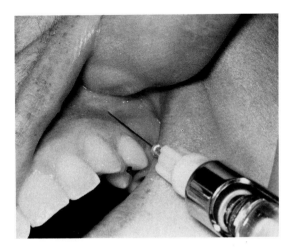

Fig. 1–18. Anesthetic test: anesthetize a single tooth at a time until pain disappears.

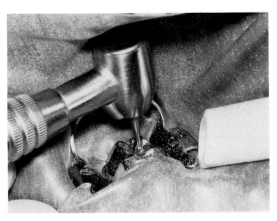

Fig. 1–19. Test cavity: When drilling through the dentino-enamel junction of an unanesthetized tooth, a painful sensation indicates some vitality present in the pulp.

persists when the tooth has been fully anesthetize, anesthetize the next tooth mesial to
it, and continue to do so until the pain disappears. If the source of the pain cannot be
determined, whether in maxillary or mandibular teeth, an inferior alveolar (mandibular block) injection should be given. Cessation of pain naturally indicates
involvement of a mandibular tooth, and
localization of the specific tooth is done by
the intraligament injection, when the anesthetic has spent itself. This test is obviously
a last resort and has an advantage over the
"test cavity," during which iatrogenic damage is possible.

Test Cavity

This test allows one to determine pulp
vitality (Fig. 1–19). It is performed when
other methods of diagnosis have failed. The
test cavity is made by drilling through the
enamel-dentin junction of an unanesthetized
tooth. The drilling should be done at slow
speed and without a water coolant. Sensitivity or pain felt by the patient is an indication
of pulp vitality; no endodontic treatment is
indicated. A sedative cement is then placed
in the cavity, and the search for the source
of pain continues. If no pain is felt, cavity
preparation may be continued until the pulp
chamber is reached. If the pulp is completely
necrotic, endodontic treatment can be continued painlessly in many cases without
anesthesia.

BIBLIOGRAPHY

1. Abou-Rass, M.: Quint. Int., *14*:437, 1983.
2. Bender, I.: J. Endod., *8*:161, 1982.
3. Bender, I., and Seltzer, S.: J. Am. Dent. Assoc., *62*:152, 1961.
4. Brynolf, I.: Swed. Dent. J., *63*:415, 1970.
5. Brynolf, I.: Odontol. Revy, *18(Suppl. 11),* 1967, and personal communication, 1977.
6. Dachi, S.F., et al.: Oral Surg., *24*:687, 1967.
7. Degering, C.I.: J. Dent. Res., *41*:695, 1962.
8. Dowden, W.E., et al.: Oral Surg., *55*:408, 1983.
9. Dummer, P.M., et al.: Int. Endod. J., *13*:27, 1980.
10. Ehrmann, E.: Fifth International Conference on Endodontics. Philadelphia, University of Pennsylvania, 1973, p. 171.
11. Fulling, H.J., and Andreasen, J.O.: Scand. J. Dent. Res. *84*:291, 1976.
12. Fuss, Z., et al.: J. Endod., *10*:147, 1985, and J. Dent. Res., *64*:240, 1985 (abstract).
13. Gelfand, M., et al.: J. Endod., *9*:71, 1983.
14. Goldman, M., et al.: Oral Surg., *33*:432, 1972.
15. Harris, W.E.: J. Endod., *8*:171, 1982.
16. Ingram, T.A., and Peters, D.D.: J. Endod., *9*:266, 1983.
17. Klein, H.J.: Am. Soc. Dent. Child., *45*:23, 1978.
18. Leff, G.S., et al.: J. Endod., *10*:188, 1984.
19. Mumford, J.: Br. Dent. J., *115*:338, 1964.
20. Mumford, J., and Bjorn, H.: Int. Dent. J., *12*:161, 1962.
21. Nielsen, J.: J. Dent. Res., *58*:2296, 1979 (abstract).
22. Peters, D.D., et al.: J. Endod., *9*:219, 1983.
23. Pitt Ford, T.R.: J. Dent. Res., *62*:417, 1983.
24. Priebe, W.A., et al.: Oral Surg., *7*:979, 1954.
25. Ravn, J.J.: Scand. J. Dent. Res., *89*:117, 1981.
26. Rickoff, B., et al.: J. Endod., *10*:139, 1985, and J. Dent. Res., *64*:310, 1985 (abstract).
27. Roit, C., and Gröndahl, H.: Swed. Dent. J., *8*:1, 1984.
28. Schwartz, S.F., and Foster, J.K.: Oral Surg., *32*:606, 1971.
29. Stafne, E.C.: J. Am. Dent. Assoc., *21*:1822, 1934.
30. Suzuki, A.: Shikwa Gakuho, *60*:37, 1960.
31. Teitler, D., et al.: Oral Surg., *34*:649, 1972.

2 Endodontic Emergencies

No one is a stranger to pain, and thus sympathy is aroused when a person appears for emergency treatment. The reason for endodontic emergency treatment is pain and, at times, swelling ensuing from pulpoperiapical pathosis. Because dental pain has many causes, the adept clinician must diagnose the origin of the pain as quickly as possible, to render rapid and effective relief. Knowing what to do and when to do it are as important as knowing how to do it.

Most dental emergencies are unscheduled intrusions into the routine of daily practice. Nevertheless, the dentist must provide speedy and effective relief because such care is an essential part of daily practice. As a result, the diagnosis and treatment are performed under stressful circumstances for both patient and dentist.

The following classification of emergencies and procedures is designed to simplify the selection of an effective method of treatment.

ACUTE REVERSIBLE PULPITIS

Acute reversible pulpitis (hyperemia) can be treated successfully by palliative procedures. Locating the involved tooth is usually a simple process; the patient can identify the tooth by pointing to it. The diagnosis and origin of the condition can be confirmed by visual, tactile, thermal, and radiographic examination of the isolated tooth.

If a recent restoration has a premature contact point, recontouring this high spot will usually relieve the pain and will allow the pulp to recuperate. If persistent painful episodes occur following cavity preparation, chemical cleansing of the cavity, or leakage of the restoration, one should remove the restoration and replace it with a sedative cement such as zinc oxide-eugenol cement. The same method can be used if recurrent decay under an old restoration has not caused pulp exposure. The best treatment is prevention: one should place a pulp-protective base under all restorations, avoid marginal leakage, reduce occlusal trauma if present, properly contour all restorations, and avoid injuring the pulp with excessive heat while preparing or polishing a metallic restoration. Following palliative treatment, such as the application of a zinc oxide-eugenol cement as a temporary sedative filling, the pain should disappear within several days. If it persists or worsens, then the pulp should be extirpated.

ACUTE IRREVERSIBLE PULPITIS

The preferable emergency treatment for both types of acute irreversible pulpitis (abnormally responsive to cold or to heat) is pulpectomy. Teeth affected by either acute reversible pulpitis or irreversible pulpitis are abnormally responsive to cold and have many similar symptoms. It is therefore essential that they be distinguished from one another because the emergency procedure for each is different. If a patient describes pain that lasts for minutes to hours, or is spontaneous, or disturbs sleep, or occurs when bending over, most likely that patient will require pulpectomy of the affected tooth rather than palliative therapy for relief of the painful symptoms.

The technique for pulpectomy is as follows:

1. Anesthetize the affected tooth.
2. Apply the rubber dam.
3. Prepare an access cavity into the pulp chamber.
4. Remove the pulp from the chamber with excavators or curettes.
5. Irrigate and debride the pulp chamber.
6. Locate the root canal orifices and explore the root canals.
7. Extirpate the pulp by sequentially instrumenting with reamers or files to within 1 mm of the radiographic root apex.
8. Irrigate with sterile saline solution, anesthetic solution, or sodium hypochlorite solution.

9. Debride with a barbed broach, fitted loosely so it can be rotated in the root canal without binding, usually following instrumentation with at least a No. 25 reamer or file to the root apex.

10. Dry the root canal with sterile absorbent points.

11. Insert a medicated cotton pledget, moistened with an obtundent such as eugenol, into the pulp chamber.

12. Place a temporary filling such as Cavit or fast-setting zinc oxide-eugenol cement over the medicated dressing and seal the access cavity.

13. Relieve any occlusal trauma.

14. Prescribe an analgesic for use only if pain recurs. Premedication or post-treatment medication with antibiotics is indicated only if the patient's condition is medically compromised or if systemic toxicity occurs subsequently.

15. Consult with the patient to alleviate any anxiety concerning the emergency procedure or potential postoperative reaction, and assure the patient of your availability.

On some occasions, the dentist does not have sufficient time to complete total extirpation of the pulp and instrumentation of the root canal. Under such circumstances, emergency pulpotomy, including debridement, drying, and sealing of a medicated dressing in the pulp chamber usually suffices. Although emergency pulpotomy is not as effective as pulpectomy, it relieves the patient of pain for several days. The patient should be rescheduled as soon as possible for additional treatment.

ACUTE ALVEOLAR ABSCESS

An acute alveolar abscess (acute periapical abscess, acute apical pericementitis, phoenix abscess) is a localized collection of pus in the alveolar bone at the root apex of a tooth following death of the pulp, with extension of the infection through the apical foramen into the periapical tissue. It is accompanied by a severe local reaction and, at times, a general reaction of systemic toxicity such as elevated temperature, gastrointestinal disturbance, malaise, nausea, dizziness, and other symptoms related to continuous pain and lack of sleep (Fig. 2–1).

The acute episode may result from pulpitis that progressively developed into pulp necrosis affecting the periapical tissues; it may

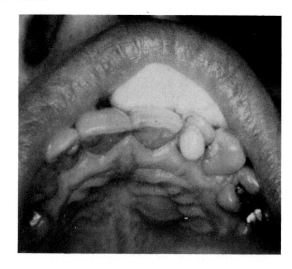

Fig. 2–1. Palatal swelling originating from acute alveolar abscess of maxillary left lateral incisor; penetration into the pulp chamber using high-speed burs resulted in immediate drainage of pus.

be an exacerbation of a chronic periapical lesion; or it may be caused by an endodontic-periodontic lesion when the periodontal abscess secondarily affects the pulp through the lateral root canals or a deep infrabony pocket that extends to or beyond the root apex. To relieve this constant pain, one should establish drainage through the root canal, preferably, and through the soft tissue and bone, if necessary (Fig. 2–2).

The emergency treatment of acute alveolar abscess differs from that of acute irreversible pulpitis. Because the pulp is necrotic, local anesthesia is not needed routinely. In fact, local anesthesia is frequently contraindicated in acutely inflamed tissue because the injection of an infiltration anesthetic does not anesthetize the tissue. Acutely inflamed tissue has a localized pH that is acidic in spite of the body's natural buffering action. Local anesthetics are effective in tissue with a more alkaline pH and, as a result, are ineffective when injected into acutely inflamed tissue. In addition, insinuating a needle and forcing anesthetic solution into an acutely infected and swollen area may increase pain and may spread infection.

Conduction anesthesia may be administered to reduce the pain of acute alveolar abscess, as long as the injection route is distant from the inflamed area. A mandibular block or an infraorbital injection can be used effectively when needed for the few isolated cases in which some pulp vitality persists. Because most of the pain that occurs during

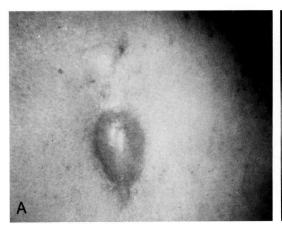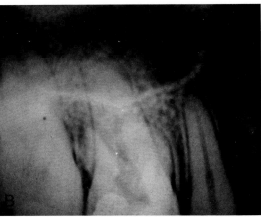

Fig. 2—2. *A,* Sinus tract forming on patient's face. *B,* Origin of sinus tract is maxillary right first molar; after completion of endodontic treatment, sinus tract disappeared permanently.

access-cavity preparation is caused by tooth movement resulting from vibration of the high-speed bur, one should stabilize the tooth with finger pressure so penetration into the pulp chamber will be painless. The value of the test cavity in treating teeth with acute alveolar abscess is twofold. First, it tests for any remaining vital pulp that could require anesthesia; and second, it initiates emergency therapy quickly, because the pulp chamber can be penetrated painlessly without delay, waiting for anesthesia to take effect.

To complete the emergency treatment of an acute alveolar abscess, the following procedure is recommended:

1. Place the rubber dam over the infected tooth.
2. Complete the access opening painlessly by bracing the tooth with finger pressure.
3. Irrigate profusely, debride the pulp chamber, but avoid forcing any solution or debris into the periapical tissue.
4. Using a No. 10 or No. 15 file or reamer as an explorer, locate the root canal orifices and instrument each root canal within 1 mm of the root apex.
5. Continue to debride and to irrigate while enlarging each root canal, but keep all instruments and irrigants within the root canals.
6. Frequently, a purulent exudate escapes into the chamber and indicates that the root canal is patent and draining; relief follows quickly. If no evidence of drainage appears, leave the tooth open, its root canals patent, and expect relief within a short time.

7. Advise the patient to use hot saline rinses for 3 min each hour.
8. Prescribe analgesics or antibiotics if indicated and necessary.

In mild cases of acute alveolar abscess, the tooth may be sealed with an antiseptic, obtundent medicament after biomechanical preparation of the chamber and root canals. Leaving the tooth open for drainage, however, reduces the possibility of continued pain and swelling. The open-drainage technique is preferable to one in which the prepared root canals are sealed, followed by incision of the soft tissue and artificial fistulation of the bone to establish drainage. Open root canals permit drainage and frequently eliminate the need for a surgical incision as well as the routine administration of oral antibiotics and analgesics.

Nevertheless, some clinicians suggest that all acutely abscessed teeth be sealed with an intracanal medicament after initial emergency instrumentation. They claim that leaving a tooth open continues the bacteriologic contamination and increases the risk of adverse reaction when the tooth is resealed. In addition, they claim that the bacterial contamination prolongs the treatment time needed to overcome the resulting infection. August found that only 3% of 311 abscessed teeth that had been left open for drainage reacted adversely after cleaning, irrigating, and resealing with an antiseptic dressing.[1] Finally, the same clinicians who advocate sealing acutely abscessed teeth admit that the teeth should be reopened for drainage if symptoms persist or worsen.

The pain of an acutely abscessed tooth,

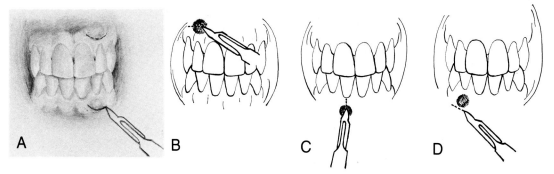

Fig. 2–3. *A,* Correct incisions at most dependent portion of swelling. *B* to *D,* Incorrect incisions. *B,* Incision at midportion of swelling. *C,* A vertical incision would leave an unsightly "V"-shaped break in the gingiva. *D,* Incision not made in the most dependent portion of the swelling.

whether of periapical or periodontal origin, is frequently accompanied by swelling. If the swelling is slight and is localized, it will disappear 24 to 48 hours after drainage has been established. Routinely, hot saline rinses should be prescribed to assist drainage. If the swelling is extensive, soft, and fluctuant, an incision through the soft tissue to the bone may be necessary (Fig. 2–3). One should first dry the mucosa over the affected area, then spray the tissue with a refrigerant topical anesthetic such as ethyl chloride. The intraoral incision is made through the soft, fluctuant swelling to the cortical bone plate. A rubber dam or gauze drain may be inserted for several days. If the swelling is hard, it can be converted to a soft, fluctuant state by rinsing with hot saline solution 3 to 5 min at a time, repeated every hour. Antibiotics and analgesics can be prescribed as needed. Finally, the tooth should be disoccluded slightly if it is extruded from its socket. This procedure eliminates pain caused by contact with teeth in the apposing arch.

ACUTE PERIODONTAL ABSCESS

An acute periodontal abscess causes pain and swelling. It is often mistaken for an acute alveolar abscess. Although the acute periodontal abscess (parietal abscess) can occur with either vital or necrotic pulp, its origin is usually an exacerbation of infection with pus formation in an existing deep infrabony pocket. If the pulp tests indicate pulp vitality within the normal range, then emergency treatment consists of curettage, debridement, and establishment of drainage of the infrabony pocket through the sulcular crevice. At times, incision of the soft tissue is necessary.

If the pulp is affected, it must be extirpated

as well. When the pulp is abnormal and vital, the tooth is treated as if for acute irreversible pulpitis. If the pulp is necrotic, the tooth should be treated as if for acute alveolar abscess. In any case, emergency periodontal treatment must be done simultaneously; otherwise, the patient will not be relieved of the pain and swelling.

EMERGENCIES DURING TREATMENT

Endodontic emergencies can occur during the course of endodontic treatment. They are usually caused by instrumentation beyond the root apex, with resultant trauma to the periapical tissue, or when debris and microorganisms are forced through the apical foramen into the periapical tissue and cause an infectious reaction. Other causes may be chemical irritants, such as irrigating solutions or intracanal medicaments, penetrating the periapical tissue, incomplete or inadequate debridement of all root canals, lost or depressed access-cavity seals, with resulting recontamination of the root canals, or overfilled root canals with subsequent periapical inflammation. These emergencies can be avoided if instruments, irrigating solutions, medicaments, cements, and filling materials are confined to the root canals themselves, and teeth under treatment are properly sealed between visits and are recontoured to prevent trauma.

With proper care during treatment, fewer than 10% of teeth react adversely. Oliet reported that 3% of 387 teeth, treated in 1 or 2 visits, were severely painful, up to 8% were moderately painful, and the remainder caused slight or no discomfort.[14] Ideally, an endodontic emergency should not occur during treatment; however, it does occur occasionally. Patients should be warned during endodontic instrumentation that a reaction may occur within the next few days and that, if it does, it can be controlled by medication, usually a mild analgesic such as aspirin. This warning will prevent an unnecessary telephone call from or complaint by the patient and will spare the dentist an unnecessary emergency treatment.

When severe periodontitis is present, the patient's pain can be relieved by reopening the tooth under the rubber dam, removing the sealed medicament, carefully wiping the root canal dry with sterile absorbent points, and resealing the root canal with a cotton pellet from which a mild obtundent, such as eugenol or cresatin, has been expressed. The occlusion should be adjusted if necessary.

If pain or swelling occurs, the sealed medicament should be removed and the tooth opened for drainage. Analgesics should be prescribed, opioid or nonopioid, depending on the severity of the reaction. If indicated, antibiotics may be prescribed as well. Incision and drainage of a soft, fluctuant swelling should be considered when drainage is insufficient or when severe pain persists.

When the root canals have already been filled and discomfort is present, the occlusion should be checked and the completed treatment and root canal fillings re-evaluated. Slight overfilling of the root canals with either the core or cement often causes a transient discomfort, but it may persist in some cases. When relieving the occlusion has not had the desired effect after a week or so, a prescription for a corticosteroid and antibiotic may be given to the patient, such as dexamethasone (Decadron) (0.50 mg) and erythromycin (250 mg) each taken 4 times a day for 4 to 5 days. The routine use of an antibiotic is contraindicated, however, and a corticosteroid should not be prescribed for patients with hypertension, gastric or duodenal ulcers, or diabetes. At times, the root canal filling must be removed, to relieve the pain and to establish drainage. In such cases, treatment should be as for an acute alveolar abscess.

When a post-crown restoration cannot be removed and an acute abscess is present, an incision and drainage should be considered if the swelling is soft and fluctuant, and an antibiotic should be prescribed. If the swelling is hard, hot mouth rinses should be recommended, and an antibiotic should be prescribed to control the infection. In some cases, if relief is not obtained, trepanation (artificial fistulation) of the bone over the root apex may be necessary.

CROWN FRACTURE

A traumatic injury to a tooth can cause a cracked crown, a fractured crown, or a fractured root and may result in pain. A cracked tooth can elicit bizarre symptoms such as sharp, piercing pain, especially during mastication. At times, thermal changes cause fleeting painful reactions. Observation of a hairline crack in a tooth confirms the diagnosis, but the crack may be difficult to detect. Transillumination or a dye can be used to disclose the crack line in the tooth (Fig. 2–4). A rubber polishing disc can be used to confirm the presence of a cracked crown. When the patient bites on the disc, it acts as a wedge on the cracked tooth and causes pain (Fig. 2–5).

When a visible crack is found, lateral pressure, either digital or from the handle of an operative instrument, is applied along the cusp on the occlusal surface. If the crown segment shears off and if the pulp is not exposed, the pain will usually disappear. The emergency treatment is completed by covering the exposed dentin with a sedative dressing and cementing a stainless steel band in place. If the pulp is exposed, a band should be cemented in place, and a pulpectomy should be performed.

If a greenstick fracture of the crown is present and the crown segment does not shear off under pressure, one should cement a stainless steel band around the tooth. Adjust the provisional restoration to eliminate any occlusal trauma to the tooth. This procedure should eliminate the pain and should allow the dentist time to re-evaluate the status of the tooth at a later date.

All the foregoing procedures are predicated on the presence of a vital pulp. Because any traumatic accident can temporarily affect the usual responses to the electric pulp test, cold test, and test cavity, negative test responses for pulp vitality are nondiagnostic and should not be the basis for selecting endodontic emergency treatment. It is wiser to assume that the pulp is vital because vital pulp in the root canal of a fractured tooth can enhance the prognosis for healing. If later evidence indicates the presence of pulp inflammation or necrosis, the pulp can be ex-

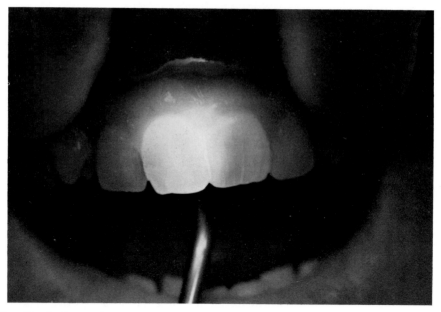

Fig. 2–4.   Transillumination can be used to locate a crack line in a tooth.

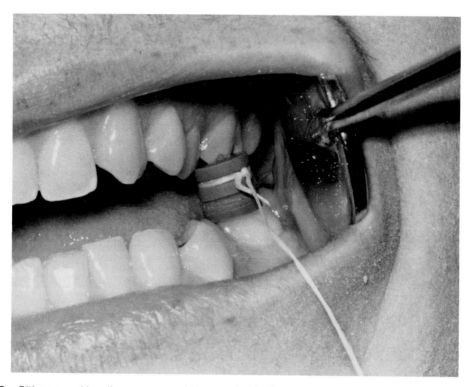

Fig. 2–5.   Biting on a rubber disc can cause pain in a cracked tooth.

tirpated at that time without altering the healing potential of the tooth.

FRACTURED ROOT

A fractured root is an endodontic emergency if the tooth is painful and, especially, if the incisal segment is mobile. The prognosis for a horizontally fractured root depends on the location and direction of the fracture. A horizontal fracture above the alveolar crest has an excellent prognosis because the tooth can be restored after endodontic treatment. The closer the root fracture is to the root apex, the more favorable the prognosis; sufficient root will remain even if the fractured segment has to be removed later.

Emergency treatment for a horizontally fractured root consists of stabilization by ligation of the tooth and adjacent teeth if mobility is present. Treat any soft-tissue lacerations. Assume that the pulp is vital, albeit "stunned" and unresponsive to tests for vitality, and do not extirpate it. If the pulp is vital, it will usually respond to tests for vitality within 6 weeks. A fractured root that contains a vital pulp has a better prognosis for root repair than one in which the pulp has died or has been extirpated.

Unfortunately, traumatic injury to a tooth may cause pulpal death. When a fractured root with a necrotic pulp requires emergency care, treatment consists of ligation for stabilization, root canal therapy including instrumentation, irrigation, debridement, and intracanal medication. If pain and swelling are present, the root canals may be left open for drainage. If the tooth is not strategic or restorable, it should be extracted as soon as possible.

A horizontal fracture at the midroot, level with or below the crest of alveolar bone, has a guarded-to-poor prognosis unless it is amenable to orthodontic root extrusion. Usually, the extra-alveolar segment, that is, incisal segment, is mobile and requires extraction. When the remaining apical root segment is long enough to retain a functional post-core crown, and has sufficient bony support, the emergency treatment for this segment is pulpectomy. If the pulp is necrotic and the tooth causes moderate-to-severe pain or swelling, then the root should be treated as if for an acute alveolar abscess.

A tooth with a vertical or longitudinal fracture of the root has a hopeless prognosis. The usual emergency treatment is extraction. On occasion, a multirooted tooth with a vertical fracture of a root can be hemisected, and the fractured root can be removed. Then the emergency treatment is removal of the fractured segment and pulpectomy of the retained segment of the tooth.

TOOTH AVULSION

The avulsed or luxated tooth is both a dental and an emotional problem. It is usually the result of trauma to an anterior tooth of a child or young adult. The shock and pain of the injury and the loss of a tooth needed for eating, speaking, and smiling, often lead to emotional upheaval in patient and parent. The situation is compounded by the need for emergency treatment, to enhance the prognosis. The longer the luxated tooth is out of its socket, the less likely it will remain in a healthy, functional state after replantation.

The following instructions should be given to the parent or patient as soon as the dentist has been informed of the accident and in preparation for an imminent visit:

1. Wash the tooth in running water without brushing or cleaning it, and examine it to be certain that the tooth is intact.
2. Have the patient rinse mouth. Replace tooth in its socket using gentle, steady finger pressure. If the patient is cooperative and able, have the patient gently close the teeth together to force the tooth back into its original position.
3. Take the patient to the dentist immediately.

If the patient or parent cannot replace the tooth in its socket, then care in transporting that tooth to the dentist becomes essential. The tooth must be carried in a moist vehicle to maintain the viability of the torn periodontal ligament. The most readily available vehicle is the patient's mouth, in which the tooth is bathed in saliva at body temperature. If this cannot be safely done, such as if the patient is too young, then one should place the tooth in a container of milk, if available, for transport to the dentist. The tooth should not be wrapped in a dry handkerchief or tissue because the periodontal ligament will become dehydrated.

Because several studies have shown that extraoral time for an avulsed tooth optimally should not exceed 30 min, the patient must be taken to the dentist immediately.[3–5,10,13]

The sooner the replantation, the better the prognosis.

On the patient's arrival at the dentist's office, the following procedure obtains:

1. If the tooth is in its socket, ligate, stabilize, and disocclude the replanted tooth. If the tooth is out of its socket or is improperly positioned, replant the tooth properly before ligation.
2. Take a radiograph to verify the position of the tooth in its socket and to examine it for any root or alveolar bone fracture. Check the adjacent teeth for possible root fracture.
3. Do not attempt endodontic treatment at this time unless the tooth requires venting (drainage). In that case, open the pulp chamber, debride it and the root canals, insert an intracanal medicament, and seal the access cavity. Endodontic treatment should be completed at a later date.

REFERRED PAIN

Accurately determining the origin of the patient's pain is the first step in emergency endodontic treatment. Although the most frequent cause of dental pain is pulpoperiapical pathosis, the astute clinician knows that pain can originate from many other sources. Referred pain may be initiated from an inflamed pulp to other parts of the body, usually on the same side and in close proximity to the tooth, or from other sources that cause pain that simulates the painful symptoms of pulpoperiapical disease.

According to Hurwitz, dental pain can have its origin in trigeminal neuralgia, atypical facial neuralgia, migraine, cardiac pain, or temporomandibular arthrosis.[11] Sinusitis or a head cold may cause pain referred to the maxillary posterior teeth. Pain arising from periodontal problems, such as periodontal abscess, occlusal trauma, muscle spasm, bruxism and clenching, and pericoronitis is often mistaken for pulpoperiapical pain.

Spicer reported pain referred to a lower molar from a basilar artery aneurysm that produced pressure in the trigeminal nerve.[17] Verbin and colleagues described odontalgia in a maxillary lateral incisor due to herpes zoster of the maxillary division of the fifth cranial nerve (trigeminal).[18] The pain subsided spontaneously following the disappearance of the mucocutaneous eruption. Sakurai and Richardson described vascular

neck pain referable to the mandibular posterior teeth.[16]

Otitis media can refer pain to the mandibular molars. Temporomandibular joint dysfunction may cause a toothache. A toothache on the left side of the mouth can be due to myocardial infarction or angina pectoris, especially if the pain occurs while the patient is exercising. A word of caution: if in the course of a dental examination any finding causes concern about the patient's health, the patient should be referred for medical examination as soon as possible.

Harris reported a case in which pain was referred to the opposite side of the mouth;[9] however, such an occurrence is rare. Other causes of referred or unusual pain include intensive radiation, systemic diseases (malaria, typhoid, influenza, anemia, hypertension, or neurasthenia), menstrual onset, neurologic diseases of the central nervous system, and some malignant diseases and tumors.

Conversely, ocular pain may be caused by disease of the pulp or periodontium of anterior teeth. Maxillary posterior teeth may refer pain to the maxillary sinus and to the back and side of the head. Pain from mandibular molars can be referred to the ear or the back of the head. Duquette and Goebel reported that pulpitis can cause temporomandibular joint pain and may be mistaken for myofascial pain dysfunction.[7] Obviously, if the pain does not originate from pulpoperiapical disease, emergency endodontic treatment will not relieve it.

ANALGESICS AND ANTIBIOTICS

The use of analgesics and antibiotics is important in endodontic emergency treatment. Because their role is essential and supportive to the previously described emergency procedures, every clinician should be familiar with their mode of action, dosage, toxicity, route of administration, indications, contraindications, and interactions with other drugs. The following description of the analgesics and antibiotics used in emergency endodontic procedures is limited in scope and is presented for orientation only. The reader is referred to pharmacologic textbooks that describe these and similar drugs in detail.

Analgesics

Analgesics are pain relievers. Generally, the narcotic analgesics are used to relieve acute, severe pain and the non-narcotic or mild analgesics are used to relieve slight-to-moderate pain. The clinician's therapeutic judgment determines which analgesic should be prescribed. He must decide the strength of the drug, whether it is to be used alone or in compound form, the frequency of use, and so on. The drugs used most often are the mild, nonopioid analgesics.

Deuben described a possible mode of action of the nonopioid analgesics as interference with membrane phospholipid metabolism.[6] When tissues are damaged, arachidonic acid is enzymatically released from the phospholipid component of the injured cellular membranes. Cyclo-oxygenase acts on the arachidonic acid to form prostaglandins, prostacyclics, and thromboxanes. Mild analgesics interfere with this cycle at the cyclo-oxygenase level and reduce the synthesis of prostaglandins; the result is the reduction or elimination of pain.

The more frequently used non-narcotic analgesics are aspirin, acetaminophen (Tylenol), diflunisal (Dolobid) naproxen (Naprosyn), and ibuprofen (Motrin). Aspirin, alone or in compound form, is used most often. In addition to relieving pain, aspirin has anti-pyretic and anti-inflammatory properties. It is effective against mild-to-moderate pain. Beaver demonstrated that 600 mg aspirin was superior to 30 mg codeine for relief of pain.[2] In spite of its widespread use and availability, aspirin should be taken with caution. It can cause an anaphylactoid reaction in an allergic person or an adverse reaction in persons with gastric ulcers. In addition, aspirin is contraindicated in patients receiving anticoagulant therapy, in patients undergoing antineoplastic chemotherapy, in diabetics, and in those suffering from gouty arthritis.

Acetaminophen, the second most commonly used analgesic, is as effective as aspirin for relief of mild-to-moderate pain. It has a lower incidence of side effects than aspirin and is effective in smaller doses. It lacks the anti-inflammatory effect of aspirin. Acetaminophen is recommended when prescribing analgesics for children and is available in liquid form.

In a double-blind study, Forbes and associates found diflunisal as effective as an acetaminophen-codeine compound, and its analgesic effect was of longer duration, up to 12 hours.[8] Diflunisal is prescribed as follows: 500 mg stat followed by 500 mg every 12 hours. This drug is contraindicated in patients with asthma, urticaria, and peptic ulcer.

Naproxen, like diflunisal, is a long-lasting analgesic. It is prescribed in 275-mg tablets, to be taken twice daily. Both naproxen and ibuprofen are proprionic acid derivatives, but their potencies differ. Ibuprofen, prescribed in doses of 300 to 400 mg 4 times daily, is more effective for severe pain relief than the daily therapeutic dose of aspirin, 3600 mg. Ibuprofen should not be used in patients with a history of peptic ulcer or aspirin intolerance.

Moore and Deuben stated that narcotic analgesics control pain better than other drugs currently available.[12] These workers postulate the mode of action of opioid analgesics as an inhibition of neurotransmission along central pain pathways by inhibiting the release of an excitatory pain transmitter. Some of these narcotic analgesics are:

morphine: not administered orally

meperidine, 50 to 100 mg (Demerol), 1 tab q4h p.r.n.

codeine, 30 mg, 1 tab q4h p.r.n.

oxycodone, 5 mg, with acetaminophen, 325 mg (Percocet-5), 1 tab q4h p.r.n.

hydrocodone, 5 mg, with acetaminophen, 500 mg (Vicodin), 1 tab q6h p.r.n.

dihydrocodeine, 16 mg, with aspirin, 356.4 mg, and caffeine, 30 mg (Synalgos-DC),1 tab q4h p.r.n.

acetaminophen, 300 mg, with codeine, 30 mg (Tylenol No. 3), 1 tab q4h p.r.n.

aspirin, 325 mg, with codeine, 30 mg (Empirin No. 3), 1 tab q4h p.r.n.

acetaminophen, 650 mg, with propoxyphene napsylate, 100 mg (Darvocet-N 100), 1 tab q4h p.r.n.

Each of these drugs must be used with caution. Narcotic analgesics may depress the central nervous system. They can interact adversely, sometimes fatally, with alcohol, antihistamines, barbiturate, local anesthetics, phenothiazines, tricyclic antidepressants, and monoamine oxidase inhibitors by enhancing the depression of the central nervous system. All opioid analgesics may be abused and should be prescribed with discretion.

Much has been written about the placebo effect of drug administration. Undoubtedly, this response can enhance the effect of all analgesics up to 40% of the time. Prensky has commented that: "pain is not merely the result of a simple stimulus-response effect. Rather it is a complex experience that goes beyond the pure sensory component. Pain involves emotional, cognitive, motivational and cultural aspects of behavior."[15] In other words, pain relief can occur following emergency treatment and the use of prescribed medication and is enhanced by the placebo effect induced by the patient's confidence in the clinician.

Antibiotics

Antibiotics are life saving therapeutic agents of inestimable value. They are used for prophylactic coverage of the medically compromised patient and, in special circumstances, an adjunctive treatment of acute periapical or periodontal infection. These drugs must be administered with care and discretion. Their future value for treating life-threatening infectious disease may be diminished or eliminated if they are used indiscriminately. One must not prescribe an antibiotic without being certain that the patient is not allergic to that antibiotic.

Ideally, the selection of a prescribed antibiotic should be based on the result of susceptibility tests that indicate effectiveness against the infecting microorganisms. The more lethal the antibiotic, the less likely resistant microorganisms will develop to it. Practically, this testing is rarely done during endodontic emergencies because susceptibility tests require several days to complete. The decision to administer antibiotics for an endodontic emergency, excluding prophylactic coverage of the medically compromised patient, depends on symptoms of systemic toxicity, such as elevated temperature, or on localized symptoms of extensive swelling or cellulitis, and the selection of antibiotic is usually empiric. Because these symptoms are usually absent in patients with pulpitis, antibiotics are rarely needed for treatment of these diseases. The use of antibiotics should be limited to adjunctive treatment of acute periapical and periodontal disease, and then only when truly needed.

The most effective antibiotic for use in endodontic emergencies is penicillin. Its mode of action is by inhibition of cell-wall synthesis during multiplication of microorganisms. Its antimicrobial action is bactericidal.

The penicillins are effective against gram-positive cocci, especially the viridans strain, rod-like bacteria, and many anaerobes involved in endodontic infections. The acid-stable penicillin V (phenoxymethyl penicillin) is the antibiotic of choice for oral administration for the medically compromised patient. The recommended standard regimen for dental procedures is: penicillin V, 2.0 g orally 1 hour before the procedure, then 1.0 g 6 hours later. In case of allergy to penicillin, erythromycin may be prescribed: 1.0 g orally 1 hour before, then 500 mg 6 hours later. Penicillin should not be prescribed for a patient with a history or suspicion of penicillin allergy.

Erythromycin's mode of action is inhibition of protein synthesis; however, its antibacterial spectrum is similar to that of penicillin. Resistant forms can occur and have been reported for staphylococci, streptococci, and enterococci. Because erythromycin is acid labile, it should be taken with food. It can be administered in tablets having an acid-insoluble coating, to ensure effective blood levels and to prevent inactivation by stomach acids.

Other antibiotics useful for treating endodontic emergencies are cephalexin (Keflex), 250 to 500 mg every 6 hours, clindamycin phosphate (Cleocin HCl), 150 to 300 mg every 6 hours, and tetracycline hydrochloride (Achromycin V), 250 to 300 mg every 6 hours. Tetracycline is the least effective of all the antibiotics listed for endodontic emergencies.

BIBLIOGRAPHY

1. August, D.S.: J. Endod., *8*:364, 1982.
2. Beaver, W.T.: Arch. Intern. Med., *141*:293, 1981.
3. Blomlöf, L.: J. Dent. Res., *62*:912, 1983.
4. Coccia, C.T.: J. Endod., *6*:413, 1980.
5. Cvek, M., et al.: Odontol. Revy, *25*:43, 1974.
6. Deuben, R.R.: Dent. Clin. North Am., *28*:401, 1984.
7. Duquette, P., and Goebel, W.M.: J. Am. Dent. Assoc., *87*:1237, 1973.
8. Forbes, J.A., et al.: JAMA, *248*:2139, 1982.
9. Harris, V.E.: J. Endod., *8*:171, 1982.
10. Hines, F.B.: J. Orthod., *75*:1, 1979.
11. Hurwitz, L.J.: Br. Dent. J., *124*:167, 1968.
12. Moore, P.A., and Deuben, R.R.: Dent. Clin. North Am., *28*:413, 1984.
13. Nasjleti, C.E.: Oral Surg., *53*:557, 1982.
14. Oliet, S.: J. Endod., *9*:147, 1983.
15. Prensky, H.D.: Contin. Ed., *1*:357, 1980.
16. Sakurai, E.H., and Richardson, J.H.: Oral Surg., *25*:553, 1968.
17. Spicer, G.H.: Oral Surg., *19*:411, 1965.
18. Verbin, R.S., et al.: Oral Surg., *26*:441, 1965.

3 The Dental Pulp and the Periradicular Tissues

Part 1 Embryology

DEVELOPMENT OF THE DENTAL LAMINA AND DENTAL PAPILLA

The dental pulp has its genesis about the sixth week of uterine life, during the initiation of tooth development[5] (Fig. 3(1)–1). Tooth development starts when the oral stratified squamous epithelium, which covers in a horseshoe-shaped pattern the primordia of the future maxillary and mandibular processes, begins to thicken and to form the dental lamina[31] (Fig. 3(1)–2). The cuboidal basal layer of the dental lamina begins to multiply and to thicken in five specific areas in each quadrant of the jaw, to mark the position of the future primary teeth. The stratified squamous oral epithelium covers an embryonic connective tissue that is called ectomesenchyme because of its derivation from neural crest cells. By a complex interaction with the epithelium, this ectomesenchyme initiates and controls the development of the dental structures. The ectomesenchyme below the thickened epithelial areas that mark the future primary teeth proliferates and begins to form a capillary network to support further nutrient activity of the ectomesenchyme-epithelium complex. This condensed area of ectomesenchyme is the future dental papilla and subsequently the pulp.

The thickened epithelial areas continue to proliferate and to migrate into the ectomesenchyme and form a bud enlargement, the enamel organ. This point is considered the bud stage of development.

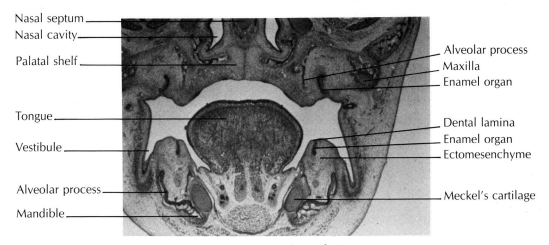

Nasal septum
Nasal cavity
Palatal shelf
Tongue
Vestibule
Alveolar process
Mandible

Alveolar process
Maxilla
Enamel organ
Dental lamina
Enamel organ
Ectomesenchyme
Meckel's cartilage

Fig. 3(1)–1. A 68-mm porcine embryo. (Courtesy of Dr. Frank Weaker, San Antonio, Texas.)

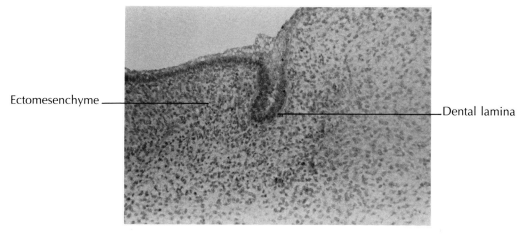

Ectomesenchyme _____   _____ Dental lamina

Fig. 3(1)–2. Invagination of the dental lamina from oral stratified squamous epithelium into the ectomesenchyme. (Courtesy of Dr. Frank Weaker, San Antonio, Texas.)

The enamel organ continues to proliferate into the ectomesenchyme with an uneven rhythmic cell division producing a convex and a concave surface characteristic of the cap stage of development. The convex surface consists of cuboidal epithelial cells and is called the outer enamel epithelium. The concave surface, called the inner enamel epithelium, consists of elongated epithelial cells with polarized nuclei that later histodifferentiate into ameloblasts. A distinct basement membrane separates the outer and inner enamel epithelium from the ectomesenchyme. In the region of the inner enamel epithelium, a cell-free or acellular zone also separates the enamel organ from the ectomesenchyme. This acellular zone contains extracellular matrix, where the future predentin will be deposited. Between the inner and the outer enamel epithelium, the cells begin to separate by the deposition of intercellular mucoid fluid rich in glycogen that forms a branch reticular arrangement called the stellate reticulum.

The ectomesenchyme, which is partially enclosed by the inner enamel epithelium, continues to increase its cellular density. The cells are large and round or polyhedral with a pale cytoplasm and large nuclei. This structure is the dental papilla, which histodifferentiates into the dental pulp.

When the ectomesenchyme surrounding the dental papilla and the enamel organ condenses and becomes more fibrous, it is called the dental follicle or dental sac, the precursor of the cementum, periodontal ligament, and alveolar bone (Fig. 3(1)–3). The dental lamina continues to proliferate at the point

where it joins the deciduous enamel organ and thereby produces the permanent bud lingual to the primary tooth germ (Fig. 3(1)–3).

The cell of the inner enamel epithelium continues to divide and thus increases the size of the tooth germ. During this growth, the inner enamel epithelium invaginates deeper into the enamel organ, and the junction of the outer and the inner enamel epithelium at the rim of the enamel organ becomes a distinct zone called the cervical loop. The deep invagination of the inner enamel epithelium and the growth of the cervical loop partially enclosing the dental papilla start to give the crown its form. This point is called the bell stage of development (Fig. 3(1)–3).

During this stage, the dental lamina that migrated into the ectomesenchyme degenerates, the primary and permanent buds are thus separated from the oral epithelium, and the distal portion of the dental lamina proliferates to form the buds of the permanent molars, which have no primary predecessors (Fig. 3(1)–3).

As development progresses, several layers of squamous cells between the stellate reticulum and the inner enamel epithelium form the stratum intermedium. This layer of cells is limited to the area of the inner enamel epithelium and seems to be involved with enamel formation.

In a complex series of events, the inner enamel epithelium exerts an inductive influence on the ectomesenchyme to begin dentinogenesis, and consequently, dentinogenesis has an inductive influence on the inner enamel epithelium to start amelogenesis.

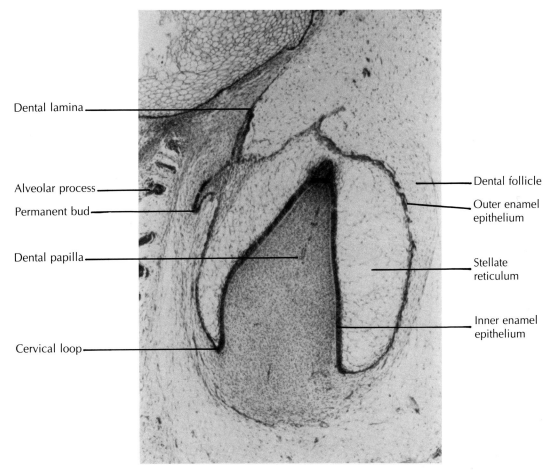

Dental lamina

Alveolar process

Permanent bud

Dental papilla

Cervical loop

Dental follicle

Outer enamel epithelium

Stellate reticulum

Inner enamel epithelium

Fig. 3(1)–3. Bell stage of development. Note the disintegration of the dental lamina. (Courtesy of Dr. Frank Weaker, San Antonio, Texas.)

This series of events begins in the area of the future cusp tips and continues to the cervical loop, the future cementoenamel junction.

DENTINOGENESIS

The periphery of the adjacent dental papilla consists of polymorphic mesenchymal cells that develop into cuboidal cells and align themselves parallel to the basement membrane of the inner enamel epithelium and the acellular zone. These cuboidal cells stop dividing and develop into columnar cells with polarized nuclei away from the basement membrane of the inner enamel epithelium. At this stage, these cells are called preodontoblasts.[37]

The preodontoblasts mature into odontoblasts by elongating themselves, by contacting adjacent odontoblasts through an increase in size, and by sending cytoplasmic processes into the acellular zone. These odontoblastic processes continue to elongate and move the odontoblast cell body toward the center of the dental papilla. During this movement, large-diameter collagen fibers known as von Korff fibers are deposited at right angles to the basement membrane in the extracellular matrix of the acellular zone. This process creates the organic matrix of the first-formed dentin or mantle dentin. As more collagen fibrils are deposited, the inner enamel epithelium basement membrane starts to disintegrate. Vesicles carrying apatite crystals bud off from the odontoblastic processes, and the crystals are deposited in the organic matrix for the initiation of mineralization. The dental papilla becomes the pulp at the moment of mantle-dentin formation.

After the deposition of mantle dentin, the odontoblasts continue to move toward the center of the pulp and to leave the odontoblastic processes behind. Organic matrix or predentin is deposited around the odonto-blastic processes. The predentin later calci-fies and thereby forms the dentinal tubules (Fig. 3(1)–4). This primary dentin is formed in increments of 4 to 8 μm per day and is continually deposited until the end of tooth development.[5] Primary dentin differs from mantle dentin in that the matrix originates solely in the odontoblasts; the collagen fibers are smaller, they are more closely packed, and they are at right angles to the tubules and are interwoven. Mineralization of primary dentin originates from the previous miner-alized dentin.

As the incremental deposition of dentin continues toward the center of the pulp, the diameter of the odontoblast processes is re-duced peripherally. Along with this reduc-tion in size is the circumferential deposition of dentin in the walls of the dentinal tubules. This dentin, which is more mineralized and is harder than primary dentin, is called peri-tubular dentin.

AMELOGENESIS

Concomitant with dentinogenesis, the cells of the inner enamel epithelium cease to divide. These cells are elongated epithelial cells called preameloblasts. The preamelo-blasts differentiate into tall columnar epithe-lial cells with their nuclei polarized toward the stratum intermedium, the ameloblasts. While the ameloblasts are differentiating, the basement membrane of the inner enamel epi-thelium is being resorbed, and dentin is being deposited to follow the contour estab-lished by the basement membrane. This proc-ess forms the future dentinoenamel junction. The ameloblasts begin to secrete enamel ma-trix against, and to follow the contour of, the already deposited dentin. The deposition of the enamel matrix causes the ameloblasts to migrate peripherally and to form conic pro-jections called Tomes' processes on their se-cretory surfaces. The migration of the ame-loblasts peripherally as they secrete enamel outlines the crown of the tooth, but blocks the source of nutrition from the dental pulp. To gain a new source of nutrition, the outer enamel epithelium becomes a flattened layer of cells that folds because of the loss of the intracellular material of the stellate reticu-lum. This change brings the capillary net-work of the dental follicle, the new source of nutrition, closer to the ameloblasts.

The orderly deposition of enamel contin-ues until the form of the crown is fully de-veloped. At this time, the ameloblasts lose their Tomes' processes, and the outer enamel epithelium, stellate reticulum, and stratum intermedium form a protective layer of strat-ified epithelium around the newly formed crown. This marks the beginning of enamel maturation or the higher mineralization of the existing enamel. This maturation process begins in the dentinoenamel junction and progresses peripherally to the enamel sur-face. During the final phase of the maturation process, the ameloblasts join the stratified epithelium to form the reduced enamel epi-

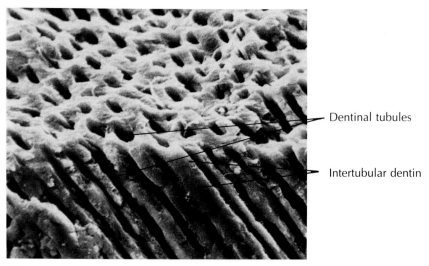

Dentinal tubules

Intertubular dentin

Fig. 3(1)–4. Scanning electron micrograph of dentin, showing intertubular dentin and tubules in the pulpal side. Mag-nification ×840. (Courtesy of Dr. Theodore Zislis, United States Army Institute of Dental Research.)

thelium, to cover and protect the enamel until eruption of the tooth.

DEVELOPMENT OF THE ROOT

On completion of the crown, the cervical loop, formed by the union of the inner and the outer enamel epithelium, proliferates to form Hertwig's epithelial root sheath, which determines the size and shape of the root of the tooth. The tip of the epithelial root sheath proliferates horizontally between the dentinal papilla and the dental follicle; this process partially encloses the dental papilla and delineates the apical foramen or foramina. This proliferation is called the epithelial diaphragm. In single-rooted teeth, the epithelial diaphragm has a single opening, which guides the formation of the root, root canal, and apical foramen. In double-rooted teeth, the diaphragm evaginates in two predetermined places that come together and form two openings; and in three-rooted teeth, evagination occurs in three predetermined places to form three openings. In multirooted teeth, the epithelial diaphragm guides the formation of the furca, roots, root canals, and apical foramina.

The vertical section of the epithelial root sheath continues to grow in an apical direction and forces the fully formed crown toward the oral cavity while maintaining the epithelial diaphragm in a stable position in the jaw. This process marks the beginning of tooth eruption.

The inner enamel epithelium below the future cementoenamel junction induces the peripheral mesenchymal cells of the dental papilla to differentiate into odontoblasts. Matrix formation and mineralization of the dentin occur as previously described. As dentin is formed, the basement membrane of the inner enamel epithelium disintegrates, and the epithelial cells lose their continuity. The disintegration of the basement membrane and the loss of continuity of the epithelial cells allow the mesenchymal cells from the dental follicle to penetrate the newly deposited dentin. These mesenchymal cells differentiate into cementoblasts, which are round, plump cells that have basophilic cytoplasm with an open nucleus in the active phase of cementogenesis and a closed nucleus and reduced cytoplasm during the resting phase. Collagen fibers followed by ground substance elaborated by the cementoblasts are deposited between the epi-

thelial cells. The cluster of cells left behind from the epithelial root sheath migrates toward the dental follicle, the future periodontal ligament. This cluster of epithelial cells comprises the cell rests of Malassez, dormant in the mature periodontal ligament and with the potential of proliferating into periradicular cysts if stimulated by chronic inflammation. When some matrix production has taken place, mineralization of the cementum starts by the spread and deposition of hydroxyapatite crystals from the dentin into the collagen fibers and the matrix. As dentinogenesis progresses in incremental phases, the apical foramen or foramina are formed by an apposition of dentin and cementum that reduces the size of the opening of the epithelial diaphragm.

Accessory canals, which are an inefficient source of collateral circulation for the pulp, are formed during the development of the root. A defect in the epithelial root sheath, a failure in the induction of dentinogenesis, or the presence of a small blood vessel produces a gap that results in the formation of an accessory canal. Accessory canals are more prevalent in the apical third of the root (Fig. 3(1)–5).[29] Sometimes, the inner enamel epithelium, which induces the cells of the dental papilla to form odontoblasts during root formation, differentiates into ameloblasts and forms enamel pearls on the root.[29]

Two kinds of cementum are laid down on the root. If the cementoblasts retract as the cementum is laid, it will be acellular cementum. If, on the other hand, the cementoblasts do not retract and are surrounded by the new cementum, the tissue formed will be cellular cementum, and the trapped cementoblasts are called cementocytes. The acellular cementum is found adjacent to the dentin. The cellular cementum is found usually in the apical third of the root overlying acellular cementum and in alternating layers with it. Cementocytes receive their nutrients from the periodontal ligament; cementum is completely avascular. Because cementum is deposited in layers throughout the life of the tooth, cementocytes are separated from the periodontal ligament, their source of nutrition, and die, leaving empty lacunae in the cementum.

Cementum is deposited in a thin layer at the cementoenamel junction to form a butt joint (30%), an overlap joint (60%), or a gap between cementum and enamel (10%).[44]

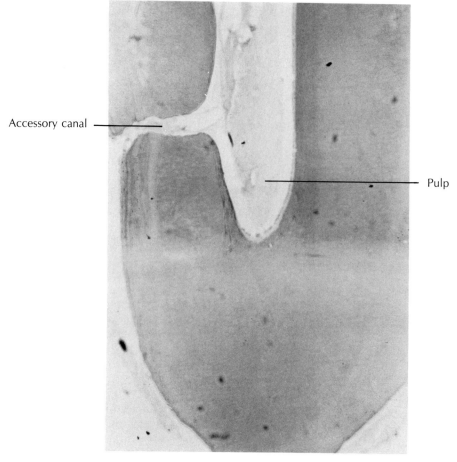

Fig. 3(1)–5. Accessory canal in apical third of root. (Courtesy of Dr. Steve Senia, San Antonio, Texas.)

This gap may produce cervical sensitivity, or it may predispose the tooth to cervical caries.

The incremental deposition of cementum continues throughout the life of the tooth, leaves rest lines on the tooth's surface, and makes the layer of cementum on the apical third of the root thicker than on the cervical third. This continued incremental deposition of cementum in the apical third maintains the length of the tooth, constricts the apical foramen, and deviates the apical foramen from the center of the apex.

DEVELOPMENT OF THE PERIODONTAL LIGAMENT AND ALVEOLAR BONE

The periodontal ligament and the alveolar bone develop at the same time as the root of the tooth. As the mesenchymal cells of the dental follicle adjacent to the tooth differentiate into cementoblasts, the cells in the periphery of the follicle differentiate into osteoblasts to form the bony crypt or alveolus of the tooth, and the mesenchymal cells of the center of the follicle differentiate into fibroblasts. These fibroblasts deposit obliquely oriented collagen fibrils that develop into fiber bundles. These obliquely oriented fiber bundles become entrapped in bone and cementum as they are deposited and thereby give rise to the periodontal ligament fibers. Deposition of bone to form the alveolus and deposition of cementum to cover the dentin of the root give form to the attachment apparatus, the periodontium. The surface of the bony crypt becomes known as the lamina dura radiographically.

CIRCULATION AND INNERVATION

The blood vessels of the pulp originate from an oval or circular reticulated plexus[12] (Fig. 3(1)–6). When fully developed, this plexus encircles the enamel organ and the dental papilla in the region of the dental follicle. A series of vessels arises from this

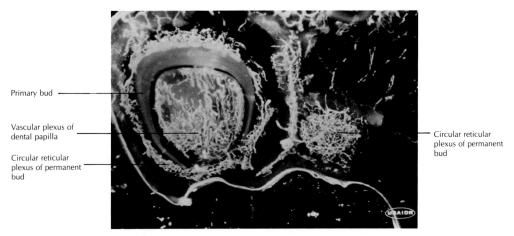

Primary bud

Vascular plexus of
dental papilla

Circular reticular
plexus of permanent
bud

Circular reticular
plexus of permanent
bud

Fig. 3(1)–6. Vascular plexus of tooth buds. Note the vessels from the circular reticular plexus entering the dental papilla to form a vascular plexus in the primary bud. (From Cutright, D.: The morphogenesis of the vascular supply to the permanent teeth. Oral Surg., *30*:284, 1970.)

plexus and grows into the dental papilla. At the beginning of dentinogenesis, vessels that have penetrated the dental papilla give rise to a vascular subodontoblastic plexus, which follows the shape of the newly formed dentin. This subodontoblastic plexus atrophies as soon as the mature thickness of dentin is established and leaves the vessels that connect with the circular reticulated plexus to form the pulpal vessels. As the tooth matures, the circular reticulated plexus develops into the periodontal plexus. The formation of the root elongates the pulpal vessels, causes the reappearance of the subodontoblastic plexus, and constricts the pulpal vessels into a small apical foramen. In multirooted teeth, the epithelial diaphragm divides the pulpal vessels randomly into the different foramina.

In the early stages of tooth development, nerve fibers can be seen in the dental follicle. At the beginning of dentinogenesis, some of the nerve fibers from the dental follicle migrate into the dental papilla. Not until the beginning of root formation does nerve proliferation of the pulp begin. Sensory nerve fibers traverse the dental papilla and, on reaching the coronal pulp, branch toward the periphery to form a plexus of nerves. This plexus of Raschkow is located in the subodontoblastic zone of the coronal pulp. These sensory nerve fibers are myelinated; therefore, they are enclosed in a sheath made of Schwann's cells. A number of nerves leave the plexus and extend into the odontoblastic layer. Some contact the odontoblasts, whereas others lose their myelin sheath and enter the predentin and the dentinal tubules. The unmyelinated nerve fibers that enter the dentinal tubules lie in the proximity of the odontoblastic processes.[23]

The blood vessels entering the dental papilla during the development bring with them sympathetic nerve fibers, which are unmyelinated. These sympathetic nerve fibers play a role in the vasoconstriction of the blood vessels.[5]

As the apical foramen matures and reduces the size of its opening, the myelinated nerve fibers form bundles located in the center of the pulp in conjunction with the blood vessels. The formation of the apical foramen is completed during the final stage of eruption of the tooth into the oral cavity, when the tooth contacts its antagonist. The completion of the apical foramen marks the end of pulp development and the beginning of secondary dentin formation by the pulp.[44]

Part 2 Normal Pulp

The dental pulp consists of vascular connective tissue contained within rigid dentinal walls. Although similar to other connective tissues in the human body, it is specialized, owing to its functions and milieu.

The elaboration of dentin to form the tooth and to protect against and to repair the effects of noxious stimuli is the primary function of the pulp. Intimately related to these formative and protective functions is a nutritive function concerned with preserving the vitality of all the cellular elements. Moreover, a sensory function allows the perception of stimuli.

The elaboration of dentin creates a special environment for the pulp. The pulp space becomes limited by dentin formation to an average volume of 0.024 ml in permanent adult human teeth.[5] This volume is continuously reduced by the deposition of secondary dentin throughout the life of the pulp, as well as by the deposition of reparative dentin in response to noxious stimuli. The encasement of the pulp in dentin creates an environment that allows only small amounts of intercellular accommodation of exudate during inflammatory reactions. This inability of the pulp to swell creates abnormally high pressure in an area of inflammation, with interruption of blood flow due to the collapse of the pulpal veins, possibly resulting in anoxia and localized necrosis.[46]

The anatomic limitation of encasement of dentin on the pulp makes the pulp an organ of terminal circulation, with limited portals of entry and exit: the apical and accessory foramina. This feature limits the vascular supply and drainage of the pulp and thereby limits its collateral circulation.

Starting at the periphery, the pulp is divided into the odontoblastic zone, which surrounds the periphery of the pulp, the cell-free zone, the cell-rich zone, and the central zone (Fig. 3(2)–1).

ODONTOBLASTIC ZONE

As discussed previously, the odontoblasts consist of cell bodies and their cytoplasmic processes (Fig. 3(2)–2). The odontoblastic cell bodies form the odontoblastic zone, whereas the odontoblastic processes are located within the predentin matrix and the dentinal tubules, extending into the dentin. In this odontoblastic zone, capillaries and unmyelinated sensory nerves are found around the odontoblastic cell bodies.

The primary function of the odontoblasts throughout the life of the pulp is the production and deposition of dentin. Because of the important and close relationship between odontoblasts and dentin, these structures are discussed together.

In histologic sections, the odontoblasts appear to be lined up in a palisading arrangement at the periphery of the pulp. The cell bodies of the odontoblasts have junctional complexes, such as gap junctions, that unite the cells and allow an interchange of metabolites.[44] These cytoplasmic bridges among odontoblasts may explain the palisading formation and the action in unison of these cells. These cell bodies vary in size, shape, and arrangement from the coronal pulp to the apical pulp. In the coronal pulp, the odontoblasts are tall, columnar cells with a nucleus polarized toward the center of the pulp. They change shape gradually to flattened cells in the apical third, and their arrangement changes from a six-to-eight-cell layer in the pulp horns to a one-cell layer in the apical pulp.

The crowded arrangement of the coronal odontoblasts is due to the rapid reduction of the pulp chamber by the deposition of dentin, which compresses the existing cells to a stratified layer. This crowding of odontoblasts produces more cells per unit area and, therefore, more dentinal tubules (45,000/mm^2) in the pulpal side than in the enamel side (20,000/mm^2).[15] As a result of this phenomenon, the configuration of the dentinal tubules in these areas is "S" shaped (Fig. 3(2)–3). Reduction of odontoblasts per unit area produces fewer tubules and results in a straighter course, as seen in the cervical third of the root or beneath the incisal edges or cusps. Further reduction in the number of cells and, consequently, in the number of dentinal tubules produces dentin typically found in the apical third. The presence of "S"-shaped tubules is a consideration in clinical endodontic practice. Operative procedures in areas with such tubules produce inflammatory changes in the odontoblastic

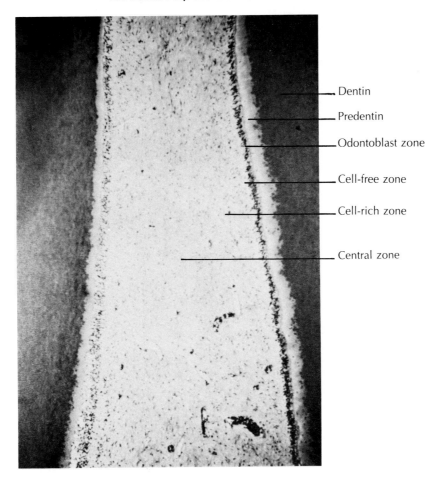

— Dentin
— Predentin
— Odontoblast zone
— Cell-free zone
— Cell-rich zone
— Central zone

Fig. 3(2)–1. Normal pulp.

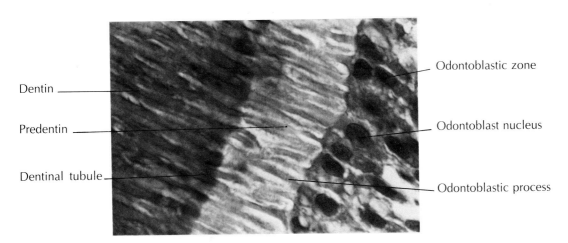

Dentin

Predentin

Dentinal tubule

Odontoblastic zone

Odontoblast nucleus

Odontoblastic process

Fig. 3(2)–2. Odontoblast and its processes.

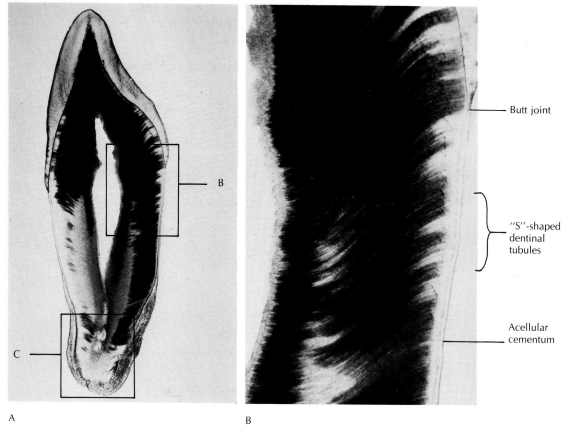

Fig. 3(2)–3. *A*, Ground section of central incisor. Note the eccentric position of the foramen and the thickness of the cementum in the apical third, as compared to the cervical third. *B*, Higher magnification of the cervical third.

layer further apically than expected. Endodontic fillings in anterior teeth must be placed 2 to 3 mm below the free margin of the gingiva, to prevent the loss of translucency in the gingival third of the crown.

Predentin Layer

Dentinogenesis includes the production, deposition, and calcification of a matrix. This matrix is the predentin layer deposited around the odontoblastic processes and is found between the calcified dentin and the odontoblastic zone (see Fig. 3(2)–2). This predentin layer, elaborated by odontoblasts, is a protein carbohydrate complex consisting of proteoglycans, phosphoproteins, plasma proteins, glycoproteins, and collagen fibrils.[38] Calcium and phosphorus salts are deposited into this matrix to produce the mineralized structure known as dentin. The pattern of calcification around the odontoblastic processes forms the dentinal tubules, and the dentin between these tubules is called intertubular dentin (Fig. 3(2)–5).

Odontoblastic Processes

The extent of the odontoblastic processes in dentin has not been determined. During the early stages of development, the processes extend into the entire thickness of the dentin. Studies in adult teeth have given conflicting information on the extent of the processes. Some studies claim that these processes extend into one-third of the thickness of the dentin (0.7 mm),[7] whereas others claim that the processes extend through the thickness of the dentin and reach the dentinoenamel junction (Fig. 3(2)–4).[1,26] The space around the odontoblastic processes, the periodontoblastic space, and the space peripheral to the end of the odontoblastic processes are filled with extracellular fluid. This fluid originates from capillary transudate and plays an important role in sensory transmission. Unmyelinated nerves for sensory perception are also found in the pulpal end of the periodontoblastic space of the dentinal tubules.

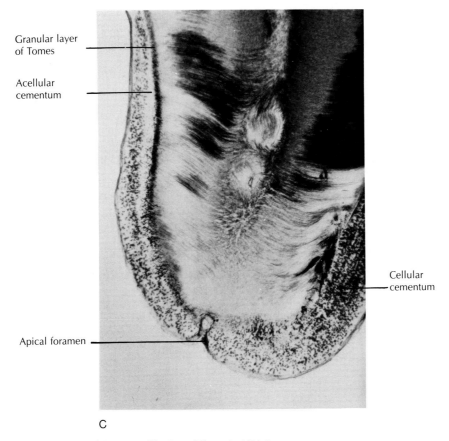

Granular layer of Tomes

Acellular cementum

Cellular cementum

Apical foramen

C

Fig. 3(2)–3. (Continued) *C,* Higher magnification of the apical third.

Incremental Lines

During dentinogenesis, there are periods of activity and periods of rest. These periods are demarcated by the presence of lines, called incremental lines. These lines are accentuated during periods of illness, by deficiencies in nutrition, and at birth. The accentuated incremental line that occurs at birth is called the neonatal line. In some areas in the mature dentin, the matrix has not calcified or is hypocalcified. These areas are called interglobular dentin. One also sees spaces in the root dentin near the cementodentinal junction, the granular layer of Tomes (see Fig. 3(2)–3). Incremental lines represent rest periods in dentinogenesis, whereas interglobular dentin and the granular layer of Tomes probably represent a defect in matrix formation.

Dentinal Tubules

The dentinal tubules extend from the predentin border to the dentinoenamel and dentinocemental junctions. They are conical in shape, with a 2.5-μm mean diameter in the pulpal wall and a 0.9-μm mean diameter in the dentinoenamel or dentinocemental junctions, because of the deposition of peritubular dentin (Fig. 3(2)–5).[15] As the dentinal tubules approach the dentinoenamel junction, they branch and increase the ratio per unit area over that of the middle third of the dentin (Fig. 3(2)–6). The branching of the dentinal tubules occurs during the beginning of dentinogenesis. Each preodontoblast sends various cytoplasmic processes into the acellular zone and thereby produces several future dentinal tubules. As the fully mature odontoblast migrates pulpally, the processes unite to form a single dentinal tubule with terminal branches at the dentinoenamel junction. This branching may explain the extreme sensitivity of the dentinoenamel junction.

Because peritubular dentin has an organic matrix with fewer collagen fibers than intertubular dentin, it is more mineralized and is harder. As the pulp ages, the continuous deposition of peritubular dentin may obliterate the dentinal tubules peripherally. This oblit-

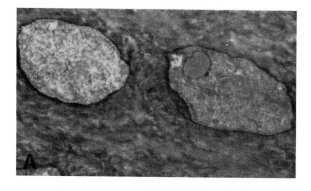
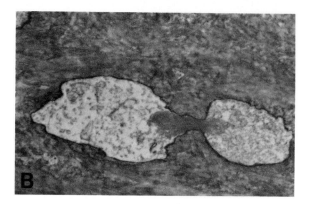
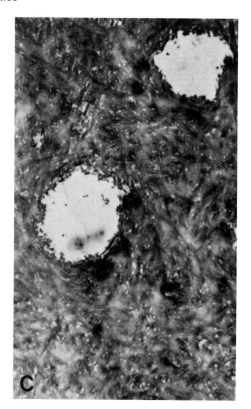

Fig. 3(2)–4. Electron micrograph of dentinal tubules with odontoblastic processes in the pulpal side of the dentin (*A*, magnification ×5000). Note the connection between the dentinal tubules (*B*, magnification ×5000). Empty dentinal tubules are 200 μm from the cementodentinal junction (*C*, magnification ×4000). (Courtesy of Dr. R. White, San Antonio, Texas.)

eration of tubules results in the formation of sclerotic dentin, which has a glassy appearance under transmitted light. Sclerosis reduces the permeability of the dentin and may serve as a pulp-protective mechanism. A mild stimulus of short duration may accelerate the production of peritubular dentin, may produce sclerosis peripherally, and may thus reduce the permeability of dentin and enhance pulp protection.[45]

By dentinogenesis, the odontoblasts are involved in the formation of the teeth and the protection of the pulp from noxious stimuli. To fulfill the formative and protective functions of the pulp, the odontoblasts deposit primary, secondary, and reparative dentin.

Primary Dentin

Primary dentin is elaborated before the teeth erupt and is divided into mantle and circumpulpal dentin (Fig. 3(2)–7).[44] Mantle dentin, the first calcified layer of the dentin deposited against the enamel, forms the dentinal side of the dentinoenamel junction. Cir-

cumpulpal dentin is the dentin formed after the layer of mantle dentin. Primary dentin fulfills the initial formative function of the pulp.

Secondary Dentin

Secondary dentin is elaborated after eruption of the teeth (Fig. 3(2)–7).[44] It can be differentiated from primary dentin by the sharp bending of the tubules producing a line of demarcation, according to Provenza.[36] It is deposited unevenly on primary dentin at a low rate and has incremental patterns and tubular structures less regular than those of primary dentin. For example, secondary dentin is deposited in greater quantities in the floor and roof of the pulp chamber than on the walls.[23] This uneven deposition explains the pattern of reduction of the pulp chamber and pulp horns as teeth age. This deposition of secondary dentin protects the pulp.

Reparative Dentin

Reparative dentin, also known as irregular or tertiary dentin, is elaborated by the pulp as a protective response to noxious stimuli

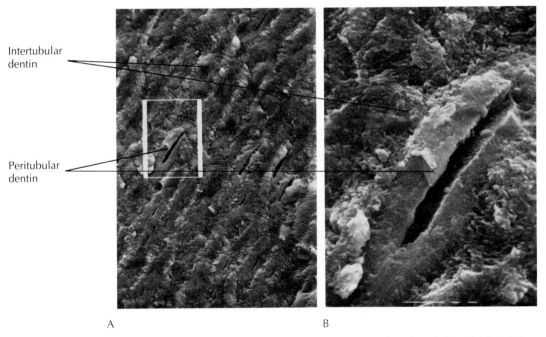

Intertubular dentin

Peritubular dentin

A   B

Fig. 3(2)–5. Scanning electron micrograph of dentin, showing a longitudinal section of a tubule and intertubular and peritubular dentin. (*A*, magnification ×1010; *B*, magnification ×4400.) (Courtesy of Dr. Theodore Zislis, United States Army Institute of Dental Research.)

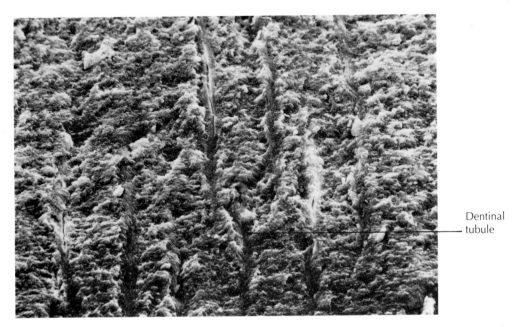

Dentinal tubule

Fig. 3(2)–6. Scanning electron micrograph of a branching dentin tubule near the dentinoenamel junction. Magnification ×1800. (Courtesy of Dr. Theodore Zislis, United States Army Institute of Dental Research.)

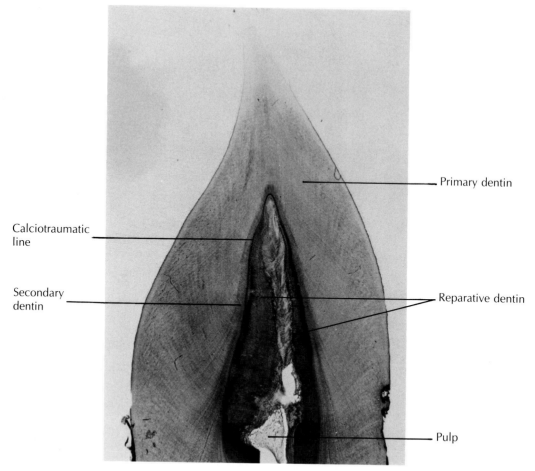

Fig. 3(2)–7. Maxillary central incisor of 48-year-old man, showing primary, secondary, and reparative dentin. (Courtesy of Dr. B. Orban.)

(Fig. 3(2)–7).[44] These stimuli can result from caries, operative procedures, restorative materials, abrasion, erosion, or trauma. The reparative dentin is deposited in the affected area at an increased rate that averages 1.5 μm per day.[40] The rate, the quality, and the quantity of reparative dentin deposited depends on the severity and duration of the injury to the odontoblasts and is usually produced by "replacement" odontoblasts.

When a mild stimulus is applied to the odontoblasts for a prolonged period of time, such as abrasion, reparative dentin may be deposited at a slower rate. This tissue is characterized by slightly irregular tubules. On the other hand, an aggressive carious lesion or other abrupt stimulus stimulates the production of reparative dentin with fewer and more irregular tubules. If the odontoblast is injured beyond repair, the degenerated odontoblasts will leave empty tubules, called dead tracts,

that allow bacteria and noxious products to enter the pulp. Reparative dentin is deposited on the pulpal wall of a dead tract unless the pulp is too atrophic. Because reparative dentin has fewer tubules, although it is less mineralized, it blocks the ingress of noxious products into the pulp. As the caries progresses and as more odontoblasts are injured beyond repair, the layers of reparative dentin become more atubular and may have cell inclusions, that is, trapped odontoblasts. Cellular inclusions are uncommon in human teeth. On removal of the caries, the mesenchymal cell of the cell-rich zone differentiates into odontoblasts to replace those that have necrosed. These newly formed odontoblasts can produce well-organized dentin or an amorphous, poorly calcified, permeable dentin. The demarcation zone between secondary and reparative dentin is called the calciotraumatic line (Fig. 3(2)–7).

CELL-FREE ZONE

The cell-free zone, or zone of Weil, is a relatively acellular zone of the pulp, located centrally to the odontoblast zone (see Fig. 3(2)–1). This zone, although called cell-free, contains some fibroblasts, mesenchymal cells, and macrophages. Fibroblasts are involved in the production and maintenance of the reticular fibers found in this zone. When odontoblasts are destroyed by noxious stimuli, mesenchymal cells and fibroblasts differentiate into new odontoblasts. Macrophages are present for phagocytosis of debris.

The main constituents of this zone are a plexus of capillaries, the nerve plexus of Raschkow, and the ground substance. The capillary plexus is involved in the nutrition of the odontoblasts and the cells of the zone and is conspicuous only during periods of dentinogenesis and inflammation. The unmyelinated nerve plexus of Raschkow is involved in the neural sensation of the pulp and can only be seen if stained with a special silver stain. The ground substance is involved in the metabolic exchanges of the cells and limits the spread of infection because of its consistency. The zone of Weil is more prominent in the coronal pulp, but it may be completely absent during periods of dentinogenesis.

CELL-RICH ZONE

The cell-rich zone is located central to the cell-free zone (see Fig. 3(2)–1). Its main components are ground substance, fibroblasts with their product the collagen fibers, undifferentiated mesenchymal cells, and macrophages.

Ground Substance

Ground substance, the main constituent of the pulp, is the part of the matrix that surrounds and supports the cellular and vascular elements of the pulp. It is a gelatinous substance composed of proteoglycans, glycoproteins, and water. The proteoglycans or mucopolysaccharides are hyaluronic acid, chondroitin sulfate, dermatan sulfate, and heparin sulfate.[38] Ground substance serves as a transport medium for metabolites and waste products of cells and as a barrier against the spread of bacteria. Age and disease may change the composition and function of the ground substance.

Fibroblasts

The fibroblasts are the predominant cells of the pulp. They may originate from undifferentiated mesenchymal cells of the pulp or from the division of existing fibroblasts. Fibroblasts are stellate in shape, with ovoid nuclei and cytoplasmic processes. As they age, they become rounder, with round nuclei and short cytoplasmic processes. The change in shape is due to a reduction in activity of the cells because of aging.

The function of the fibroblasts is elaboration of ground substance and collagen fibers, which constitute the matrix of the pulp. Fibroblasts are also involved in the degradation of collagen and the deposition of calcified tissue. They can elaborate denticles and can differentiate to replace dead odontoblasts, with the potential for reparative dentin formation. Although fibroblasts are present in the cell-free and central zones of the pulp, they are concentrated in the cell-rich zone, especially in the coronal portion.

In the pulp are two types of fibers: elastic fibers found in the walls of arterioles and collagenous fibers found in the body of the pulp. The collagenous fibers are secreted by fibroblasts, to form a reticular network to support the body of the pulp, and by odontoblasts as part of the dentinal matrix.

When seen through the electron microscope, the pulp collagen fibers have the periodicity of 640-Å cross banding characteristics of collagen.[5] In young pulp, the collagen fibers are small and occur in diffuse patterns throughout the pulp. These fibers have an affinity to silver stain (argyrophilic) because of a carbohydrate component.[29] In older pulp, the collagen fibers are found in large bundles, usually concentrated in the central region. These older fibers lose their argyrophilic properties.

As compared to the coronal third, the apical third of the mature pulp contains more collagen fibers, is therefore more fibrous, and has a whitish coloration. This fibrous characteristic of the apical third protects the neurovascular bundle from injury and is of clinical significance because it facilitates the removal of the pulp during pulpectomy. Because of the reduction of the pulp space through the continuous deposition of secondary dentin and because of the increased deposition of collagen, the pulp becomes more fibrous with age. Concomitantly, one sees a decrease in cellular elements and a reduction in the reparative potential of the pulp.

Undifferentiated Mesenchymal Cells

The undifferentiated mesenchymal cells are derived from the mesenchymal cells of the dental papilla. Because of their function in repair and regeneration, they retain pluripotential characteristics and can differentiate into fibroblasts, odontoblasts, macrophages, or osteoclasts. They resemble fibroblasts in that they are stellate in shape, with a large nucleus and little cytoplasm. These cells, if present, are usually located around blood vessels in the cell-rich zone and are difficult to recognize.

Macrophages, Lymphocytes, and Plasma Cells

Macrophages are found in the cell-rich zone, especially near blood vessels. These cells are blood monocytes that have migrated into the pulp tissue. Their function is to phagocytize necrotic debris and foreign materials.

Lymphocytes and plasma cells, if present in the normal pulp, are found in the coronal subodontoblastic region. The function of these cells in the normal pulp may be immune surveillance.

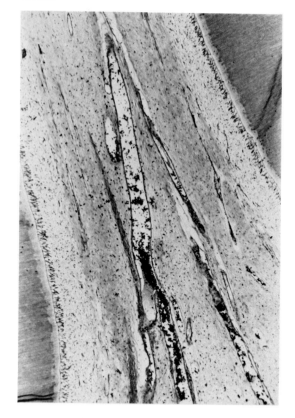

Fig. 3(2)–8. Centrally located blood vessels of the pulp.

CENTRAL ZONE

The central zone or pulp proper contains blood vessels and nerves that are embedded in the pulp matrix together with fibroblasts (see Fig. 3(2)–1). From their central location, blood vessels and nerves send branches to the periphery of the pulp (Figs. 3(2)–8 to 3(2)–10).

The neurovascular bundle enters the pulp through the apical foramina. It consists of one or two arterioles with their sympathetic nerve fibers and myelinated and unmyelinated sensory nerves entering the pulp, and two or three venules and lymphatic vessels exiting the pulp. In some teeth, accessory foramina may serve as portals of entry and exit for blood vessels only.

Circulation

The afferent circulation of the pulp consists of arterioles entering the apical foramen. As these vessels traverse the center of the pulp, they branch into terminal arterioles, metarterioles, precapillaries, and finally capillaries. The capillaries end in the cell-poor zone and form a rich subodontoblastic plexus

(Figs. 3(2)–9 and 3(2)–11). This plexus may send capillary loops that pass between the odontoblasts.[42]

The efferent circulation consists of postcapillary venules and collecting venules, which empty into two or three venules that exit through the apical foramina and empty into the vessels in the periodontal ligament.[42] Lymphatic vessels follow this same pattern[29,38] (see Fig. 3(2)–9).

The function of the blood vessels is to transport nutrients, fluids, and oxygen to the tissues and to remove metabolic waste from the tissues by maintaining an adequate flow of blood through the capillaries. This metabolic exchange occurs in the capillary bed. This exchange of nutrients and metabolic waste is accomplished by a series of mechanisms. The sympathetic nerves that accompany the arterial blood vessels are able to contract the smooth muscle in the middle layer of the arterioles, the smooth muscle fibers that encircle part of the walls of the metarterioles, and the precapillary muscle sphincters. The contraction and relaxation of the smooth muscle regulate the size of the lumen of the vessels and thereby control the

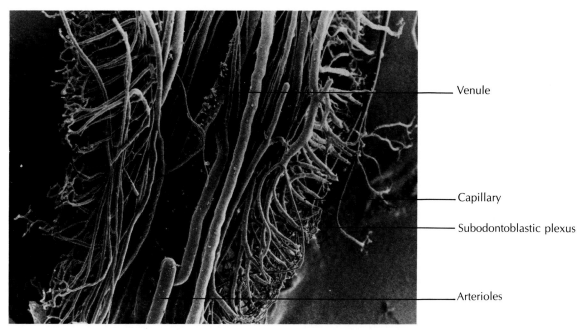

Venule

Capillary

Subodontoblastic plexus

Arterioles

Fig. 3(2)–9. Scanning electron micrograph of a corrosion resin cast of dog pulpal vasculature. Note the central location of venules and arterioles, the lateral branching of the arterioles into capillaries to form the subodontoblastic plexus, and the continuous round connection between capillaries and postcapillary venules. (From Takahashi, K., Kishi, Y., and Kim, S.: A scanning electron microscope study of the blood vessels of dog pulp using corrosion resin casts. J. Endodont., 8:131, 1982.)

flow of blood to the tissues. The decrease in the diameter of the vessel, or vasoconstriction, and the increase in the diameter of the vessel, or vasodilation, explain the prominence of the capillary bed during periods of high metabolic activity such as dentinogenesis or inflammation and the almost complete disappearance of the capillary bed during periods of metabolic inactivity. Vasoconstriction and vasodilation can be mediated by humoral agents. Epinephrine elaborated by the adrenal medulla constricts the smooth muscle of the blood vessels. Acetylcholine liberated by the parasympathetic nerves dilates the blood vessels.[21]

Another mechanism increases or decreases the flow of blood to the capillary bed. This is a direct connection between the arterioles and venules called an arteriovenous anastomosis, or shunt. This anastomosis can decrease blood flow to the capillaries by diverting it from the arterioles to the venules thus bypassing the capillary bed. This mechanism may decrease or stop the flow of blood to an area of injury and may prevent hemorrhage and thrombosis.[21]

The transfer of nutrients and metabolic waste through the capillary walls is controlled by the laws of hydrostatics and osmo-

sis. The walls of the capillaries consist of a single layer of endothelial cells covered with a layer of glycoproteins inside the lumen, with a basement membrane in the periphery (Fig. 3(2)–11). The walls of the capillaries are an average of 0.5 μm thick and serve as a permeable membrane that permits the exchange of fluids.[38] Although uncommon, intercellular fenestrations or pores are also found in the capillary walls. These pores, which are covered with a diaphragm of plasma membrane, are used for the rapid transfer of fluids and nutrients. The water-soluble nutrients in plasma filter through the capillary walls into the pulp tissues when the intravascular pressure in the arterial capillaries is higher than the osmotic pressure of the pulpal tissue. The absorption of metabolic wastes from the pulpal tissues into the capillary venules and lymphatic vessels occurs when the tissues' osmotic pressure is higher than the intravascular pressure of the postcapillary venules and lymphatic vessels. The absorption of metabolic wastes and fluids prevents their accumulation in the pulpal tissues and also precludes increases in the pulpal tissue pressure.[17]

In areas of pulpal injury, the permeability of the capillary walls permits the seepage of

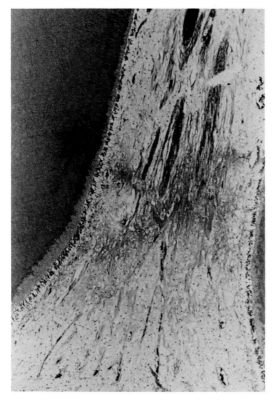

Fig. 3(2)–10. Centrally located nerves of the pulp.

blood proteins into the pulpal tissues and increases the tissues' osmotic pressure of the area. This increase in osmotic pressure attracts more fluid to the area; the result is the stagnation of fluid known as edema.[17]

Lymphatic System

Lymphatic vessels are present in the pulp (Fig. 3(2)–12). Their fine endothelial structure makes them difficult to see. The function of these lymphatic vessels is the removal of interstitial fluid and metabolic waste products, to maintain the intrapulpal tissue pressure at a normal level. These lymphatic vessels follow the course of the venules toward the apical foramen.[29,38]

Interstitial Fluid

Interstitial fluid bathes all the pulpal tissues and fills the dentinal tubules in their distal extension and around the odontoblastic processes. The interstitial fluid that fills the dentinal tubules is called dentinal fluid. As previously discussed, the encasement of the pulp in dentin produces a limited environment permitting only a small amount of interstitial fluid. The presence of this fluid in the pulpal cavity produces an average in-

trapulpal pressure of approximately 10 mm Hg. Because of the rigid encasement, a small increase in intrapulpal pressure to 13 mm Hg during inflammatory changes causes reversible changes in the pulp, but increases to 35 mm Hg produce irreversible changes. Owing to the structural makeup of the matrix, in which the ground substance is reinforced by collagen fibers, the pulp seems to be able to limit the area of increased intrapulpal pressure during periods of inflammation.

Innervation

The sensory mechanism of the pulp is composed of sensory afferent and autonomic efferent systems. The afferent system conducts impulses perceived by the pulp from a variety of stimuli to the cortex of the brain, where they are interpreted as pain, regardless of the stimulus. The efferent system conducts impulses from the central system to the smooth muscle of the arterial vessels to regulate the volume and rate of the blood flow. By regulating blood circulation to the pulp, the efferent system controls the intrapulpal blood pressure and possibly dentin formation.[5]

The sensory afferent impulses originate in unmyelinated nerve endings. In the odontoblast layer in the predentin, these nerve endings run either straight or spirally, terminating in multiple ending-like enlargements and may penetrate the dentin by a few microns. Only 10 to 20% of the dentinal tubules in the coronal dentin contain nerve endings, with almost none in the radicular dentin.[48]

Approximately 80% of the nerves of the pulp are C-type fibers, and the rest are A-delta fibers. The C fibers are unmyelinated and have a diameter of 0.3 to 1.2 μm and a conduction velocity of 0.4 to 2 m/sec.[48] The conduction of these fibers, which are of smaller diameter than A-delta fibers, is slow. These fibers are probably distributed throughout the pulp tissue; therefore, they conduct throbbing and aching pain associated with pulp tissue damage.[48]

The A-delta fibers are myelinated and have a diameter of 2 to 5 μm and a conduction velocity of 6 to 30 m/sec.[48] The A-delta fibers, with a larger diameter than that of the C fibers, conduct impulses at a higher velocity. These impulses are interpreted as sharp and pricking pain.[48] The A-delta fibers are distributed in the odontoblastic and subodonto-

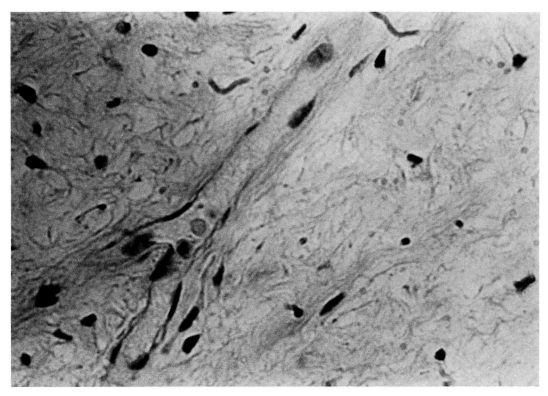

Fig. 3(2)–11. Capillary in the cell-free zone during a period of inflammation. (Courtesy of Dr. Steve Senia, San Antonio, Texas.)

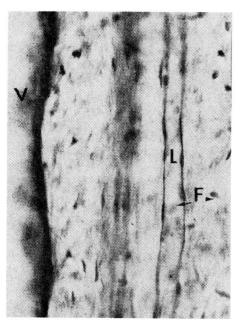

Fig. 3(2)–12. The lymphatic vessel (L) consists of endothelial lining surrounded by scattered fibroblasts (F). V, Vein, (From Bernick, S.: Lymphatic vessels of the human dental pulp. J. Dent. Res., 56:70, 1977.)

blastic zones and are associated with dentinal pain.

The impulse travels from C- or A-delta-fiber nerve endings, through the plexus of Raschkow, to the nerve trunk in the central zone of the pulp (see Fig. 3(2)–10). The A-delta fibers are enclosed in myelin sheaths while traversing the plexus of Raschkow.

The nerve trunk is composed of myelinated A-delta fibers in the periphery and unmyelinated C fibers in the center. This arrangement may protect the unmyelinated nerve fibers. Neural impulses travel through the nerve trunk and exit the tooth through the apical foramen. In the periapical area, the nerve trunk joins the maxillary or mandibular division of the fifth cranial nerve. The nerve impulses travel through the fifth cranial or trigeminal nerve, to the pons, to the thalamus, and finally to the cortex, where they are interpreted as pain.

The efferent motor pathway in the dental pulp consists of sympathetic fibers from the cervical ganglion that enter through the apical foramina in the outer layer of the arterioles, the tunica adventitia. The nerves travel with the vessels and terminate in the smooth muscle of the tunica media of the arterioles, metarterioles, and precapillaries. As discussed previously, the sympathetic nerves provide vasomotor control to circulation and therefore regulate blood flow in response to stimuli. Some evidence suggests that the parasympathetic nerve fibers that accompany the trigeminal nerve are involved in the control of dentinogenesis.

The excitation of C fibers, associated with tissue injury, can be readily explained by the action of the increased tissue pressure or by the action of the chemical mediators of inflammation in the nerve endings; the result is pain. The excitation of A-delta fibers, associated with dentin sensitivity, is more difficult to explain because no direct connection between the periphery of the dentin and the nerve endings has been found. Three theories have been proposed to explain the sensitivity of dentin. First is the direct stimulation of the nerve endings of the pulp; the lack of nerve endings at the periphery of the dentin negates this theory. The second theory proposes that the odontoblasts function as nerve endings. This theory cannot be accepted, however, because no one knows for certain how far the odontoblastic processes extend in the dentinal tubules, and no evidence indicates that the odontoblasts are able to function as nerve endings. The third theory, the hydrodynamic theory, takes into consideration the length of the odontoblastic processes, the length of the nerve fibers, and the fluid-filled dentinal tubules. It states that any fluid movement in the dentinal tubules and around the odontoblasts as the result of a stimulus excites the nerve endings and produces an impulse. This theory is the most tenable of the three.

The hydrodynamic theory explains the painful reaction of the pulp to heat, cold, cutting of the dentin, and probing of the dentin. Heat expands the dentinal fluid, cold contracts the dentinal fluid, cutting the dentinal tubules allows the dentinal fluid to escape, and probing the cut or exposed dentinal surface may deform the tubules and produce fluid movement. All these stimuli produce movement of the dentinal fluid and excitation of the nerve endings.

Mineralizations

Other histologic structures found in the dental pulp are mineralizations. Although their presence has been related to age and disease, they are found also in young normal dental pulps. They are present as nodules called denticles or pulp stones and diffuse calcifications. Denticles predominate in the pulp chamber, whereas diffuse calcifications are predominantly found in the root canals.

Denticles are either true or false denticles, according to their histologic structure. True denticles are uncommon, are usually found near the apex, and are composed of dentin or dentinal-type calcifications with tubules, surrounded by odontoblast-like cells. False denticles are of two types histologically: (1) round or ovoid with concentric calcified layers and smooth surfaces; and (2) amorphous without lamination and rough surfaces. The calcific tissue is usually deposited around collagen fibers, necrotic cell debris, or thrombi. These denticles can be found free in pulp tissue, attached to the dentinal walls, or embedded in dentin (Fig. 3(2)–13).

Diffuse calcifications usually follow the trajectory blood vessels, nerves, and the collagen fiber bundles (Fig. 3(2)–14). They are most often found in the walls of blood vessels. Diffuse calcifications seem to be related to aging because their incidence increases with age.

The origin of pulp calcification is controversial. The occurrence of this phenomenon in young and old dental pulps prevents the exposition of a reasonable theory.

Radiographs may show denticles in the coronal chamber. This finding should alert the clinician to the possible need for removal of the denticles, to obtain access into the orifices of the root canals. Calcifications in the root canals usually are not seen radiographically, but they are detectable during exploration of the root canal. This type of calcification may prevent the clinician from reaching the apical foramen and may therefore prevent complete instrumentation of the root canal. Pulpalgia has been attributed to the presence of denticles. No correlation has been established between calcification and pulpalgia.

Aging

Age causes important changes in the pulp. The continuous deposition of secondary dentin throughout the life of the pulp and the deposition of reparative dentin in response to stimuli reduce the size of the pulp chambers and root canals and thereby decrease the pulp volume. This diminution of the pulp is called atrophy. A concomitant decrease in the diameter of the dentinal tubules by the continuous deposition of peritubular dentin also occurs. Some of these tubules close completely and form sclerotic dentin. One also

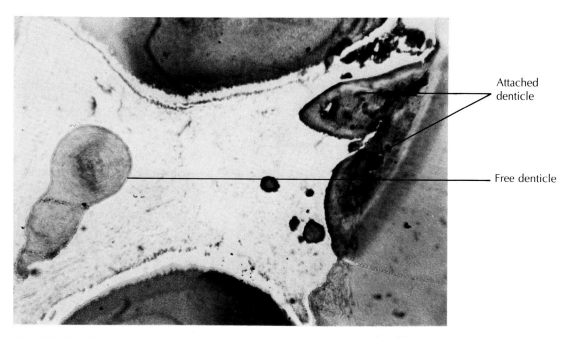

Attached
denticle

Free denticle

Fig. 3(2)—13. False denticles in the pulp chamber. Note the concentric layers of calcification in the free denticle. (Courtesy of Dr. Steve Senia, San Antonio, Texas.)

sees a reduction in the fluid content of the dentinal tubules. All these changes make the dentin less permeable and more resistant to external stimuli.

The decrease in pulp volume reduces the cellular, vascular, and neural content of the pulp. The odontoblasts seem to atrophy and may disappear completely under areas of sclerotic dentin.

The fibroblasts are reduced in size and numbers, but the collagen fibers are increased in number and in size, probably because of the decrease in the collagen solubility and turnover with advancing age. This change is referred to as fibrosis. Fibrosis is more evident in the radicular portion of the pulp than elsewhere.

The blood vessels decrease in number, and arteries undergo arteriosclerotic changes. Calcific material is deposited in the tunica adventitia and tunica media. These changes reduce the blood supply to the pulp. The number of nerves is also reduced. The ground substance undergoes metabolic changes that predispose it to mineralization. Changes in the blood vessels, nerves, and ground substance predispose the pulp to dystrophic calcifications.[38]

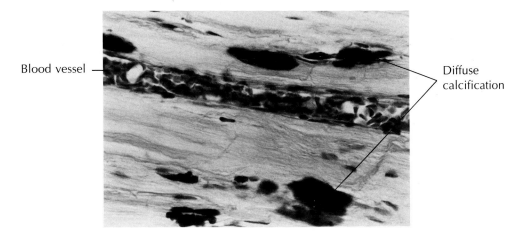

Blood vessel

Diffuse
calcification

Fig. 3(2)—14. Diffuse calcifications following the path of a blood vessel.

Part 3   Normal Periradicular Tissues

The periradicular tissues consist of the cementum, which covers the roots of the teeth, the alveolar process, which forms the bony troughs containing the roots of the teeth, and the periodontal ligament, whose collagen fibers, embedded in the cementum of the roots and in the alveolar processes, attach the roots to the surrounding tissues (Fig. 3(3)–1). In this area, portals of entry and exit between root canals and surrounding tissue are located, and pathologic reactions to diseases of the pulp are manifested.

CEMENTUM

Cementum is bone-like calcified tissue that covers the roots of the teeth (see Fig. 3(2)–3). As previously discussed, it is derived from mesenchymal cells of the dental follicle that differentiate into cementoblasts. The cementoblasts deposit a matrix, called cementoid, that is incrementally calcified and produces two types of cementum: acellular and cellular. Chronologically acellular cementum is deposited first against the dentin forming the cementodentinal junction, and as a rule, it covers the cervical and middle thirds of the root. Cellular cementum is usually deposited on acellular cementum in the apical third of the root and alternates with layers of acellular cementum. Cellular cementum is deposited at a greater rate than acellular cementum and thereby entraps the cementoblasts in the matrix. These entrapped cells are called cementocytes. The cementocytes lie in crypts of cementum known as lacunae.

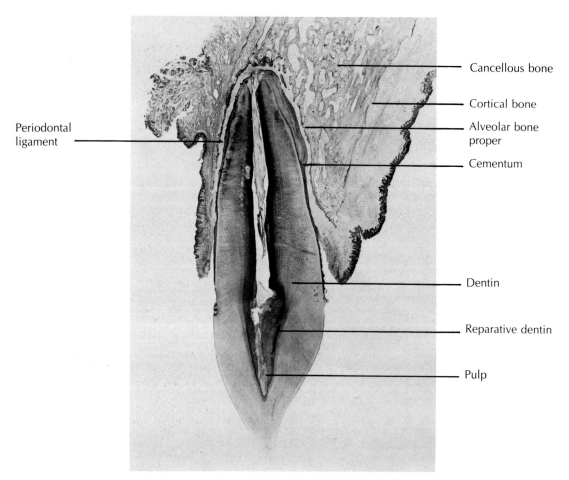

Periodontal ligament

Cancellous bone

Cortical bone

Alveolar bone proper

Cementum

Dentin

Reparative dentin

Pulp

Fig. 3(3)–1.   Cross section of a 48-year-old man's maxillary central incisor, showing the periradicular area. (Courtesy of Dr. B. Orban.)

From the lacunae, canals, called canaliculi, which contain protoplasmic extensions of the cementocytes and serve as pathways for nutrients to the cementocytes, interlace with other canaliculi of other lacunae to form a system comparable to the haversian system of bone. Because cementum is avascular, its nutrition comes from the periodontal ligament. As incremental layers of cementum are deposited, the periodontal ligament may be further displaced, and some cementocytes may die as a result and may leave empty lacunae.[5,29,34,44]

The thickness of cementum reflects one of its functions. Cementum is about 20 to 50 μm thick at the cementoenamel junction and 20 to 150 μm thick in the apical third of the root (Fig. 3(3)–1).[44] The greater thickness of cementum at the apex is due to its continuous deposition during the eruptive life of the tooth to preserve its height in the occlusal plane. The continuous deposition of cementum also gives form to the mature apical foramen. The foramen, as it matures, becomes conical, with the apex of the cone, called the minor diameter (constricture), facing the pulp and the base, called the major diameter, facing the periodontal ligament (Fig. 3(3)–2).[22] The continuous deposition of cementum increases the major diameter and results in an average deviation of the apical foramen of 0.2 to 0.5 mm from the center of the root apex.[16] The minor diameter dictates the apical termination of root canal instrumentation and obturation and is located an average of 0.5 mm from the cemental surface in young teeth and 0.75 mm from the surface in mature teeth.[22] Although the cementodentinal junction may coincide with the minor diameter, cementum may grow unevenly and may alter this relationship (Fig. 3(3)–2).

The fibers of the periodontal ligament occur between the osteoblasts and cementoblasts and are embedded into the bone and

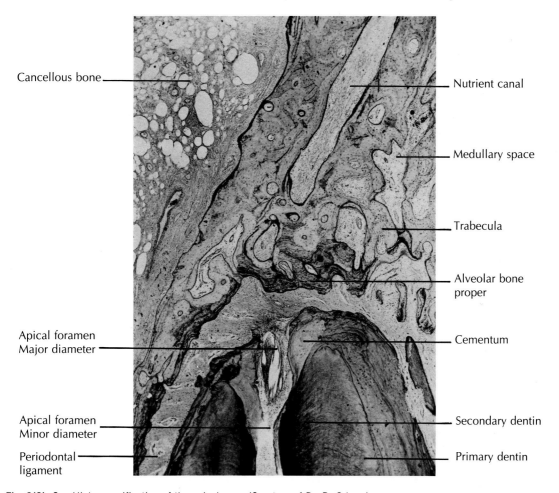

Fig. 3(3)–2. High magnification of the apical area. (Courtesy of Dr. B. Orban.)

cementum, respectively. These embedded fibers, called Sharpey's fibers, attach the periodontal ligament to bone and cementum.[44]

Repair is another function of the cementum. Root fractures and resorptions are usually repaired by cementum.[11] The closing of immature roots by apexification procedures is accomplished by deposition of cementum or cementum-like tissue.[11] Cementum also has a protective function. It is more resistant to resorption than bone, probably because of its avascularity. As a result, orthodontic movement of roots can usually be performed with a minimum of resorptive damage.[44] Other functions are the maintenance of the periodontal width by the continuous deposition of cementum and the sealing of accessory and apical foramina after root canal therapy.

PERIODONTAL LIGAMENT

The periodontal ligament is a dense, fibrous connective tissue that occupies the space between the cementum and the alveolar bone (Figs. 3(3)–1 to 3(3)–3). It surrounds the necks and roots of the teeth and is continuous with the pulp and gingiva. The periodontal ligament is composed of ground substance, interstitial tissue, blood and lymph vessels, nerves, cells, and fiber bundles.[44]

The width of the periodontal ligament varies from 0.15 to 0.38 mm.[44] Variations in width occur from tooth to tooth and in different areas of the ligament in the same root. The periodontal ligament is thinner at the rotational fulcrum of the teeth.[5] Teeth with heavy occlusal loads have wider periodontal ligaments than teeth with minimal occlusal loads, in which periodontal ligaments are thinner. With advancing age, the width of the periodontal ligament is reduced.

Interstitial Tissue

The interstitial tissue is the loose connective tissue that surrounds blood and lymphatic vessels, nerves, and the fiber bundles. This tissue contains collagen fibers independent of the fiber bundles of the periodontal ligament. Changes in its configuration are due to continuing changes in the fiber bundles. The spaces in the periodontal ligament, filled with interstitial tissue, blood vessels, lymph vessels, and nerves, are called interstitial spaces (Fig. 3(3)–3).[5]

Circulation and Lymphatic System

The ligament is richly supplied with blood vessels that provide nutrients for osteogenic, cementogenic, and fibrogenic activities. The alveolar artery branches into the dental and interalveolar arteries. In posterior teeth, it also branches into interradicular arteries. The dental artery enters the floor of the bony crypt, and before it penetrates the apical foramen, it branches into arterioles and capillaries that form a plexus to supply the apical area of the periodontal ligament.[44]

The interalveolar artery branches from the alveolar artery and coronally traverses the cancellous bone of the lateral wall of the bony crypt; its lateral branches, called perforating arteries, enter through the cribriform plate into the lateral periodontal ligament (Fig. 3(3)–3). The perforating arteries in the periodontal ligament branch into arterioles and capillaries forming a rich plexus. The dental and interalveolar arterial plexus are more prominent in the bone side of the ligament because of the constant remodeling activity of bone. The interalveolar artery exits through the crest of the alveolar process and forms the gingival branches. These gingival branches supply the gingiva and the coronal part of the periodontal ligament.

The posterior teeth also have interradicular arteries that traverse the cancellous bone of the interradicular septum. These arteries form perforating branches that supply the periodontal ligament in the root furcations.

The interdental, interradicular, and dental veins drain into the alveolar vein. Also present is a network of lymphatic vessels that follows the venous drainage into the alveolar lymph channels.[44]

The blood vessels of the periodontal ligament provide two important functions: a nutritive function to the periodontal ligament cells; and a protective function. Arteriovenous anastomoses and glomeruli-like structures between arteries and veins are present in the periodontal vasculature and regulate the blood pressure and tissue fluid pressure; they thereby provide a hydraulic mechanism for support of the teeth during function.[5]

Innervation

The alveolar nerves, which originate in the trigeminal nerve, innervate the periodontal ligament. They are divided into ascending periodontal or dental, interalveolar, and interradicular nerves. The nerves of the periodontal ligament, as in any other connective

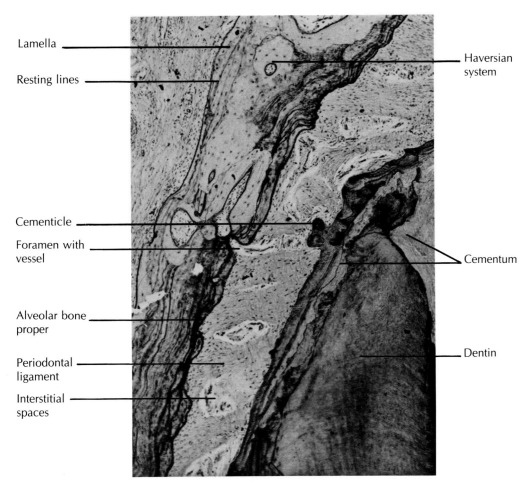

Lamella

Resting lines

Cementicle

Foramen with vessel

Alveolar bone proper

Periodontal ligament

Interstitial spaces

Haversian system

Cementum

Dentin

Fig. 3(3)–3. High magnification of the periodontal ligament. (Courtesy of Dr. B. Orban.)

tissue, follow the distribution of the arteries. The alveolar branches innervate the apical region, the interalveolar branches innervate the lateral periodontal ligament, and branches of the interradicular nerve innervate the furcal periodontal ligament of the posterior teeth.[5,44]

The nerves end in fibers of small or large diameter. The small-diameter fibers, whether myelinated or unmyelinated, terminate as free endings in the interstitial spaces and are associated with pain. The large-diameter fibers are myelinated, terminate in knob-like or spindle-like specialized endings near the principal fibers of the periodontal ligament, and are mechanoreceptors associated with touch, pressure, and proprioception.[5,44]

Sympathetic nerves accompany the arterial blood vessels in the periodontal ligament. These nerves are associated with the vasomotor control of blood flow in the arteries and capillaries.

The nerve endings of the periodontal ligament enable one to perceive pain, touch, pressure, and proprioception. Proprioception, which gives information on movement and position in space, enables one to perceive the application of forces to the teeth, movement of the teeth, and the location of foreign bodies on or between the surfaces of the teeth. This proprioceptive sense may trigger a protective reflex mechanism that opens the mandible to prevent injury to the teeth or periodontal ligament when one bites into a hard object. Proprioception permits the localization of areas of inflammation in the periodontal ligament. Such inflammatory reactions in the periodontal ligament can be identified by percussion and palpation tests.[5,29]

Cells of the Periodontal Ligament

The active cells of the periodontal ligament are the fibroblasts, osteoblasts, and cementoblasts.[5,44] The fibroblasts are spindle-shaped cells with oval nuclei and long cytoplasmic processes. They are usually aligned parallel to the collagen fibers, with their processes wrapped around the fiber bundles. Fibroblasts synthesize collagen and matrix and are involved in the degradation of collagen for its remodeling. The result is a constant remodeling of the principal fibers and maintenance of a healthy periodontal ligament. Because of these important functions, the fibroblasts are the most important cells of the periodontal ligament.

The osteoblasts or bone-forming cells are found in the periphery of the periodontal ligament lining the bony socket. They are usually seen in various stages of differentiation. If active, they are cuboidal in shape and may have deposited a layer of matrix, called osteoid, between them and mature bone. When inactive, they appear as flattened cells and may resemble fibroblasts. The function of osteoblasts is the deposition of collagen and matrix, which is deposited on the surface of the bone and to which Sharpey's fibers are attached. Calcification of the osteoid anchors Sharpey's fibers. The constant remodeling of bone provides for the continued renewal of the attachment of the periodontal ligament to bone.

Osteoclasts or bone-resorbing cells are found in the bone periphery during periods of bone remodeling (Fig. 3(3)–4). Osteoclasts are multinucleated cells with a ruffle or striated border toward the area of bone resorption. As the osteoclasts demineralize and disintegrate the matrix, scooped-out areas in the bone, called Howship's lacunae, are formed (Fig. 3(3)–4). Osteoclasts are usually found in these lacunae. This pattern of resorption gives the border of the bone an irregular shape. As resorption ceases, bone apposition begins and leaves lines of demarcation called reversal lines (Fig. 3(3)–4).

Cementoblasts, as previously discussed, are aligned in the periphery of the periodontal ligament opposite the cementum. The cementoblasts, with cytoplasmic processes, appear cuboidal if in a single layer, or squamous if in multiple layers. Their function is the deposition of a matrix consisting of collagen fibrils and ground substance called cementoid. Cementoid is found between calcified cementum and the layer of cementoblasts that thickens in periods of activity. The fibers of the periodontal ligament

are found between cementoblasts and are entrapped in the cementoid. As the cementoid calcifies, the fibers of the periodontal ligament become anchored in the newly formed cementum and are called Sharpey's fibers, the same as periodontal ligament fibers anchored in bone. Cementoid may protect the cementum against erosion.

Cementoclasts, or cementum-resorbing cells, are not found in the normal periodontal ligament because cementum does not normally remodel. They are only found in patients with certain pathologic conditions.

Other cells present in the normal periodontal ligament are the epithelial cell rests of Malassez, undifferentiated mesenchymal cells, mast cells, and macrophages. The epithelial cell rests of Malassez are remnants of Hertwig's epithelial root sheath. These cells are located in the cementum side of the periodontal ligament. Their function is unknown, but they can proliferate to form cysts in the presence of noxious stimuli.

The undifferentiated mesenchymal cells are usually stellate cells with large nuclei located near the blood vessels. These cells may differentiate into fibroblasts, odontoblasts, or cementoblasts.

Mast cells, found near blood vessels, are large, round or oval cells with round, centrally located nuclei. Their cytoplasm is characterized by numerous red granules that may obscure the nuclei. These granules contain heparin, a blood coagulant, and histamine, which can increase capillary permeability. Histamine, which is released through the degranulation of mast cells caused by acute inflammatory reactions, contracts the endothelial cells in vessel walls with resulting intercellular gaps and vascular permeability.

Macrophages are also present near blood vessels. They resemble fibroblasts in form, but with shorter processes and smaller, darkly stained nuclei. Their function is the phagocytosis of cellular debris and foreign bodies. Macrophages have digestive vacuoles containing lysosomal enzymes that process ingested materials.

Periodontal Fibers

The periodontal fibers are the principal structural components of the periodontal ligament.[5,44] Two types are known: collagen and oxytalan fibers. Collagen fibrils are organized into fibers, which, in turn, are organized into bundles. The fibers that constitute the bundles are not continuous from

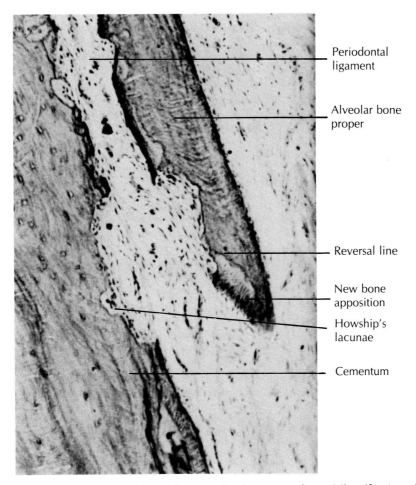

Periodontal ligament

Alveolar bone proper

Reversal line

New bone apposition

Howship's lacunae

Cementum

Fig. 3(3)—4. High magnification of the periodontal ligament, showing an area of remodeling. (Courtesy of Dr. B. Orban.)

bone to cementum, but consist of strands that can be continually and individually remodeled by fibroblasts without causing loss of the continuity of the bundles. The terminal fibers of the bundles insert into cementum on one side and bone on the other side. These terminal fibers are called Sharpey's fibers regardless of cementum or bone insertion. The fibers are arranged in bundles with a definite functional arrangement. These bundles follow an undulating course that allows some movement of the tooth in its alveolar socket.

The fiber bundles are arranged into principal fiber groups: transseptal, alveolar crest, horizontal, oblique, apical, and interradicular. The transseptal group is embedded into the cementum of adjacent teeth traversing the alveolar crest interproximally. The alveolar crest group is embedded into the cementum below the cementoenamel junction, is situated obliquely, and ends in the alveolar crest. The horizontal group is embedded into the cementum apical to the alveolar crest group and moves horizontally into the alveolar bone. The oblique group is embedded into the cementum apically to the horizontal group and travels obliquely in a coronal direction, to be embedded into the alveolar bone. The apical group is embedded into the apical cementum and the fundus of the alveolar socket. The interradicular group is embedded in cementum and alveolar bone of the furca of multirooted teeth.

The functions of the fibers of the periodontal ligament are to attach the tooth to its alveolar socket, to suspend it in its socket, to protect the tooth and the alveolar socket from masticatory injuries, and to transform vertical masticatory stresses into tension on the alveolar bone.

The oxytalan fibers, believed to be immature elastic fibers, traverse the periodontal ligament in an axial direction. One end of these fibers may be embedded in cementum or bone, and the other in the wall of the blood vessels. Their function is unknown, although they may support the blood vessels.

Calcifications

Cementicles may be found in the periodontal ligament (see Fig. 3(3)–3).[5] These calcifications are attached to cementum, embedded in it, or free in the periodontal ligament near the cemental border. Epithelial cells may form the nidus for these calcifications.

Diseases of the pulp are manifested in the periodontal ligament. Inflammatory reactions, ranging from abscesses to granulomas and cysts, may destroy and replace the periodontal ligament.

ALVEOLAR PROCESS

The alveolar process is divided into the alveolar bone proper and the supporting alveolar bone[5,6,44] (Figs. 3(3)–1 to 3(3)–3, 3(3)–5, and 3(3)–6).

Alveolar Bone Proper

The alveolar bone proper is the bone that lines the alveolus or the bony sockets that house the roots of the teeth. The alveolar bone proper is part of the periradicular tissues. It begins its formation by intramembranous ossification at the initial stage of root formation. The osteoblasts at the periphery of the periodontal ligament deposit an organic matrix called osteoid, which consists of collagen fibrils and ground substance that contains glycoproteins, phosphoproteins, lipids, and proteoglycans. As the osteoblasts deposit the matrix, some are trapped in it; these cells are called osteocytes. The matrix is calcified by the deposition of hydroxyapatite crystals consisting principally of calcium and phosphates.

The osteocytes in calcified bone lie in oval spaces called lacunae, which communicate with each other by means of canaliculi. This system of canals brings nutrients into the osteocytes and removes their metabolic waste products.

Bone deposited incrementally during periods of osteoblastic activity forms leaves of bone called lamellae (see Fig. 3(3)–3). Resting periods are demarcated by dark lines called resting lines, which run parallel to the surface of the bone. Osteocytes in their la-

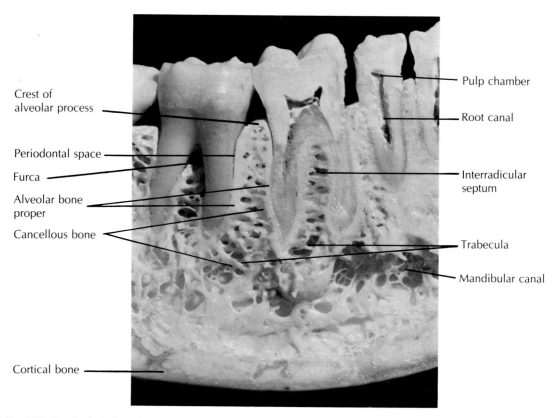

Crest of alveolar process

Periodontal space

Furca

Alveolar bone proper

Cancellous bone

Cortical bone

Pulp chamber

Root canal

Interradicular septum

Trabecula

Mandibular canal

Fig. 3(3)–5. Sagittal view of the alveolar process.

Buccal

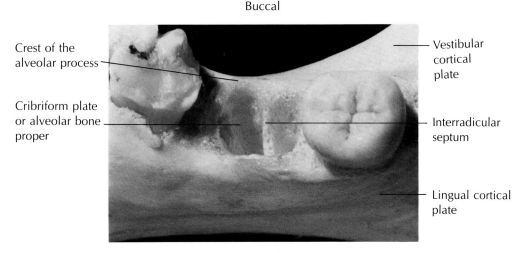

Crest of the alveolar process

Cribriform plate or alveolar bone proper

Vestibular cortical plate

Interradicular septum

Lingual cortical plate

Lingual

Fig. 3(3)–6. Alveolus of the alveolar process.

cunae are evenly distributed throughout the surface of the lamellae. The lamellae, resting lines, lacunae with their osteocytes, and canaliculi give bone its histologic characteristics.

The alveolar bone proper consists of bundle bone in the periphery of the alveoli and lamellated bone toward the center of the alveolar process. The peripheral bone is called bundle bone because Sharpey's fibers of the periodontal ligament are embedded in it. Because the peripheral Sharpey's fibers may be calcified, and because lamellae are almost indistinct, this bone is thick and has a more radiopaque appearance in radiographs than cancellous bone or periodontal ligament spaces. The radiographic image of the alveolar bone proper is called the lamina dura.

The alveolar bone proper can also be referred to as the cribriform plate (Fig. 3(3)–6). This term refers to the many foramina that perforate the bone. These foramina contain vessels and nerves that supply teeth, periodontal ligament, and bone.

Supporting Alveolar Bone

Adjacent to the alveolar bone proper is a diploë of cancellous (spongy) bone covered by two outer tables of compact bone (see Figs. 3(3)–1, 3(3)–5, and 3(3)–6). One of the outer tables of compact bone is vestibular, and the other is lingual or palatal. The cancellous bone consists of lamellated bone arranged in branches called trabeculae (see Fig. 3(3)–2). Between the trabeculae are medullary spaces, filled with marrow. Marrow can be fatty or hematopoietic. In adults, the marrow in the mandible and maxilla is usually fatty, but hematopoietic tissue is found in certain locations such as the maxillary tuberosity, maxillary and mandibular molar periradicular areas, and premolar periradicular areas. Hematopoietic marrow spaces appear radiolucent in radiographs.

Also present in cancellous bone are nutrient canals (see Fig. 3(3)–2). These canals contain vessels and nerves. They usually terminate in the alveolar crest in small foramina through which vessels and nerves enter the gingiva.

The amount of cancellous bone varies among areas of the maxilla and mandible and depends on the width of the alveolar process and the size and shape of the root of the teeth.

Cortical (compact) bone covers the cancellous bone and is formed by lamellated bone. This lamellated bone has lacunae arranged in concentric circles around central canals called the haversian system (see Fig. 3(3)–3). Cortical bone comes together with the alveolar bone proper to form the alveolar crest around the necks of the teeth.

Bone serves as the calcium reservoir of the body. The body, under hormonal control, regulates and maintains calcium metabolism. Therefore, constant physiologic remodeling of bone by osteoclastic and osteoblastic activity occurs. This activity can be seen more readily in the trabeculae. The trabecular pattern is constantly altered in response to occlusal forces. In the trabeculae are resting lines (see Fig. 3(3)–3), which are characteristic of periods of osteoblastic activity, and resorptive lines (see Fig. 3(3)–4), which are characteristic of periods of osteoclastic activity. Resting lines are characteristically dark lines parallel to the surface, whereas resorptive lines are scalloped and point to the areas of resorption known as Howship's lacunae.

Diseases of the pulp can affect the tissues of the periradicular area. Acute inflammatory changes in the periodontal ligament that originate in the pulp produce extrusion of the tooth. Chronic inflammatory changes of pulpal origin in the periodontal ligament can cause resorption of the lamina dura, external root resorption, areas of bone resorption, or areas of bone condensation. Systemic diseases may also produce bony changes in the periradicular area. These pathologic changes are discussed in Chapters 4 and 5.

The reader is advised that the discussions in the chapter on embryology, the normal pulp, and normal periradicular tissues are intended as a review of embryology, physiology, and histology as it applies to the clinical science of endodontics. The reader is referred to standard textbooks on these subjects for more comprehensive and detailed discussion.

BIBLIOGRAPHY

1. Aubin, J.E.: J. Dent. Res., 64:515, 1985.
2. Avery, J.R.: Oral Surg., 32:113, 1971.
3. Baume, L.J.: The Biology of Pulp and Dentin. Basel, S. Karger, 1980.
4. Bernick, S.: J. Dent. Res., 43:406, 1964.
5. Bhaskar, S.N.: Orban's Oral Histology and Embryology, 9th Ed. St. Louis, C.V. Mosby, 1980.
6. Bhaskar, S.N.: Synopsis of Oral Histology. St. Louis, C.V. Mosby, 1962.
7. Brännström, M., and Garberoglio, R.: Acta Odontol. Scand., 30:291, 1972.
8. Byers, M.R.: J. Comp. Neurol., 191:413, 1980.
9. Carranza, F.A.: Glickman's Clinical Periodontology, 6th Ed. Philadelphia, W.B. Saunders, 1984.
10. Cohen, B., and Kramer, I.R.H.: Scientific Foundation of Dentistry. Chicago, Year Book Medical Publishers, 1976.
11. Cohen, S., and Burns, R.C.: Pathways of the Pulp, 3rd Ed. St. Louis, C.V. Mosby, 1984.
12. Cutright, D.E.: Oral Surg., 30:284, 1970.
13. Fearnhead, R.W.: Proc. R. Soc. Med., 54:877, 1961.
14. Finn. S.B.: Biology of the Dental Pulp Organ: A Symposium. Alabama. University of Alabama Press, 1968.
15. Garberoglio, R., and Brännström. M.: Arch. Oral Biol., 21:355, 1976.
16. Green. D.: Morphology of the Endodontic System. New York. David Green. 1969.
17. Heyerass, K.J.: J. Dent. Res., 64:585. 1985.
18. Holland. G.R.: J. Dent. Res., 64:499. 1985.
19. Ingle. J.I., and Taintor, J.F.: Endodontics. 3rd Ed. Philadelphia, Lea & Febiger. 1985.
20. Johnsen. D.C.: J. Dent. Res., 64:555. 1985.
21. Kim, S.: J. Dent. Res., 64:590, 1985.
22. Kuttler. Y.: J. Am. Dent. Assoc.. 50:544. 1955.
23. Linde, A.: Dentin and Dentinogenesis. Vols. I and II. Boca Raton, FL. CRC Press, 1984.
24. Linde, A.: J. Dent. Res., 64:523. 1985.
25. Lindhe, J.: Textbook of Clinical Periodontology. Copenhagen, Munksgaard, 1984.
26. Maniatopoulos, C., and Smith. D.C.: Arch. Oral Biol., 28:701. 1983.
27. Mjör, I.A.: J. Dent. Res., 64:621. 1985.
28. Mjör, I.A.: Reaction Patterns in Human Teeth. Boca Raton, FL, CRC Press, 1983.
29. Mjör, I.A., and Fejerskon, A.: Histology of the Human Tooth, 2nd Ed. Copenhagen, Munksgaard, 1979.
30. Närhi. M.V.O.: J. Dent. Res., 64:564. 1985.
31. Nery, E.B., et al.: Arch. Oral Biol., 15:1315. 1970.
32. Olgart, L.M.: J. Dent. Res., 64:572. 1985.
33. Oor, T.: Human Tooth and Dental Arch Development. Tokyo, Ishiyaka, 1981.
34. Osborn, J.W., and Ten Cate, A.R.: Advanced Dental Histology, 3rd Ed. Bristol, England, J. Wright and Sons, 1976.
35. Pashley, D.H.: J. Dent. Res., 64:613,1985.
36. Provenza, D.V.: Fundamentals of Oral Histology and Embryology. Philadelphia, J.B. Lippincott, 1972.
37. Ruch, J.V.: J. Dent. Res., 64:489. 1985.
38. Seltzer, S., and Bender, I.B.: The Dental Pulp, 3rd Ed. Philadelphia, J.B. Lippincott, 1984.
39. Siskin, M.: The Biology of the Human Dental Pulp. St. Louis, C.V. Mosby, 1973.
40. Stanley, H.R.: Human Pulp Response to Restorative Dental Procedures, Rev. Ed. Gainesville, FL, Storter Printing, 1981.
41. Takahashi, K.: J. Dent. Res., 64:579. 1985.
42. Takahashi, K., Kishi, Y., and Kim, S.: J. Endod., 8:131, 1982.
43. Ten Cate, A.R.: J. Dent. Res., 64:549. 1985.
44. Ten Cate, A.R.: Oral Histology: Development, Structure and Function. St. Louis, C.V. Mosby, 1980.
45. Thomas, H.F.: J. Dent. Res., 64:607. 1985.
46. Van Hassel, H.J.: Oral Surg., 32:126, 1971.
47. Veis, A.: J. Dent. Res., 64:552. 1985.
48. Weine, F.S.: Endodontic Therapy, 3rd Ed. St. Louis, C.V. Mosby, 1982.
49. Yamamura, T.: J. Dent. Res., 64:530. 1985.

4 Diseases of the Dental Pulp

The pulp is the formative organ of the tooth. It builds primary dentin during the development of the tooth, secondary dentin after tooth eruption, and reparative dentin in response to stimulation as long as the odontoblasts remain intact. The pulp responds to heat and cold stimuli which are perceived only as pain. Heat, at temperatures between 60° F (16° C) and 130° F (55° C) when applied directly to an intact tooth surface, is usually well tolerated by the pulp, but foodstuffs and beverages above and below this temperature range can also be endured. Cavity preparation also produces temperature changes, with an increase of 20° C in temperature during dry cavity preparation 1 mm from the pulp and a 30° C increase 0.5 mm from the pulp.[99] A theoretic model has shown that the sensory reaction to thermal stimulation is registered before a temperature change occurs at the pulpodential junction, where the nerve endings are located.[111] The sensation of pain, a warning signal that the pulp is endangered, is a protective reaction, as it is elsewhere in the body.

The pulp has been described both as a highly resistant organ and as an organ with little resistance or recuperating ability. Its resistance depends on cellular activity, nutritional supply, age, and other metabolic and physiologic parameters. This variability has led to the remark that: "Some pulps will die if you look crossly at them, while others can't be killed with an ax." The poor recuperative ability of the pulp may be due to high plasminogen activity, which rapidly breaks down the fibrin following injury.[7] On the whole, the resistance of the pulp to injury is slight, but evidence of unusual persistence of vitality following injury has been reported.[9,27,40]

The desirability of maintaining a vital pulp and of protecting it from injury was recognized by the earliest practitioners of dentistry. In the development of the dental art, the integrity of the pulp was frequently violated in the execution of a technically satisfactory mechanical restoration. Tooth structure was sacrificed, at times indiscriminately, to provide the patient with a filling or bridge that occasionally suggested the grossly ornamental rather than the functional. As a result, the pulp often suffered, dying some time after the restoration was placed. In other instances, the pulp was intentionally removed. The value of the pulp as an integral part of the tooth, both anatomic and functional, was recognized by many dentists, however, and efforts were made to conserve it. Today, history seems to be repeating itself. Restorative dentistry has made radical demands on the integrity of the pulp. Mouth reconstruction has imposed responsibilities on the dentist that are not always met, with detriment to the pulp. Moreover, although high-speed cavity and crown preparation with an adequate stream of water directed on the tooth will cause no permanent damage to the pulp if the procedure is carefully executed, speedy but dry preparation or continuous low-speed preparation may cause irreparable damage. Careful cavity preparation and the use of cavity linings or cements in deep cavities, in addition to periodic prophylactic and home care, help to maintain the integrity and vitality of the pulp.

CAUSES OF PULP DISEASE

The causes of pulp disease are physical, chemical, and bacterial. They may be grouped as in Table 4–1.

Physical Causes

Physical causes include mechanical, thermal, or electrical injuries.

Mechanical Injuries

These injuries are usually due to either trauma or pathologic wear of teeth.

Trauma. Traumatic injury may or may not be accompanied by fracture of the crown or root. Trauma is less frequently the cause of pulp injury in adults than in children. Trau-

Table 4–1. Causes of Pulp Disease

I. Physical
  A. Mechanical
    1. Trauma
      a. Accidental (contact sports)
      b. Iatrogenic dental procedures (wedging of teeth, cavity or crown preparation, etc.)
    2. Pathologic wear (attrition, abrasion, etc.)
    3. Crack through body of tooth (cracked tooth syndrome)
    4. Barometric changes (barodontalgia)
  B. Thermal
    1. Heat from cavity preparation, at either low or high speed
    2. Exothermic heat from the setting of cement
    3. Conduction of heat and cold through deep fillings without a protective base
    4. Frictional heat caused by polishing a restoration
  C. Electrical (galvanic current from dissimilar metallic fillings)
II. Chemical
  A. Phosphoric acid, acrylic monomer, etc.
  B. Erosion (acids)
III. Bacterial
  A. Toxins associated with caries
  B. Direct invasion of pulp from caries or trauma
  C. Microbial colonization in the pulp by blood-borne microorganisms (anachoresis)

matic injury of the pulp may be due to a violent blow to the tooth during a fight, sports, automobile accident, or household accident. Habits such as opening bobby pins with the teeth, compulsive bruxism, nail biting, and thread biting by seamstresses may also cause pulpal injury that may lead to death of the pulp (Fig. 4–1).

In addition, certain dental procedures occasionally injure the pulp. Some are avoidable; others are not. Accidental exposure of the pulp during excavation of carious tooth structure, too-rapid movement of the teeth during orthodontic treatment, rapid separation of teeth by means of a mechanical separator, the use of pins for mechanical retention of amalgam or other restoration, and malleting of gold-foil filling without adequate cement base are among the iatrogenic causes of dental injuries. During cavity preparation, the remaining dentin thickness should be between 1.1 and 1.5 mm, to protect the pulp against inflammation and bacterial access.[87] Dehydration of the pulp by a continuous air stream may cause aspiration of odontoblastic nuclei.[13,20] Dehydration may also be caused by restorative materials such

as Cavit, which is hydrophilic and absorbs fluid from the dentinal tubules as it sets.[46]

Cutting of the odontoblastic processes during cavity preparation may cause degeneration of the odontoblastic layer on the surface of the pulp in the region of the preparation, and hemorrhages may occur in the body of the pulp, if the peripheral injury is severe enough.[30] In most cases, secondary dentin forms and walls off the injured tract of dentin. If the injury is continued, however, or if irritating fluids gain access to the dentinal tubules, serious and more permanent damage to the pulp may occur.

Pathologic Wear. The pulp may also become exposed or nearly exposed by pathologic wear of the teeth from either abrasion or attrition if secondary dentin is not deposited rapidly enough. Occlusal trauma may also injure the pulp because of repeated irritation to the neurovascular bundle in the periradicular area.

Cracked Tooth Syndrome. Incomplete fractures through the body of the tooth may cause pain of apparently idiopathic origin. This is referred to as the "cracked tooth syndrome."[18] The patient usually complains of pain, ranging from mild to excruciating, at the initiation or the release of the biting pressure.[100] The most reliable diagnostic method is to try to reproduce the pain. When the patient bites on a cotton applicator or rubber wheel, the fracture segments may separate, and the pain may be reproduced at the initiation or release of the biting pressure. Close examination of the crown of the tooth may disclose an enamel crack, which may be better visualized by using a dye or by transilluminating the tooth with a fiberoptic light. Removal of intracoronal restoration in suspected teeth may reveal a crack in the enamel running into the dentin. Such teeth may be sensitive for years because of an incomplete fracture of enamel and dentin that produces only mild pain; eventually, this pain becomes severe when the fracture involves the pulp chamber.

The pulp in these teeth may become necrotic. Some of these cracked teeth fracture completely, and the patient will then be free of symptoms. If the patient has an incomplete fracture of only the enamel and dentin, a full-crown restoration immobilizing the fragments may be successful.

Radiation. Laser radiation sufficient to cause cavitation in teeth also causes severe degenerative changes in the pulp.[1,107] On the

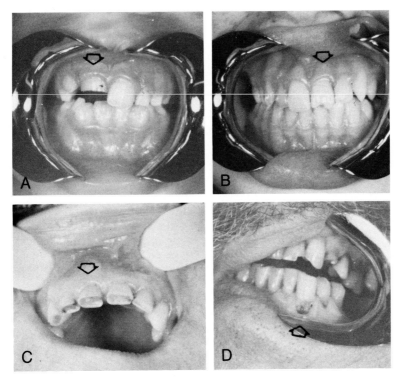

Fig. 4–1. *A,* Fracture of an upper incisor. *B,* Incisal notch from biting of threads by a seamstress; the result was death of the pulp. *C,* Attrition resulting in death of the pulp, maxillary right incisor. *D,* Abrasion or erosion causing sensitivity of lower cuspid tooth and requiring endodontic treatment.

other hand, cobalt radiation had no visible effect on pulps of monkeys, as compared with control subjects in one study.[43]

Pulpal Reaction to Fillings. Fillings made of silver amalgam, copper amalgam, silicate composites, and even oxyphosphate-of-zinc cement produce some pulp reaction when they are inserted into cavities prepared in dentin. The deeper the cavity, the greater is the damage caused, but in most cases the pulp recovers from the injury.

Thermal Injury

Thermal causes of pulp injury are uncommon.

Heat from Cavity Preparation. The chief offender is heat developed by a bur or diamond during cavity preparation. High-speed engines and carbide burs may reduce operating time, but they may also accelerate pulp death if they are used without a coolant. The heat generated may be sufficient to cause irreparable pulp damage.

In experimental studies on monkeys, dental pulp recovered from a rise in temperature of 10° F, it did not usually recover when the rise was between 10 and 20° F, and it did not

recover from a temperature rise of 20° F or more.[117] In another study, in cavities prepared at low speed with a coolant and without a coolant, and at high speed with a coolant and without a coolant, the only increase in intrapulpal temperature occurred when low speed was used without a coolant. At all other times, under the conditions of the experiment, the temperature dropped. In fact, the deeper the cavity, the greater was the drop in temperature, up to 8° C when used with a coolant.[6] Langeland has stated, however, that "no conclusions as to the innocuousness of a preparation and filling procedure can be drawn from the temperature measurements."[56]

Special care must be exercised when the cavity is large, or when the tooth is being prepared for a cast or jacket crown, because cutting of dentin is extensive, and many dentinal tubules are exposed.

Studies of sound human teeth in which cavity preparations were done at 50,000 rpm or higher with an air turbine, with adequate water cooling of the tooth, showed less injury to the pulp tissue than when cavities were prepared at speeds between 6,000 and 20,000 rpm, without a coolant. Damage and abscess formation of the pulp occurred when a water spray was not used.[102]

Evidence suggests that pulpal damage is repaired more rapidly when cavity preparation is done under a water spray.[64] When a cavity is prepared with an air turbine and water spray, the pulp shows little or no response to the cutting. The dentinal tubules remain open or are unaffected for a longer period of time. In comparison with preparation at low speed, it takes longer for reparative or secondary dentin to develop, if it develops at all. The application of sterilizing agents following high-speed preparation may cause greater pulpal irritation because the dentinal tubules are open.

In an evaluation of the effect of high speed on the dental pulp, Zander stated that "all research on pulp reaction to high speed instrumentation has been conducted on sound teeth while in actual practice some type of pulp reaction has already occurred. . . . Any injury, then, produced by high speed is superimposed upon already existing alterations in the pulp."[118]

Extensive research studies on high-speed preparation have shown that: (1) the stream of water or air-water spray must be directed at the dentin directly under the bur for maximum cooling; (2) the water stream is deflected in a centripetal direction by the rotation of the bur; (3) burns in the dentin may occur from overheating because of malfunction of the water spray or stream, with a corresponding reaction in the pulp; (4) "aspiration of odontoblast nuclei" occurs with inadequate water spray; (5) dry cavity preparation not only causes burns in dentin, but also "migration of odontoblasts, the migration of erythrocytes, and hyperemia" of the pulp.[54–56,58] It was found experimentally that the greater the length of time the dentin was dried, the greater was the severity of odontoblast displacement.[21]

Frictional Heat during Polishing. Enough heat may also be generated during polishing of a filling or during setting of cement to cause at least transient pulp injury.

Heat Conduction by Fillings. Metallic fillings close to the pulp without an intermediate cement base may conduct temperature changes rapidly to the pulp and may eventually destroy it. Sudden changes in temperature from foodstuffs, such as eating ice cream and drinking coffee, or chewing ice cubes, may also contribute to pulp injury.

Barodontalgia

The list of physical causes of pulp injury would not be complete without a consideration of high-altitude changes on the pulp. Barodontalgia, also known as aerodontalgia, denotes toothache occurring at low atmospheric pressure experienced either during flight or during a test run in a decompression chamber. Barodontalgia has generally been observed in altitudes over 5,000 feet, but it is more likely to occur at 10,000 feet or above. A tooth with chronic pulpitis can be symptomless at ground level, but it may cause pain at high altitude because of reduced pressure.[81] Lining the cavity with a varnish or a base of zinc-phosphate cement, with a subbase of zinc-oxide-eugenol cement in deep cavities, helps to prevent barodontalgia.

Chemicals

Chemical causes of pulp injury are probably the least common, although at one time the presence of arsenic in silicate-cement powder and the use of a desensitizing paste containing paraformaldehyde accounted for many pulp deaths. Silicate restorations are the most frequent cause of pulp death in incisor teeth.[50] Polycarboxylate cement is well tolerated by the pulp.[83,91,96] The application of a cavity cleanser to a thin layer of dentin may cause inflammation of the pulp. In one study, cavity cleansers such as citric acid caused a deep inflammatory response that gradually decreased in about a month.[21] Some of the self-curing plastic materials have produced hyperemias of the pulp shortly after insertion of the filling and even pulp death a week or two after insertion.[8,34,53,57,61,88] Acid etchants, when used on exposed dentin preliminary to the application of a composite resin, irritate the pulp without necessarily causing pain.[28,63]

Reaction of the pulp to composite restorations, with or without the use of acid etchants, varies from slight to severe.[14,26,28,43,44,85,105] To protect the pulp, one should use calcium hydroxide bases in deep cavities and calcium hydroxide liner in shallow cavities.[26,28,43,105] Irritating or dehydrating chemicals used for sterilizing or drying a cavity, such as alcohol and chloroform, should be avoided. The application of a sodium-fluoride solution to prevent recurrence of decay is not dangerous to the pulp if it is applied for 5 min.[15,66,68,76] The use of an 8% stannous-fluoride solution for more than

30 sec in deep cavities is contraindicated, however.[15] Glass-ionomer cement produces about the same degree of irritation as zinc-oxide-eugenol cement.[49,109]

Slow, progressive erosion on the labial or facial surfaces at the cervices of the teeth may eventually subject the pulp to irritation and may cause permanent damage.

Bacteria

In 1894, W.D. Miller suggested that bacteria were a possible cause of inflammation in the pulp.[71] The most common cause of pulp injury is bacterial. Bacteria or their products may enter the pulp through a break in the dentin, either from caries or accidental exposure, from percolation around a restoration, from extension of infection from the gingiva, or by way of the blood. Although the circulating pathway is difficult to prove, some experimental evidence indicates that it is possible (anachoretic effect). Microorganisms play an important role in the genesis of pulpal disease. The presence or absence of bacterial irritation is the determining factor in pulp survival once the pulp has been mechanically exposed.[48] Despite food impaction, dentinal bridging has occurred in the pulps of gnotobiotic (germ-free) rats after pulp exposure. On the other hand, pulpal necrosis, abscess formation, and granulomas developed in exposed pulps of rats kept under ordinary laboratory conditions.

Once bacteria have invaded the pulp, the damage is almost always irreparable. The report on a small study of painful pulpitis stated: "pulpitis and actual pulp exposure, whether associated with deep caries, deep restorations, or other causes, go hand in hand. There was no correlation between the severity of the pain and the extent of pulp involvement."[72]

The species of bacteria recovered from inflamed or infected pulps are many and varied. Although lactobacilli (acidogenic organisms) are commonly found in carious dentin, they are seldom recovered from the pulp because of their low degree of invasiveness. Microorganisms need not be present in the pulp to produce inflammation; the by-products of bacteria in the dentin may be sufficiently irritating to cause an inflammatory reaction.[22,44,59,67]

The bacteria most often recovered from infected vital pulps are streptococci and staphylococci, but many other microorganisms, from diphtheroids to anaerobes, have

also been isolated. It is likely that the type of organism recovered depends on whether the pulp is cultured in situ or after extraction of the tooth, whether it communicates with the fluids of the mouth, whether the disease is an initial hyperemia of pulpitis, and whether the disorder has progressed to necrosis. Perhaps in many cases the organisms recovered from the pulp have nothing to do with the disease itself. The same types of organisms are generally found in both coronal and radicular portions of infected pulps. In a study using bacterial cultures of more than 700 cases, agreement regarding the presence or absence of microorganisms occurred in 77% of the cases.[37]

In another study, bacteria in infected pulps were present only in areas of necrosis or partial necrosis, and even though the area of necrosis was heavily laden with bacteria within the root canal, none were seen in the adjacent periradicular tissue.[29]

Pathways of Bacterial Invasion of the Pulp

Bacteria may enter the pulp in one of three ways: (1) direct invasion by way of the dentin, such as caries, fracture of the crown or root, exposure during cavity preparation, attrition, abrasion, erosion, or crack in crown; (2) invasion through open blood vessels or lymphatics, associated with periodontal disease, an accessory canal in the furcation area, gingival infection, or scaling of teeth; and (3) invasion through the blood, such as during infectious diseases or transient bacteremia. Bacteria may penetrate the dentin during the cutting of a cavity by contamination of the smear layer, by penetration of the bacteria in open dentinal tubules from the carious process, and by the introduction of bacteria because of unclean operative practices. Bacteria and toxins penetrate the dentinal tubules and, on reaching the pulp, produce inflammatory reactions.[11,14,43,69,85,104]

Studies have shown an anachoretic effect in lower animals.[2,23,89] Anachoresis refers to the attraction or fixation of blood-borne bacteria in areas of inflammation. Actual invasion of the pulp by way of lymphatic fluid or the blood is rare, however. It is questioned whether invasion by the lymphatic vessels occurs at all, unless an inroad is made for the bacteria by mechanical manipulation of the tissues, as by deep scaling with attendant laceration of the gingiva. It is also questioned whether invasion of the pulp by bacteria occurs through the blood, unless the pulp is already inflamed or necrotic. Even when a large area of periapical bone has been destroyed by infection from the root canal, the adjacent teeth may remain vital. Studies of the presence of viruses in the pulp and periapical tissues are few.[86,93] Viruses from these tissues have not been isolated to date.

Reaction of the Pulp to Bacterial Invasion

One should consider the mechanism of pulp injury and the resulting changes. Once the pulp is exposed, either by caries or by trauma, it may be considered infected because microorganisms gain access to it almost immediately. The invading bacteria, however, may be confined entirely to the small area of pulp exposure. At first, the infection is localized to a small area of the pulp, just as infection following a scratch of the arm is localized. Although the coronal area of the pulp may be involved by a mild or even severe infective process, the body and apical portion of the pulp may remain normal. The reaction of the pulp in the involved area is an inflammatory response. Polymorphonuclear leukocytes reach the area, and further dissemination of bacteria deeper into the pulp is prevented. Because some microorganisms enter the dentinal tubules, they may gain a foothold that is difficult to dislodge. In this respect, injury of the pulp and injury of the arm or some other part of the body differ; in the latter, microorganisms are more readily reached by tissue defenses. The reaction in an inflamed pulp also differs from that in an inflamed arm or other organ in that little or no room is provided during the inflammatory state for swelling of the pulp because the pulp is entirely enclosed in a hard, unyielding dentinal wall, except at the apical foramen. If the inflammatory process is severe, it will extend deeper into the pulp and all the symptoms of an acute reaction will be manifested. Considerable inflammatory exudate accumulates and causes pain from pressure on the nerve endings. Areas of necrosis develop, owing to disturbance in nutritional supply, many of the polymorphonuclear leukocytes die, and pus forms, further irritating nerve cells. If the process is less severe, lymphocytes and plasma cells will replace the polymorphonuclear leukocytes in numbers, and the inflammatory reaction may be confined to the surface of the pulp. Such a chronic inflammatory state may be localized for a long time unless the microorganisms penetrate deeper into the pulp and

cause an acute reaction manifested by a clinical "flare-up." On the other hand, the chronic process may continue until most of or all the pulp is involved, ultimately leading to its death. In the course of this development, the organisms may be killed, but more commonly they survive and set up a reaction in the periapical tissue by their products of metabolism.

During the inflammatory reaction, tissue pressure is increased. Stasis occurs, with resulting necrosis of the pulp. In some cases, the necrotic but sterile pulp tissue causes no symptoms and remains quiescent for years. This situation is the exception, however, because in most cases the microorganisms survive and, if virulent, multiply rapidly and reach the periapical tissue, where they continue their destruction and produce an acute alveolar abscess. If they are less virulent, the microorganisms will remain in the root canal and, by their toxic products, will gradually and quietly produce a chronic abscess without giving rise to subjective symptoms other than those associated with a sinus tract, if one develops. When the defensive forces of the periapical tissues are adequate, a ring of granulation tissue is formed to delimit the bacteria and to neutralize their toxins. In some cases, such low-grade irritation stimulates the epithelial rests and causes a cyst.

Meanwhile, during this process, the dentinal tubules may become infiltrated with products of blood decomposition, bacteria, and occasionally, food debris, and the dentin becomes discolored. Such discoloration of tooth structure is sometimes the first clinical sign that the pulp has died.

DISEASES OF THE PULP

Inflammation of the Pulp

Pulpitis or inflammation of the pulp may be acute or chronic, partial or total, and the pulp may be infected or sterile. Because the extent of inflammation, whether partial or total, at times cannot even be determined histologically, and because the bacteriologic state, whether the tissue is infected or sterile, cannot be determined except by smear or culture, the only clinical differentiation possible in pulpitis is between acute and chronic. Two types of chronic inflammation of the exposed pulp can be identified clinically: (1) chronic pulpitis of exposed pulp due to caries or trauma; and (2) chronic hyperplastic pulpitis. The acute form of pulpitis generally runs a precipitous, short, painful, and sometimes violently painful, course. The chronic forms are practically symptomless or only slightly painful and are therefore usually of longer duration.

The types of inflammation of the pulp are not always distinct. Because one type may blend into another, acute and chronic inflammation may both be present on histologic examination. The interpretation of microscopic studies of the pulp and other tissues depends on the preparation of the specimen, that is, fixation, angle at which the specimen is cut, and staining, as well as on the particular section examined microscopically. In one study, teeth were bisected, and each half was examined separately. In one tooth, half the pulp had a severe lesion, whereas the other half had only a few inflammatory cells.[96]

Clinical classification of pulpal diseases is based primarily on symptoms. No correlation exists between histopathologic findings and the existing symptoms. The value of the clinical classification lies in its use by the clinician to determine the appropriate care and treatment, the endodontic prognosis, and probably, the restorative needs of the tooth.

The demarcation between irritation of the pulp leading to productive stimulation of secondary dentin formation and that leading to hyperemia is indistinct, as is the demarcation between the degree of irritation leading to hyperemia and that leading to pulpitis. In one case, a slight degree of irritation produces a symptomless productive reaction of the pulp, in another it produces hyperemia, and in still another, acute pulpitis may result. The reaction depends not only on the degree of irritation, but also on the individual makeup and resistance of the pulp tissue to injury.

Baume found no direct correlation between clinical symptoms and histologic findings. Based on clinical symptoms, he divided diseases of the pulp into four categories: (1) "the symptomless, vital pulp which has been injured or involved by deep caries, for which pulp capping may be done; (2) pulps with a history of pain which are amenable to pharmacotherapy; (3) pulps indicated for extirpation and immediate root filling; and (4) necrosed pulps involving infection of radicular dentin accessible to antiseptic root canal therapy."[4]

Seltzer and Bender found little correlation between clinical symptoms and histologic appearance, but they stated nevertheless that a clinical classification is justified.[92] They have correlated the results of clinical tests of the pulp with the histologic diagnosis, as follows: treatable: (a) intact, uninflamed pulp, (b) transitional stage, (c) atrophic pulp, (d) acute pulpitis, and (e) chronic partial pulpitis without necrosis; and untreatable: (a) chronic partial pulpitis with necrosis, (b) chronic total pulpitis, and (c) total pulp necrosis.[92]

Garfunkel and associates found a direct correlation between clinical diagnosis and histologic examination in 49% of pulps examined and a partial correlation in 46%.[32] Wegner and Knorr compared clinical symptoms of pulpitis with histologic findings in 138 teeth.[114] The symptoms and findings agreed in only 40% of cases; in the remainder, histologic examination showed the pulpitis to be more pronounced than the clinical symptoms indicated. In an assessment of 104 teeth with pulpitis, Masacres and Bonner found a correlation between the clinical and the histologic diagnosis in almost 75% of the teeth studied.[65]

The diseases of the pulp may be clinically classified as in Table 4–2.

Reversible Pulpitis

Definition. Reversible pulpitis is a mild-to-moderate inflammatory condition of the pulp caused by noxious stimuli in which the pulp is capable of returning to the uninflamed state following removal of the stimuli. Pain of brief duration may be produced by thermal stimuli in the reversibly inflamed pulp, but the pain subsides as soon as the stimulus is removed.

Table 4–2. Diseases of the Pulp

I. Pulpitides (inflammation)
  A. Reversible
    1. Symptomatic (acute)
    2. Asymptomatic (chronic)
  B. Irreversible pulpitis
    1. Acute
      a. abnormally responsive to cold
      b. abnormally responsive to heat
    2. Chronic
      a. asymptomatic with pulp exposure
      b. hyperplastic pulpitis
      c. internal resorption
II. Pulp degeneration
  A. Calcific (radiographic diagnosis)
  B. Others (histopathologic diagnosis)
III. Necrosis

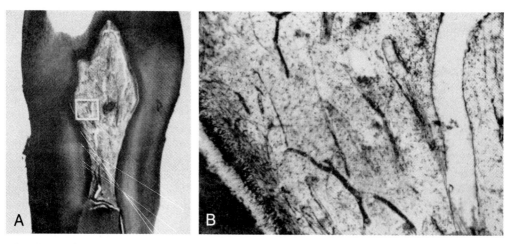

Fig. 4–2. Hyperemia of pulp. *A,* Lower magnification. *B,* High-power magnification of area outlined in *A,* showing dilated and congested blood vessels; note the dilated blood vessel on the right, with missing corpuscles. (Courtesy of the Department of Histopathology, School of Dental Medicine, University of Pennsylvania, Philadelphia.)

Histopathology. Reversible pulpitis may range from hyperemia to mild-to-moderate inflammatory changes limited to the area of the involved dentinal tubules, such as dentinal caries (Fig. 4–2). Microscopically, one sees reparative dentin, disruption of the odontoblast layer, dilated blood vessels, extravasation of edema fluid, and the presence of immunologically competent chronic inflammatory cells. Although chronic inflammatory cells predominate, one may see acute inflammatory cells.[110,111]

Cause. Reversible pulpitis may be caused by any agent that is capable of injuring the pulp. Specifically, the cause may be any of the following: trauma, as from a blow or from a disturbed occlusal relationship; thermal shock, as from preparing a cavity with a dull bur or keeping the bur in contact with the tooth for too long, or from overheating during polishing a filling; excessive dehydration of a cavity with alcohol or chloroform, or irritation of exposed dentin at the neck of a tooth; placement of a fresh amalgam filling in contact with, or occluding, a gold restoration; chemical stimulus, as from sweet or sour foodstuffs or from irritation of a silicate or self-curing acrylic filling; or bacteria, as from caries. Following insertion of a restoration, patients often complain of mild sensitivity to temperature changes, especially cold. Such sensitivity may last 2 to 3 days or a week, or even longer, but it gradually subsides. This sensitivity is symptomatic of reversible pulpitis. Circulatory disturbances, such as those accompanying menstruation or pregnancy, may also result in a transient pe-

riodic hyperemia. Local vascular congestion associated with the common cold or with sinus disease can cause a generalized transient hyperemia of the pulp of the maxillary posterior teeth. The irritant that causes hyperemia or mild inflammation in one pulp may produce secondary dentin in another, if the irritant is mild enough or if the pulp is vigorous enough to protect itself.

Symptoms. Symptomatic reversible pulpitis is characterized by sharp pain lasting but a moment. It is more often brought on by cold than hot food or beverages and by cold air. It does not occur spontaneously and does not continue when the cause has been removed. The clinical difference between reversible and irreversible pulpitis is quantitative; the pain of irreversible pulpitis is more severe and lasts longer. In reversible pulpitis, the cause of the pain is generally traceable to a stimulus, such as cold water or a draft of air, whereas in irreversible pulpitis, the pain may come without any apparent stimulus. Asymptomatic reversible pulpitis may result from incipient caries and is resolved on removal of the caries and proper restoration of the tooth.

Diagnosis. Diagnosis is by a study of the patient's symptoms and by clinical tests. The pain is sharp, lasts but a few seconds, and generally disappears when the stimulus is removed. Cold, sweet, or sour usually causes it. Pain may become chronic. Although each paroxysm may be of short duration, the paroxysms may continue for weeks or even months. The pulp may recover completely, or the pain may last longer each time, and intervals of relief may become shorter, until the pulp finally succumbs.

Because the pulp is sensitive to temperature changes, particularly cold, application of cold is an excellent method of locating and diagnosing the involved tooth. A tooth with reversible pulpitis reacts normally to percussion, palpation, and mobility, and the periapical tissue is normal on radiographic examination.

Differential Diagnosis. In reversible pulpitis, the pain is generally transitory, lasting a matter of seconds, whereas in irreversible pulpitis, the pain may last several minutes or longer. The patient's description of the pain, particularly regarding its onset, character, and duration, is often of inestimable help in arriving at a correct differential diagnosis. Thermal tests are useful in locating the affected tooth if unknown. The electric pulp test, using less current than on a control tooth, is an excellent corroborating test.

Treatment. The best treatment for reversible pulpitis is prevention. Periodic care to prevent the development of caries, early insertion of a filling if a cavity has developed, desensitization of the necks of teeth where gingival recession is marked, use of a cavity varnish or cement base before insertion of a filling, and care in cavity preparation and polishing are recommended, to prevent pulpitis. When reversible pulpitis is present, removal of the noxious stimuli usually suffices. Once the symptoms have subsided, the tooth should be tested for vitality, to make sure that pulpal necrosis has not occurred. When pain persists despite proper treatment, the pulpal inflammation should be regarded as irreversible, the treatment for which is pulp extirpation.

Prognosis. The prognosis for the pulp is favorable if the irritant is removed early enough; otherwise, the condition may develop into irreversible pulpitis.

Irreversible Pulpitis

Definition. Irreversible pulpitis is a persistent inflammatory condition of the pulp, symptomatic or asymptomatic, caused by a noxious stimulus. Acute irreversible pulpitis exhibits pain usually caused by hot or cold stimulus, or pain that occurs spontaneously. The pain persists for several minutes to hours, lingering after removal of the thermal stimulus.

Histopathology. This disorder has chronic and acute inflammatory stages in the pulp.

Irreversible pulpitis may be caused by a longstanding noxious stimulus such as caries. As it penetrates the dentin, caries causes a chronic inflammatory response previously discussed with regard to reversible pulpitis. If the caries is not removed, the inflammatory changes in the pulp will increase in severity as the decay approaches the pulp (Fig. 4–3). The postcapillary venules become congested, as previously discussed, and affect the circulation within the pulp, causing pathologic changes such as necrosis. These necrotic areas attract polymorphonuclear leukocytes by chemotaxis and start an acute inflammatory reaction. Phagocytosis by the polymorphonuclear leukocytes of the area of necrosis ensues. After phagocytosis, the polymorphonuclear leukocytes, which have a short life span, die and release lysosomal enzymes. The lysosomal enzymes lyse some of the pulp stroma and, together with the cellular debris of the dead polymorphonuclear leukocytes, form a purulent exudate (pus).

This inflammatory reaction produces microabscesses (acute pulpitis) (Fig. 4–4). The pulp, trying to protect itself, walls off the areas of the microabscesses with fibrous connective tissue. Microscopically, one sees the area of the abscess and a zone of necrotic tissue, with microorganisms present if in the late carious state, along with lymphocytes, plasma cells, and macrophages. No microorganisms are found in the center of the abscess because of the phagocytic activity of the polymorphonuclear leukocytes. If the carious process continues to advance and penetrates the pulp, the histologic picture changes. One then sees an area of ulceration (chronic ulcerative pulpitis) that drains through the carious exposure into the oral cavity and reduces the intrapulpal pressure and, therefore, the pain. Histologically, one sees an area of necrotic tissue, a zone of infiltration by polymorphonuclear leukocytes, and a zone of proliferating fibroblasts forming the wall of the lesion, where calcific masses may be present (Fig. 4–5). The areas beyond the abscess or the ulceration may be normal or may undergo inflammatory changes.

Some of the responses described may be related to an antibody-mediated hypersensitivity response. Seltzer and Bender described a possible mechanism by which high concentrations of antigen from microorganisms in the carious process may induce the formation of immunoglobulins.[92] An im-

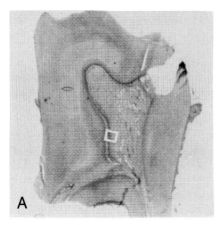
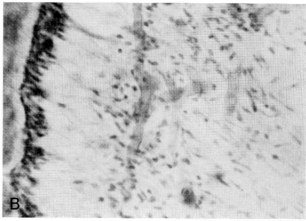

Fig. 4–3. *A,* Caries involving primary and secondary dentin; irreversible pulpitis. *B,* High-power magnification of the area outlined in *A.* Blood vessels are dilated, and the endothelial cells are swollen; serous exudate distends the tissues, particularly on the pulpal side of the odontoblasts. (Courtesy of the Department of Histopathology, School of Dental Medicine, University of Pennsylvania, Philadelphia.)

mune antigen-antibody precipitate, in the presence of complement, attracts polymorphonuclear leukocytes, followed by phagocytosis and cell degradation, with the release of lysosomes into the pulp tissue. The liberation of proteases results in the formation of a pulp abscess.

Changes in the odontoblastic layer vary from disruption to complete destruction; on the other hand, nerves seem to be resistant to inflammatory changes.[62,110,111]

Irreversible pulpitis progresses to necrosis, as discussed later in this chapter.

Cause. The most common cause of irreversible pulpitis is bacterial involvement of the pulp through caries, although any clini-cal factor, chemical, thermal, or mechanical, already mentioned as a cause of pulp disease may also cause pulpitis. As previously stated, reversible pulpitis may deteriorate into irreversible pulpitis.

Symptoms. In the early stages of irreversible pulpitis, a paroxysm of pain may be caused by the following: sudden temperature changes, particularly cold; sweet or acid foodstuffs; pressure from packing food into a cavity or suction exerted by the tongue or cheek; and recumbency, which results in congestion of the blood vessels of the pulp. The pain often continues when the cause has been removed, and it may come and go spontaneously, without apparent cause. The pa-

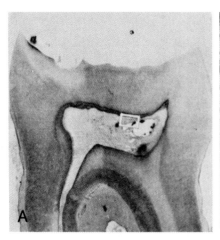
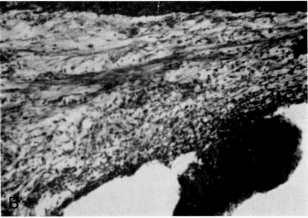

Fig. 4–4. Irreversible pulpitis. *A,* The empty space to the right of the white, rectangular area is an abscess cavity from which the fluid content (pus) has dropped out during preparation of the section. *B,* High-power magnification showing granulocytes and a clump of polymorphonuclear cells at the lower right. (Courtesy of the Department of Histopathology, School of Dental Medicine, University of Pennsylvania, Philadelphia.)

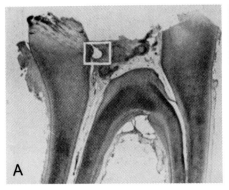
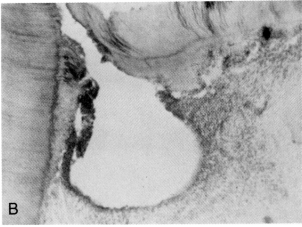

Fig. 4–5. Irreversible pulpitis. *A*, Occlusal caries with an extensive opening into the pulp. Pulp stones occupy the larger part of the pulp cavity. *B*, High-power magnification of the area outlined in *A*. Caries involves primary, secondary, and reparative dentin. An abscess cavity is present, with acute and chronic inflammation of surrounding tissues. (Courtesy of the Department of Histopathology, School of Dental Medicine, University of Pennsylvania, Philadelphia.)

tient may describe the pain as sharp, piercing, or shooting, and it is generally severe. It may be intermittent or continuous, depending on the degree of pulpal involvement and depending on whether it is related to an external stimulus. The patient may also state that bending over or lying down, that is, change of position, exacerbates the pain; changes in intrapulpal pressure may be the cause. Changes in the blood pressure of the pulp may also occur.[5,113,116] The patient may also have pain referred to adjacent teeth, to the temple or sinuses when an upper posterior tooth is involved, or to the ear when a lower posterior tooth is affected.

In later stages, the pain is more severe and is generally described as boring, gnawing, or throbbing, or as if the tooth were under constant pressure. The pulp need not be macroscopically exposed, but a slight exposure is generally present, or else the pulp is covered with a layer of soft, leathery decay. When no outlet is present, whether because of a covering of decay or a filling or because of food packed into a small exposure in the dentin, pain can be most intense. Patients are often kept awake at night by the pain, which continues to be intolerable despite all their efforts at analgesia. Pain is increased by heat and is sometimes relieved by cold, although continued cold may intensify the pain. After exposure and drainage of the pulp, pain may be slight, manifesting itself as a dull consciousness, or it may be entirely absent. Pain can return if food packs into the cavity or underneath a leaky filling; it may not be as

intense because of degeneration of the superficial nerve fibers.

Apical periodontitis is absent, except in the later stages, when inflammation or infection extends to the periodontal ligament.

Diagnosis. Inspection generally discloses a deep cavity extending to the pulp or decay under a filling. The pulp may already be exposed. On gaining access to the exposure, one may see a grayish, scum-like layer over the exposed pulp and the surrounding dentin. This layer is composed of food debris, degenerated polymorphonuclear leukocytes, microorganisms, and blood cells. The surface of the pulp is eroded. An odor of decomposition is frequently present in this area. Probing into the area is not painful to the patient until the deeper areas of the pulp are reached. At this level, both pain and hemorrhage may occur. If the pulp is not exposed by the carious process, a drop of pus may be expressed when one gains access to the pulp chamber.

Radiographic examination may not show anything of significance that is not already known clinically; it may disclose an interproximal cavity not seen visually, or it may suggest involvement of a pulp horn. A radiograph may also show exposure of the pulp, caries under a filling, or a deep cavity or filling threatening the integrity of the pulp. In the early stages of irreversible pulpitis, the thermal test may elicit pain that persists after removal of the thermal stimulus. In the late stages, when the pulp is exposed, it may respond normally to a thermal stimulus, but generally it reacts feebly to heat and cold. The electric pulp test induces a response with a marked variation in current from the normal. Results of examination for mobility and percussion and palpation tests are negative.

Differential Diagnosis. One must distinguish between reversible and irreversible pulpitis. In reversible pulpitis, pain produced by thermal stimulus disappears as soon as the stimulus is removed, whereas in irreversible pulpitis, the pain lingers after the stimulus is removed, or it can occur spontaneously.

In the asymptomatic stage of irreversible pulpitis, the exposed pulp exhibits little or no pain, except when food is packed into the cavity. More current is required to elicit a response to the electric pulp test than in a control tooth. In the early symptomatic stage, less current than normal is needed to elicit a response to the electric pulp tester, and the pulp is often abnormally responsive to cold stimulus. The induced or spontaneous pain that occurs is sharp, piercing, and readily identified with a specific tooth. Other symptoms may develop, such as diffuse, dull, constant pain, characterized by throbbing and gnawing, and the tooth may respond abnormally and severely to heat. This response generally is indicative of a later stage of irreversible pulpitis. In this stage of irreversible pulpitis, the symptoms may simulate those of an acute alveolar abscess. Such an abscess, however, causes at least some of the following symptoms, which help to differentiate it from irreversible pulpitis: swelling, tenderness on palpation, tenderness on percussion, mobility of the tooth, and lack of response to pulp-vitality tests. In addition, the patient may have symptoms of systemic toxicity such as fever and nausea.

The pain of pulpitis is easy to localize by the patient at the onset. Once discomfort increases, the patient loses the ability to identify a particular tooth in the quadrant. A previous history of pain may help one to localize the origin of the pulpalgia. When pulpal pain is difficult to localize, the application of heat with a consequent abnormal response is indicative of irreversible pulpitis in that tooth.

Treatment. Treatment consists of complete removal of the pulp, or pulpectomy, and the placement of an intracanal medicament to act as a disinfectant or obtundent, such as cresatin, eugenol, or formocresol. In posterior teeth, in which time is a factor, the removal of the coronal pulp or pulpotomy and the placement of a formocresol or similar dressing over the radicular pulp should be performed as an emergency procedure. Surgical removal should be considered if the tooth is unrestorable.

Prognosis. The prognosis of the tooth is favorable if the pulp is removed and if the tooth undergoes proper endodontic therapy and restoration.

Chronic Hyperplastic Pulpitis

Definition. Chronic hyperplastic pulpitis or "pulp polyp" is a productive pulpal inflammation due to an extensive carious exposure of a young pulp. This disorder is characterized by the development of granulation tissue, covered at times with epithelium and resulting from long-standing, low-grade irritation (Fig. 4–6).

Histopathology. Histopathologically, the surface of the pulp polyp is usually covered by stratified squamous epithelium.[45,90] The pulp polyps of deciduous teeth are more likely to be covered with stratified squamous epithelium than those of permanent teeth. Such epithelium may be derived from the gingiva or from freshly desquamated epithelial cells of the mucosa or tongue. The tissue in the pulp chamber is often transformed into granulation tissue, which projects from the pulp into the carious lesion. The granulation tissue is young, vascular connective tissue containing polymorphonuclear neutrophils, lymphocytes, and plasma cells. The pulp tissue is chronically inflamed. Nerve fibers may be found in the epithelial layer[10] (Fig. 4–7).

Cause. Slow, progressive carious exposure of the pulp is the cause. For the development of hyperplastic pulpitis, a large, open cavity, a young, resistant pulp, and a chronic, low-grade stimulus are necessary. Mechanical irritation from chewing and bacterial infection often provide the stimulus.

Symptoms. Chronic hyperplastic pulpitis is symptomless, except during mastication, when pressure of the food bolus may cause discomfort.

Diagnosis. This disorder is generally seen only in the teeth of children and young adults. The appearance of the polypoid tissue is clinically characteristic; a fleshy, reddish pulpal mass fills most of the pulp chamber or cavity or even extends beyond the confines of the tooth (see Fig. 4–6). At times, the mass is large enough to interfere with comfortable closure of the teeth, although in the

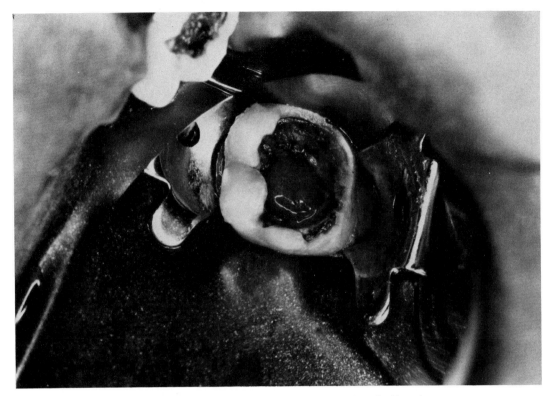

Fig. 4–6. Chronic hyperplastic pulpitis. (Courtesy of Dr. Steve Senia, San Antonio, Texas.)

early stages of development it may be the size of a pin. Polypoid tissue is less sensitive than normal pulp tissue and more sensitive than gingival tissue. Cutting of this tissue produces no pain, but pressure thereby transmitted to the apical end of the pulp does cause pain. Nerve fibers in the epithelial layer have been seen in 18 of 125 hyperplastic pulps examined histologically.[97] This tissue bleeds easily because of a rich network of blood vessels. If the hyperplastic pulp tissue extends beyond the cavity of a tooth, it may appear as if the gum tissue is growing into the cavity. To differentiate a pulp polyp from proliferating gingival tissue, one should raise and trace the stalk of the tissue back to its origin, the pulp chamber.

It should not be difficult to diagnose chronic hyperplastic pulpitis by clinical examination alone. The hyperplastic pulp tissue in the pulp chamber or cavity of a tooth is characteristic in appearance. Radiographs generally show a large, open cavity with direct access to the pulp chamber. The tooth may respond feebly or not at all to the thermal test, unless one uses extreme cold, as from an ethyl chloride spray. More current

than normal may be required to elicit a response by means of the electric pulp tester.

Differential Diagnosis. The appearance of hyperplastic pulpitis is characteristic and should be easily recognized. The disorder must be distinguished from proliferating gingival tissue.

Treatment. Efforts at treatment should be directed toward elimination of the polypoid tissue followed by extirpation of the pulp, provided the tooth can be restored. When the hyperplastic pulpal mass has been removed with a periodontal curette or spoon excavator, the bleeding can be controlled with pressure. The pulp tissue of the chamber is then completely removed, and a dressing of formocresol is sealed in contact with the radicular pulp tissue. The radicular pulp is extirpated at a later visit. If time permits, the entire procedure, pulpectomy, can be completed in a single visit.

Prognosis. The prognosis for the pulp is unfavorable. The prognosis for the tooth is favorable after endodontic treatment and adequate restoration.

Internal Resorption

Definition. Internal resorption is an idiopathic slow or fast progressive resorptive

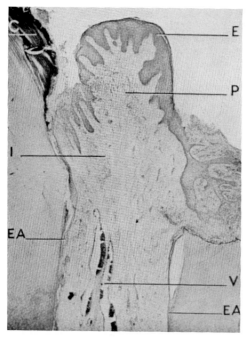

Fig. 4–7. Chronic hyperplastic pulpitis (pulp polyp) of the lower bicuspid. C, Carious dentin on the inner wall of the broken-down crown; E, stratified squamous epithelium with keratinized surface layer; P, hyperplastic pulp tissue; I, inflammatory exudate cells in the pulp tissue; V, enlarged blood vessels; EA, epithelial attachment to the wall of the root canal. (From Boulger: J. Dent. Res.)

process occurring in the dentin of the pulp chamber or root canals of teeth.

Histopathology. Unlike caries, the internal resorption is the result of osteoclastic activity. The resorptive process is characterized by lacunae, which may be filled in by osteoid tissue. The osteoid tissue may be regarded as an attempt at repair. The presence of granulation tissue accounts for profuse bleeding when the pulp is removed. Multinucleated giant cells or dentinoclasts are present. The pulp is usually chronically inflamed. Metaplasia of the pulp, that is, transformation to another type of tissue such as bone or cementum, sometimes occurs.

Cause. The cause of internal resorption is not known, but such patients often have a history of trauma.

Symptoms. Internal resorption in the root of a tooth is asymptomatic. In the crown of the tooth, internal resorption may be manifested as a reddish area called "pink spot." This reddish area represents the granulation tissue showing through the resorbed area of the crown.

Diagnosis. Internal resorption may affect either the crown or the root of the tooth, or

it may be extensive enough to involve both (Figs. 4–8 and 4–9). It may be a slow, progressive, intermittent process extending over 1 or 2 years, it may develop rapidly and may perforate the tooth within a matter of months. Although any tooth in the mouth can be involved, those most readily recognized are the maxillary anterior teeth. Usually, internal resorption is diagnosed during routine radiographic examination. The appearance of the "pink spot" occurs late in the resorptive process, when the integrity of the crown has been compromised (Fig. 4–9). The radiograph usually shows a change in the appearance of the wall in the root canal or pulp chamber, with a round or ovoid radiolucent area.

Differential Diagnosis. When internal resorption progresses into the periodontal space and a perforation of the root occurs, it is difficult to differentiate from external resorption. In internal resorption, the resorptive defect is more extensive in the pulpal wall than on the root surface; this defect usually is recognized by means of a radiograph.

Treatment. Extirpation of the pulp stops the internal resorptive process. Routine endodontic treatment is indicated, but obturation of the defect requires a special effort, preferably with a plasticized gutta-percha method. In many patients, however, the condition progresses unobserved because it is painless, until the root is perforated. In such a case, calcium-hydroxide paste is sealed in the root canal and is periodically renewed until the defect is repaired. Repair is completed when a calcific barrier is present. When repair has been completed, the canal with its defect is obturated with plasticized gutta-percha.

Prognosis. The prognosis is best before perforation of the root or crown occurs. In the event of a root-crown perforation, the prognosis is guarded and depends on the formation of a calcific barrier or access to the perforation that permits surgical repair.

Pulp Degeneration

Although degeneration of the pulp, as such, is seldom recognized clinically, the types of pulp degeneration should be included in a description of diseases of the pulp. Degeneration is generally present in the teeth of older people. Degeneration may also be the result of persistent, mild irritation in teeth of younger people, however, as in calcific degeneration of the pulp. Degeneration

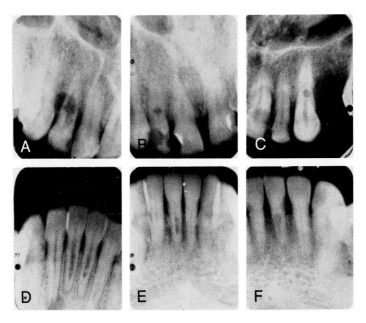

Fig. 4–8. *A to F,* Teeth showing evidence of internal resorption.

is not necessarily related to infection or caries, although a cavity or filling may be present in the affected tooth. The early stage of pulp degeneration does not usually cause definite clinical symptoms. The tooth is not discolored, and the pulp may react normally to electric and thermal tests. As degeneration of the pulp progresses, the tooth may become discolored, and the pulp will not respond to stimulation. The specific types of pulp degeneration are discussed in the following paragraphs.

Calcific Degeneration. In calcific degeneration, part of the pulp tissue is replaced by calcific material; that is, pulp stones or denticles are formed (Fig. 4–10). This calcification may occur either within the pulp chamber or root canal, but it is generally present in the pulp chamber. The calcified material has a laminated structure, like the skin of an onion, and lies unattached within the body of the pulp. Such a denticle or pulp stone may become large enough to give an impression of the pulp cavity when the calcified

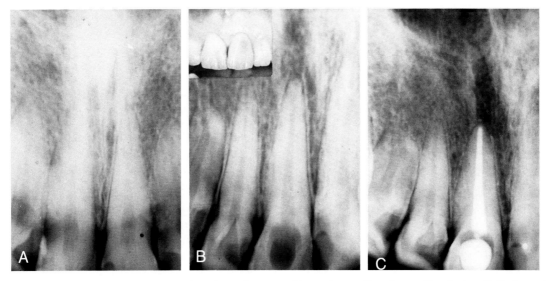

Fig. 4–9. *A,* Radiograph taken 18 months prior to the onset of internal resorption of a maxillary incisor. *B,* Radiograph showing evidence of internal resorption of the crown (inset shows external appearance). *C,* After endodontic treatment.

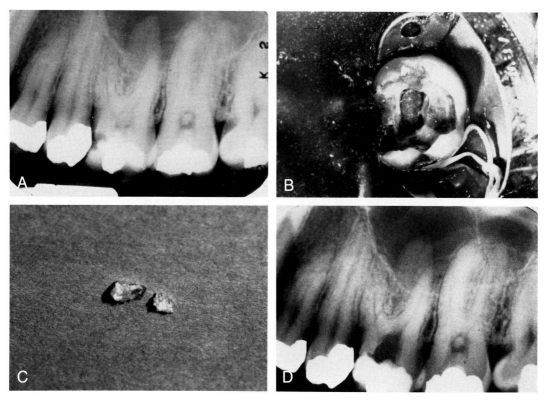

Fig. 4–10. Pulp stones. *A*, Preoperative radiograph of a maxillary first molar, *B*, Clinical photograph showing a pulp stone filling the entire pulp chamber. *C*, Pulp stone. *D*, After removal of stone. (Courtesy of Dr. M.L. Canales, San Antonio, Texas.)

mass is removed. In another type of calcification, the calcified material is attached to the wall of the pulp cavity and is an integral part of it. It is not always possible to distinguish one type from another on a radiograph.

It is estimated that pulp stones are present in more than 60% of adult teeth. They are considered to be harmless concretions, although referred pain in a few patients has been ascribed to the presence of these calcifications in the pulp.

Teeth with pulp stones have also been suspected of being foci of infection by some clinicians. No difference has been found in incidence of pulp stones between a group of arthritic patients and a normal control group of approximately the same ages.[98] The reader should refer to Chapter 3 for further information on and illustrations of calcification.

Atrophic Degeneration. In this type of degeneration, observed histopathologically in pulps of older people, fewer stellate cells are present, and intercellular fluid is increased. The pulp tissue is less sensitive than normal. So-called "reticular atrophy" is an artifact produced by delay of the fixative agent in reaching the pulp and should not be confused with atrophic degeneration. No clinical diagnosis exists.

Fibrous Degeneration. This form of degeneration of the pulp is characterized by replacement of the cellular elements by fibrous connective tissue. On removal from the root canal, such a pulp has the characteristic appearance of a leathery fiber (Fig. 4–11). This disorder causes no distinguishing symptoms to aid in the clinical diagnosis.

Pulp Artifacts. Vacuolization of the odontoblasts was once thought to be a type of pulp degeneration characterized by empty spaces formerly occupied by odontoblasts. It is probably an artifact caused by poor fixation of the tissue specimen. Fatty degeneration of the pulp, along with reticular atrophy and vacuolization, are all probably artifacts with the same cause, that is, unsatisfactory fixation.

Tumor Metastasis. Metastasis of tumor cells to the dental pulp is rare, except possibly in terminal stages. The mechanism by which such pulpal involvement takes place in most cases is direct local extension from the jaw. One report noted involvement of a

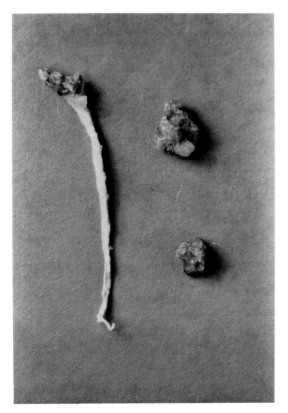

Fig. 4–11. Fibrotic radicular pulp with pulp-chamber pulp stones from a maxillary first molar. (Courtesy of Dr. G. Walters, San Antonio, Texas.)

molar pulp in an 11-year-old patient with chondromyxosarcoma of the mandible.[88] Of 39 patients with malignant tumors of the mouth studied, only in 1 were tumor cells found in the pulp.[106]

Necrosis of Pulp

Definition. Necrosis is death of the pulp. It may be partial or total, depending on whether part of or the entire pulp is involved. Necrosis, although a sequel to inflammation, can also occur following a traumatic injury in which the pulp is destroyed before an inflammatory reaction takes place. As a result, an ischemic infarction can develop and may cause a dry-gangrenous necrotic pulp.[103] Necrosis is of two general types: coagulation and liquefaction.

Types. In coagulation necrosis, the soluble portion of tissue is precipitated or is converted into a solid material. Caseation is a form of coagulation necrosis in which the tissue is converted into a cheesy mass consisting chiefly of coagulated proteins, fats, and water.

Liquefaction necrosis results when proteolytic enzymes convert the tissue into a softened mass, a liquid, or amorphous debris.

The end products of pulp decomposition are those of protein decomposition, namely, hydrogen sulfide, ammonia, fatty substances, indican, ptomaines, water, and carbon dioxide. The intermediate products, such as indole, skatole, putrecine, and cadaverine, contribute to the unpleasant odor sometimes emanating from a root canal.

Cause. Necrosis of the pulp can be caused by any noxious insult injurious to the pulp, such as bacteria, trauma, and chemical irritation.

Symptoms. An otherwise normal tooth with a necrotic pulp causes no painful symptoms. Frequently, discoloration of the tooth is the first indication that the pulp is dead. The dull or opaque appearance of the crown may be due merely to a lack of normal translucency. At other times, however, the tooth may have a definite grayish or brownish discoloration and may lack its usual brilliance and luster. The presence of a necrotic pulp may be discovered only by chance because such a tooth is asymptomatic, and the radiograph is nondiagnostic. Teeth with partial necrosis can respond to thermal changes, owing to the presence of vital nerve fibers passing through the adjacent inflamed tissue.[62,110]

Diagnosis. Radiographs generally show a large cavity or filling, an open approach to the root canal, and a thickening of the periodontal ligament. Some teeth have neither a cavity nor a filling, and the pulp has died as a result of trauma. A few patients have a history of severe pain lasting from a few minutes to a few hours, followed by complete and sudden cessation of pain. During this time, "the pulp sang its swan song" and lulled the patient into a false sense of security and well-being. In other cases, the patient is unaware that the pulp has died slowly and silently, without causing symptoms. A tooth with a necrotic pulp does not respond to cold, the electric pulp test, or the test cavity. In rare cases, however, a minimal response to the maximum current of an electric pulp tester occurs when the electric current is conducted through the moisture present in a root canal following liquefaction necrosis to neighboring vital tissue. In other patients, a few apical nerve fibers survive and respond similarly. Nerve fibers are resistant to inflammatory changes.[62,75,110] A correlation of cold

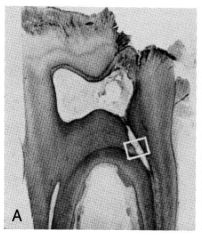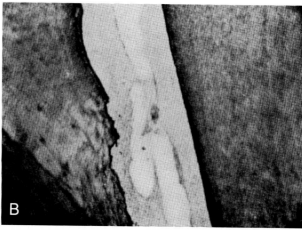

Fig. 4–12. Necrosis of the pulp. *A,* Caries involves primary and secondary dentin. The space represents a former abscess cavity. The tissue in the pulp and canals is necrotic, as shown by the higher magnification in *B.* Note that no nuclei are visible, and cell detail is lost. (Courtesy of the Department of Histopathology, School of Dental Medicine, University of Pennsylvania, Philadelphia.)

and electric tests and a history of pain, in conjunction with a thorough clinical examination, should establish a correct diagnosis.

Bacteriology. Many bacteria have been isolated from teeth with necrotic pulps. In a high percentage of these cases, the root canal contains a mixed microbial flora, both aerobic and anaerobic. For further information, see Chapter 13.

Histopathology. Necrotic pulp tissue, cellular debris, and microorganisms may be seen in the pulp cavity. The periapical tissue may be normal, or slight evidence of inflammation of the apical periodontal ligament may be present (Fig. 4–12).

Treatment. Treatment consists of preparation and obturation of the root canals.

Prognosis. The prognosis for the tooth is favorable, if proper endodontic therapy is instituted.

BIBLIOGRAPHY

1. Adrian, J.C., et al.: J. Am. Dent. Assoc., *83*:113, 1971.
2. Allard, U., et al.: Oral Surg., *48*:454, 1979.
3. Austin, L.T.: J. Am. Dent. Assoc., *17*:1930, 1930.
4. Baume, L.: SSO Schweiz. Monatsschr Zahnheilkd., *77*:1085, 1965, and Transactions of the Fourth International Conference on Endodontics. Philadelphia, University of Pennsylvania Press, 1968, p. 66.
5. Beveridge, E.E., and Brown, A.C.: Oral Surg., *19*:655, 1965.
6. Bhaskar, S.N., and Lilly, G.E.: J. Dent. Res., *44*:644, 1965.
7. Björlin, G., et al., Oral Surg., *39*:488, 1975.
8. Björn, H.: Nor. Tannlaegeforen. Tidsskr., *65*:487, 1955.
9. Boulger, E.P.: J. Am. Dent. Assoc., *15*:1778, 1928.
10. Boyd, W.: A Textbook of Pathology, 8th Ed. Philadelphia, Lea & Febiger, 1970.
11. Brännström, M.: Dentin and Pulp in Restorative Dentistry. Nacka, Sweden, Dental Therapeutics, 1981.
12. Brännström, M.: Oral Surg., *21*:517, 1966.
13. Brännström, M.: Acta Odontol. Scand., *18*:235, 1960.
14. Brännström, M., and Nordenwall, K.J.: J. Dent. Res., *57*:3, 1978.
15. Brännström, M., and Nyborg, H.: J. Dent. Res., *50*:1548, 1971.
16. Burke, G.H.: J. Endod., *2*:87, 1976.
17. Burket, L.W.: Yale J. Biol. Med., *9*:271, 287, 1937.
18. Cameron, C.E.: J. Am. Dent. Assoc., *68*:406, 1964, and *93*:971, 1976.
19. Cotton, W.R.: J. Dent. Child., *38*:85, 1971.
20. Cotton, W.R.: Oral Surg., *24*:78, 1967.
21. Cotton, W.R., and Siegel, R.L.: U.S. Navy Med., *68*:27, 1977.
22. Crane, F.L.: Int. Dent. J., *18*:451, 1968.
23. Csernyei, J.: J. Dent. Res., *18*:527, 1939.
24. Cvek, M.: Odontol. Revy, *24*:343, 1973.
25. Dellow, P.G., and Roberts, M.L.: Aust. Dent. J., *11*:384, 1966.
26. Dickey, D.M., et al.: J. Am. Dent. Assoc., *88*:108, 1974.
27. Ehrich, W., and Harris, T.N.: J. Exp. Med., *76*:335, 1942.
28. Eriksen, H.M.: J. Dent. Res., *55*:281, 1976.
29. Figg, W.A., et al.: J. Dent. Res., *23*:214, 1944.
30. Fish, E.W.: Experimental Investigation of Enamel, Dentine, and the Dental Pulp. London, John Bale, Sons and Daniellson, 1932, p. 70.
31. Fulghum, R.S., et al.: J. Dent. Res., *52*:637, 1973.
32. Garfunkel, A., et al.: Oral Surg., *35*:110, 1973.
33. Grossman, L.I.: J. Dent. Res., *46*:551, 1967.
34. Grossman, L.I.: J. Am. Dent. Assoc., *46*:265, 1953.
35. Grossman, L.I.: Ann. Dent., *1*:121, 1942.
36. Grossman, L.I.: Unpublished data.
37. Grossman, L.I., and Oliet, S.: Oral Surg., *25*:235, 1968.

38. Harris, R., and Griffin, C.J.: Aust. Dent. J., *18*:88, 1973.
39. Heithersay, G.S.: J. Br. Endod. Soc., *7*:74, 1975.
40. Hess, W.: Z. Stomatol., *35*:82, 1937.
41. Hey, R.J., et al.: J. Oral Pathol., *6*:317, 1977.
42. Hutton, M., et al.: Oral Surg., *38*:279, 1974.
43. Inokoshi, S., et al.: J. Dent. Res., *61*:1014, 1982.
44. Iserman, G.T.: Oral Surg., *48*:353, 1979.
45. Janksy, Z.: Rev. Stomatol., *51*:432, 1950.
46. Johnson, G.J.: J. Prosthet. Dent., *26*:307, 1971.
47. Johnson, R.H., et al.: J. Am. Dent. Assoc., *81*:108, 1970.
48. Kakehashi, S., et al.: Oral Surg., *20*:340, 1965.
49. Kawahara, H., et al.: J. Dent. Res., *58*:1080, 1979.
50. Kaye, M.A.: Br. Dent. J., *125*:59, 1968.
51. Keudell, K.: J. Endod., *2*:146, 1976.
52. Klotz, M.D., et. al.: J. Am. Dent. Assoc., *71*:871, 1965.
53. Kramer, I.R.H.: Br. Dent. J., *101*:378, 1956, and J. Dent. Res., *34*:782, 1955.
54. Langeland, K.: Oral Surg., *14*:210, 1961.
55. Langeland, K.: Odontol. Tidskr., *68*:463, 1960.
56. Langeland, K.: Oral Surg., *12*:1235, 1959.
57. Langeland, K.: Acta Odontol. Scand., *13*:239, 1956, and Nor. Tannlaegeforen. Tidsskr., *66*:304, 1956.
58. Langeland, K., and Langeland, L.K.: J. Am. Dent. Assoc., *76*:991, 1968.
59. Langeland, K.: Symposium on Operative Dentistry. Nijmegen, Netherlands, 1975.
60. Lawson, B.F., and Mitchell, D.F.: Oral Surg., *17*:47, 1964.
61. Leatherman, G.H.: Br. Dent. J., *117*:124, 1953.
62. Lin, L.L., and Langeland, K.: Oral Surg., *51*:292, 1981.
63. Macko, D.J., et al.: Oral Surg., *45*:430, 1978.
64. Marsland, E.A., and Shovelton, D.: Arch. Oral Biol., *15*:411, 1970.
65. Masacres, C., and Bonner, M.: J. Can. Dent. Assoc., *44*:65, 1978.
66. Massler, M., and Evans, J.A.: J. Dent. Res., *46*:1469, 1967.
67. Massler, M., and Pawlak, J.: Oral Surg., *43*:929, 1977.
68. Maurice, C.G., and Schour, I.: J. Dent. Res., *35*:69, 1956.
69. Majåre, B., et al.: Acta Odontol. Scand., *37*:267, 1979.
70. Menkin, V.: Biochemical Mechanisms in Inflammation. Springfield, IL, Charles C Thomas, 1956.
71. Miller, W.D.: Dent. Cosmos, *36*:505, 1894.
72. Mitchell, D., and Tarplee, R.E.: Oral Surg., *13*:1360, 1960.
73. Moist, R.R., and Yanoff, H.M.: J. Dent. Res., *44*:570, 1965.
74. Mullaney, T.P., et al.: Oral Surg., *30*:690, 1970.
75. Mullaney, T.P., et al.: Oral Surg., *21*:479, 1966.
76. Nishikawa, T., et al.: Jpn. J. Conserv. Dent., *9*:72, 1966.
77. Noyes, F.B., and Dewey, K.W.: JAMA, *71*:1179, 1918.
78. Nygaard-Ostby, B.: J. Am. Dent. Assoc., *50*:7, 1955.
79. Olsen, P.: J. Can. Dent. Assoc., *30*:771, 1964.
80. Orban, B.: J. Dent. Res., *19*:537, 1940.
81. Orban, B., and Ritchey, B.T.: J. Am. Dent. Assoc., *32*:145, 1945.
82. Paterson, R.C.: Br. Dent. J., *140*:174, 1976.
83. Plant, C.G.: Br. Dent. J., *129*:424, 1970, and *135*:317, 1973.
84. Pohto, M.: Ylipainos Suome (Helsinki), *48*:30, 1952.
85. Qvist, V.: Scand. J. Dent. Res., *83*:54, 1975.
86. Rauch, B.: J. Can. Dent. Assoc., *24*:404, 1958.
87. Reeves, R., and Stanley, H.R.: Oral Surg., *22*:59, 1966.
88. Robinson, H.B.G.: Am. J. Orthod. Oral Surg., *33*:558, 1947.
89. Robinson, H.B.G., and Boling, L.R.: J. Am. Dent. Assoc., *28*:268, 1941.
90. Rodden, H.G.: Proceedings of the Tenth Congress of the Australian Dental Association, 1939.
91. Safer, D.S., et al., Oral Surg., *33*:966, 1972.
92. Seltzer, S., and Bender, I.B.: The Dental Pulp, 3rd Ed. Philadelphia, J.B. Lippincott, 1984, p. 382.
93. Shindell, E.: Oral Surg., *15*:1382, 1962.
94. Skogedal, O., and Tronstad, L.: Oral Surg., *43*:135, 1977.
95. Smith, D.C.: Br. Dent. J., *125*:381, 1968.
96. Smulson, M.H.: Dent. Clin. North Am., *28*:699, 1984.
97. Southam, J.C., and Hodson, J.J.: Arch. Oral Biol., *18*:1255, 1973.
98. Sorrin, S.: J. Dent. Res., *20*:287, 1941.
99. Stambaugh, R.V., and Wittrock, J.W.: J. Prosthet. Dent., *37*:537, 1977.
100. Stanley, H.R.: Human Pulp Responses to Restorative Dental Procedures. Gainesville, FL, Storter Printing, 1981.
101. Stanley, H.R., and Ranney, R.R.: Oral Surg., *15*:1396, 1962.
102. Stanley, H.R.,and Swerdlow, H.: J. Am. Dent. Assoc., *58*:49, 1959.
103. Stanley, H.R., et al.: J. Dent. Res., *58*:1507, 1979.
104. Stanley, H.R., et al.: J. Endod., *4*:325, 1978.
105. Stanley, H.R., et al.: J. Am. Dent. Assoc., *91*:817, 1975.
106. Stewart, E.E., and Stafne, E.C.: Oral Surg., *8*:842, 1955.
107. Taylor, R., et al.: Oral Surg., *19*:786, 1965.
108. Thoma, K.: Dent. Items Int., *57*:28, 1935.
109. Tobias, R.S., et al., Br. Dent. J., *144*:345, 1978.
110. Torneck, C.D.: J. Endod., *7*:8, 1981.
111. Trowbridge, H.O.: J. Endod., *7*:52, 1981.
112. Trowbridge, H.O., et al.: J. Endod., *5*:405, 1979.
113. Van Hassel, H.J.: Oral Surg., *32*:126, 1971.
114. Wegner, H., and Knorr, E.: Dtsch. Stomatol., *18*:279, 1968.
115. Wittgow, W.C., and Sabistan, C.B.: J. Endod., *1*:168, 1975.
116. Wynn, W. et al.: J. Dent. Res., *42*:1169, 1963.
117. Zach, L., and Cohen, G.: Oral Surg., *19*:515, 1965.
118. Zander, H.: Transactions of the Second International Conference on Endodontics. Philadelphia, University of Pennsylvania Press, 1958, p. 20.

5 Diseases of the Periradicular Tissues

Because of the interrelationship between the pulp and the periradicular tissues, pulpal inflammation causes inflammatory changes in the periodontal ligament even before the pulp becomes totally necrotic. Bacteria and their toxins, immunologic agents, tissue debris, and products of tissue necrosis from the pulp reach the periradicular area through the various foramina of the root canals and give rise to inflammatory and immunologic reactions. Pulpal disease is only one of several possible causes of diseases of the periradicular tissues. Neoplastic disorders, periodontal conditions, developmental factors, and trauma can also cause periradicular diseases.

Periradicular diseases of pulpal origin may be classified as acute or chronic (Table 5–1).

ACUTE PERIRADICULAR DISEASES

These disorders are acute alveolar abscess, including an exacerbation of a chronic lesion and acute apical periodontitis.

Acute Alveolar Abscess

Synonyms. Acute abscess, acute apical abscess, acute dentoalveolar abscess, acute periapical abscess, and acute radicular abscess.

Definition. An acute alveolar abscess is a localized collection of pus in the alveolar

Table 5–1. Disease of the Periradicular Tissues

Acute periradicular disease
  Acute alveolar abscess
  Acute apical periodontitis
    Vital
    Nonvital
Chronic periradicular diseases with areas of rarefaction
  Chronic alveolar abscess
  Granuloma
  Cyst
Condensing osteitis
External root resorption
Diseases of the periradicular tissues of nonendodontic origin

bone at the root apex of a tooth following death of the pulp, with extension of the infection through the apical foramen into the periradicular tissues. It is accompanied by a severe local, and, at times, general, reaction. An acute abscess is a continuance of the disease process beginning in the pulp and progressing to the periradicular tissues, which, in turn, react severely to the infection.

Cause. Although an acute abscess may be the result of trauma or of chemical or mechanical irritation, the immediate cause is generally bacterial invasion of dead pulp tissue. At times, neither a cavity nor a restoration is present in the tooth, but the patient has a history of trauma. Because the pulp tissue is solidly enclosed, no drainage is possible, and the infection continues to extend in the direction of least resistance, that is, through the apical foramen, and thereby involves the periodontal ligament and periradicular bone.

Symptoms. The first symptom may be a mere tenderness of the tooth that may be relieved by continued slight pressure on the extruded tooth to push it back into the alveolus. Later, the patient has severe, throbbing pain, with attendant swelling of the overlying soft tissue. As the infection progresses, the swelling becomes more pronounced and extends beyond the original site. The tooth becomes more painful, elongated, and mobile. At times, the pain may subside or cease entirely while the adjacent tissue continues to swell. If left unattended, the infection may progress to osteitis, periostitis, cellulitis, or osteomyelitis. The contained pus may break through to form a sinus tract, usually opening in the labial or buccal mucosa. At other times, it may exit anywhere near the tooth, such as the skin of the patient's face or neck, or even the antrum or nasal cavity.

Swelling is usually seen in the adjacent tissues close to the affected tooth. When swelling becomes extensive, the resulting cellulitis may distort the patient's appearance grotesquely. At times, such swelling extends beyond the immediate vicinity of the diseased periradicular tissues. When a maxillary anterior tooth is involved, particularly a cuspid, swelling of the upper lip may extend to one or both eyelids. When a maxillary posterior tooth is affected, the cheek may swell to an immense size, distorting the patient's facial features. In the case of a mandibular anterior tooth, the swelling can involve the lower lip and chin and, in severe cases, the neck. When a mandibular posterior tooth is involved, swelling of the cheek may extend to the ear or even around the border of the jaw into the submaxillary region (Fig. 5–1). The tissue at the surface of the swelling appears taut and inflamed; pus starts to form beneath it. Such liquefaction is the result of activity of proteolytic enzymes such as trypsin and cathepsin. The surface tissues become distended from the pressure of the underlying pus and finally rupture from this pressure and from lack of resistance caused by continued liquefaction. The pus may exude through a tiny opening, which becomes larger with time, or from two or more openings, depending on the degree of softening of the tissues and on the amount of pressure from the contained pus. This process is the beginning of a chronic alveolar abscess. The sinus tract ultimately heals by granulation after the elimination of the infection in the root canal. A gutta-percha cone, placed in the sinus tract and imaged radiographically, often points to the involved tooth.

The point at which the pus breaks into the mouth depends on the thickness of alveolar bone and the overlying soft tissues. Obviously, the confined pus takes the path of least resistance. In the upper jaw, this path is generally along the labial alveolar plate, which is thinner than the palatal plate of bone. Suppuration from the upper lateral incisors or from the palatal root of a maxillary molar may occur palatally because these roots lie in closer proximity to the palatal plate of bone. In the lower jaw, swelling generally takes place in the vestibule of the mouth along the buccal alveolar plate, but it may occur along the lingual alveolar wall in the case of lower molars because of the position of the roots in their alveoli.

In addition to the localized symptoms of an acute alveolar abscess, a general systemic reaction of greater or lesser severity may occur. The patient may appear pale, irritable, and weakened from pain and loss of sleep, as well as from absorption of septic products. Patients with mild cases may have only a slight rise in temperature (99 to 100° F), whereas in those with severe cases, the temperature may reach several degrees above normal (102 to 103° F). The fever is often preceded or accompanied by chills. Intestinal stasis can occur, manifesting itself orally by a coated tongue and foul breath. The patient may complain of headache and malaise.

Diagnosis. The diagnosis is generally made quickly and accurately from the clinical examination and from the subjective history given by the patient. In the early stages, however, it may be difficult to locate the tooth because of the absence of clinical signs and the presence of diffuse, annoying pain. The tooth is easily located when the infection has progressed to the point of periodontitis and extrusion of the tooth; a radiograph may help one to determine the tooth affected by showing a cavity, a defective restoration, thickened periodontal ligament space, or evidence of breakdown of bone in the region of the root apex (Fig. 5–1). Because the lesion has been present for a short period of time and is confined to medullary bone, a radiograph does not show destruction of alveolar bone. If the acute alveolar abscess is an exacerbation of a long-standing chronic alveolar abscess, an area of periapical rarefaction will be evident on a radiograph. A diagnosis may be confirmed by means of the electric pulp test and by thermal tests. The affected pulp is necrotic and does not respond to electric current or to application of cold. The tooth may be tender to percussion, or the patient may state that it hurts to chew with the tooth, the apical mucosa is tender to palpation, and the tooth may be mobile and extruded.

Differential Diagnosis. Acute alveolar abscess should be differentiated from periodontal abscess and from irreversible pulpitis. A periodontal abscess is an accumulation of pus along the root surface of a tooth that originates from infection in the supporting structures of the tooth. It is associated with a periodontal pocket and is manifested by swelling and mild pain. On pressure, pus may exude near the edematous tissue or through the sulcus. The swelling is usually located opposite the midsection of the root and gingival border, rather than opposite the root apex or beyond it (Fig. 5–2). A periodontal abscess is generally associated with vital rather than with pulpless teeth, in con-

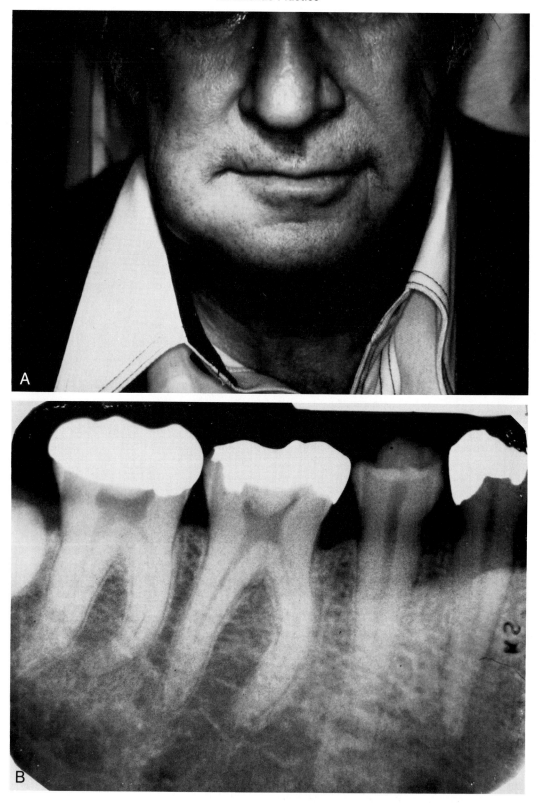

Fig. 5–1. Acute alveolar abscess of the mandibular right first premolar. *A,* The swelling extended around the border of the mandible and into the submandibular region. *B,* The radiograph shows a restoration in the mandibular right first premolar that, during preparation of the cavity, may have exposed the pulp. A diffuse rarefaction is also visible in the periradicular area of the mandibular right first premolar.

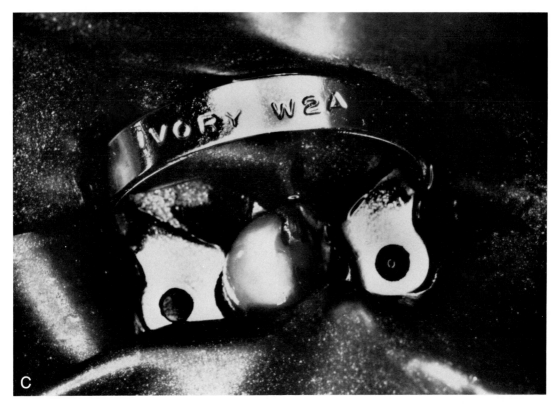

Fig. 5–1 (Continued).   *C,* Drainage was established through the root canal. (Courtesy of D.R. Anthony, Corpus Christi, Texas.)

trast to an acute alveolar abscess, in which the pulp is dead. Tests for pulp vitality are useful in establishing a correct diagnosis.

Bacteriology. In an abscess, the concentration of microorganisms is unusually large. Streptococci and staphylococci are generally recovered, but if the purulent material is collected as it drains out of the root canal, it may be sterile because it will consist chiefly of dead leukocytes and dead bacteria. An analysis of 100 consecutive cases of acute alveolar abscess failed to show a relationship between any specific type of organism and the abscess.[13] Sundqvist, in his study using anaerobic methods of cultivation, isolated Bacteroides melaninogenicus from mixed flora in every case of flare-up when a periapical area of rarefaction was present.[37] One hundred and eight varieties of microorganisms were isolated from 76 intact teeth, all of which had an acute alveolar abscess. Of the total number, 32% of these microorganisms were anaerobes in mixed culture.[24]

Histopathology. The marked infiltration of polymorphonuclear leukocytes and the rapid accumulation of inflammatory exudate in response to an active infection distend the periodontal ligament and thereby elongate the tooth. If the process continues, the periodontal fibers will separate, and the tooth will become mobile. Although some mononuclear cells may be found, the chief inflammatory cells are polymorphonuclear leukocytes. As the bony tissue in the region of the root apex is resorbed, and as more and more of the polymorphonuclear leukocytes die in their battle with the microorganisms, pus is formed. Microscopically, one sees an empty space or spaces, where suppuration has occurred, surrounded by polymorphonuclear and some mononuclear cells. The root canal itself may appear to be devoid of tissue, and instead, clumps of microorganisms and debris may be observed (Fig. 5–3).

Treatment. Treatment consists of establishing drainage and controlling the systemic reaction (see Fig. 5–1). When symptoms have subsided, the tooth should be treated endodontically by conservative means. During the first visit, if the tooth has been left open for drainage, one must perform careful and thorough debridement by instrumentation and irrigation before medicating and sealing the root canal. Once the root canal is sealed,

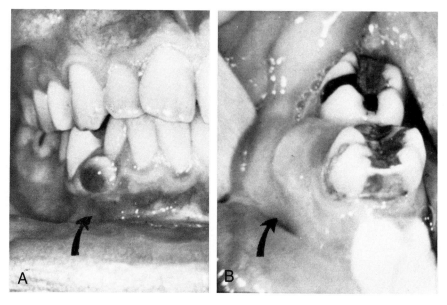

Fig. 5–2. *A*, Periodontal abscess between the right cuspid and the first premolar. *B*, Periodontal abscess of the lower right molar that might be mistaken for an acute alveolar abscess because of the severe swelling extending down to the mucobuccal fold.

endodontic treatment is completed as described in Chapters 11 and 14. Additional information on emergency cases can be found in Chapter 2.

Prognosis. The prognosis for the tooth is generally favorable, depending on the degree of local involvement and the amount of tissue destruction. Although the symptoms of an acute alveolar abscess may be severe, pain and swelling generally subside if adequate drainage is established. In most cases, the tooth can be saved by endodontic treatment, and the severity of the symptoms need not bear any relation to the ease or difficulty of treatment. When purulent material has been discharged through the gingival sulcus and the periodontium has been extensively destroyed, the prognosis is guarded. In selected cases, combined periodontal and endodontal treatment will restore the tooth to functional health.

Acute Apical Periodontitis

Definition. Acute apical periodontitis is a painful inflammation of the periodontium as a result of trauma, irritation, or infection

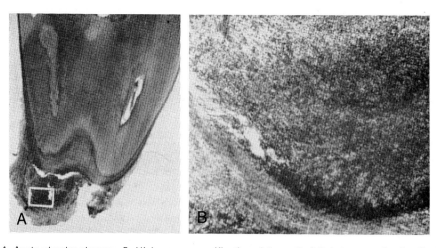

Fig. 5–3. *A*, Acute alveolar abscess. *B*, High-power magnification of the wall of the abscess, showing the inner margin of that wall on the lower left and the large aggregation of neutrophils above it. (Courtesy of the Department of Histopathology, School of Dental Medicine, University of Pennsylvania, Philadelphia.)

through the root canal, regardless of whether the pulp is vital or nonvital.

Cause. Acute apical periodontitis may occur in a vital tooth that has experienced occlusal trauma caused by abnormal occlusal contacts, by a recently inserted restoration extending beyond the occlusal plane, by wedging of a foreign object between the teeth such as a toothpick, food, or a sliver of rubber dam left by a dentist, or by a blow to the teeth.

Acute apical periodontitis may also be associated with the nonvital tooth. It may be caused by the sequelae of pulpal diseases, that is, the diffusion of bacteria and noxious products from an inflamed or necrotic pulp, or its cause may be iatrogenic, such as root canal instrumentation forcing bacteria or debris inadvertently through the apical foramen, forcing of irritating medicaments such as camphorated monochlorophenol or formocresol through the apical foramen, extension of obturating material through the apical foramen to impinge on periapical tissue, perforation of the root, or overinstrumentation during cleaning and shaping of root canals.

Symptoms. The symptoms of acute apical periodontitis are pain and tenderness of the tooth. The tooth may be slightly sore, sometimes only when it is percussed in a certain direction, or the soreness may be severe. The tooth may be extruded, making closure painful.

Diagnosis. The diagnosis is frequently made from a known history of a tooth under treatment. The symptoms are either the result of irritation originating from endodontic treatment, caused by overinstrumentation, medicinal irritants, or overfilling, in which case the tooth is pulpless, or the result of noxious stimuli irritating the periodontal ligament, in which case the pulp is vital. The tooth is tender to percussion or slight pressure, whereas the mucosa overlying the root apex may or may not be tender to palpation. Radiographic examination may show a thickened periodontal ligament or a small area of rarefaction if a pulpless tooth is involved, and it may show normal periradicular structures if a vital pulp is present in the tooth (Fig. 5–4).

Differential Diagnosis. A differential diagnosis should be made between acute apical periodontitis and acute alveolar abscess. At times, the difference is only one of degree because acute alveolar abscess represents a further stage in development, with breakdown of periapical tissue, rather than merely an inflammatory reaction of the periodontal ligament. The patient's history, symptoms, and clinical test results help one to differentiate these diseases.

Bacteriology. The pulp and periapical tissues may be sterile, if periodontitis is due to a blow, to occlusal trauma, or to chemical or mechanical irritation during endodontic treatment. Bacteria or toxic bacterial products present in the root canal may either be forced through or grow beyond the apical foramen and may irritate the apical periodontal tissues.

Histopathology. An inflammatory reaction occurs in the apical periodontal ligament. The blood vessels are dilated, polymorphonuclear leukocytes are present, and an accumulation of serous exudate distends the periodontal ligament and extrudes the tooth slightly. If the irritation is severe and continued, osteoclasts may become active and may break down the periapical bone; the next developmental stage, namely, acute alveolar abscess, may follow.

Treatment. Treatment of acute apical periodontitis consists of determining the cause and relieving the symptoms. It is particularly important to determine whether apical periodontitis is associated with a vital or a pulpless tooth. When the acute phase has subsided, the tooth is treated by conservative means.

Prognosis. The prognosis for the tooth is generally favorable. The occurrence of symptoms of acute apical periodontitis during endodontic treatment in no way affects the ultimate outcome of treatment.

Acute Exacerbation of a Chronic Lesion

Synonyms. Phoenix abscess.

Definition. This condition is an acute inflammatory reaction superimposed on an existing chronic lesion, such as a cyst or granuloma.

Cause. The periradicular area may react to noxious stimuli from a diseased pulp with chronic periradicular disease. While chronic periradicular diseases, such as granulomas and cysts, are in a state of equilibrium, these apical reactions can be completely asymptomatic. At times, because of an influx of necrotic products from a diseased pulp, or because of bacteria and their toxins, these apparently dormant lesions may react and may cause an acute inflammatory response. Lowering of the body's defenses in the presence of bacteria and the bacteria released

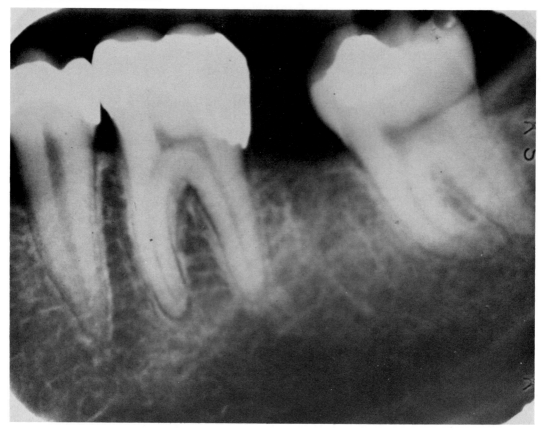

Fig. 5—4. Acute apical periodontitis of the mandibular first molar. Note the enlargement of the periodontal space on the mesial root.

from the root canal or the mechanical irritation during root canal instrumentation may also trigger an acute inflammatory response.

Symptoms. At the onset, the tooth may be tender to the touch. As inflammation progresses, the tooth may be elevated in its socket and may become sensitive. The mucosa over the radicular area may be sensitive to palpation and may appear red and swollen.

Diagnosis. The exacerbation of a chronic lesion is most commonly associated with the initiation of root canal therapy in a completely asymptomatic tooth. In such a tooth, radiographs show well-defined periradicular lesions. The patient may have a history of a traumatic accident that turned the tooth dark after a period of time or of postoperative pain in a tooth that had subsided until the present episode of pain. Lack of response to vitality tests points to a diagnosis of necrotic pulp, although, on rare occasions, a tooth may respond to the electric pulp test because of

fluid in the root canal; or in a multirooted tooth.

Differential Diagnosis. An acute exacerbation of a chronic lesion causes symptoms similar to those of an acute alveolar abscess. Because the treatment of both lesions is the same, no differential diagnosis is needed. This tooth can be distinguished from a tooth with painful pulpitis by testing for pulp vitality. A tooth with acute irreversible pulpitis responds to an electric pulp test and the application of cold, whereas a tooth with a flare-up of a chronic periradicular disease tests nonvital by such methods.

Bacteriology. An abscess usually forms as a result of microbial infection, although some abscesses, called "sterile abscesses," form in the absence of bacteria. The periradicular lesions are usually devoid of bacteria, except for transient bacteria.

Histopathology. In the granuloma or cyst and the adjacent periradicular tissues are areas of liquefaction necrosis with disintegrating polymorphonuclear neutrophils and cellular debris (pus). These areas are surrounded by infiltration of macrophages and some lymphocytes and plasma cells.

Treatment. The treatment of acute exacerbation of a chronic lesion, which is an emergency, is the same as that of an acute alveolar abscess. See Chapter 2 for more detailed information.

Prognosis. The prognosis for the tooth is good once the symptoms have subsided.

CHRONIC PERIRADICULAR DISEASES WITH AREAS OF RAREFACTION

These diseases are chronic alveolar abscess, granuloma, and radicular cyst.

Chronic Alveolar Abscess

Synonym. Chronic suppurative apical periodontitis.

Definition. A chronic alveolar abscess is a long-standing, low-grade infection of the periradicular alveolar bone. The source of the infection is in the root canal.

Cause. Chronic alveolar abscess is a natural sequela of death of the pulp with extension of the infective process periapically, or it may result from a pre-existing acute abscess.

Symptoms. A tooth with a chronic alveolar abscess is generally asymptomatic; at times, such an abscess is detected only during routine radiographic examination or because of the presence of a sinus tract (Fig. 5–5). The sinus tract usually prevents exacerbation or swelling by providing continual drainage of the periradicular lesion. A radiograph taken after the insertion of a gutta-percha cone into the sinus tract often shows the involved tooth by tracing the sinus tract to its origin (Fig. 5–5). At times, the sinus tract is several teeth removed from the cause. When an open cavity is present in the tooth, drainage may occur by way of the root canal. When no sinus tract is present, the cellular debris and bacteria are phagocytized by macrophages, and the fluids are absorbed through blood and lymph channels.

Diagnosis. A chronic abscess may be painless or only mildly painful. At times, the first sign of osseous breakdown is radiographic evidence seen during routine examination or discoloration of the crown of the tooth. The radiograph often shows a diffuse area of bone rarefaction, but the radiographic appearance of the lesion is nondiagnostic. The periodontal ligament is thickened. The rarefied area may be so diffuse as to fade indistinctly into normal bone (Fig. 5–5). When asked, the patient may remember a sudden, sharp pain that subsided and has not recurred, or he may relate a history of traumatic injury. Clinical examination may show a cavity, a composite, acrylic, or metallic restoration, or a gold or jacket crown under which the pulp may have died without causing symptoms. In other cases, the patient may complain of slight pain and awareness of the tooth, particularly during mastication. The tooth does not react to the electric pulp test or to thermal tests.

Differential Diagnosis. Clinically, it is practically impossible to establish an accurate diagnosis among the periradicular diseases with radiographs alone. Historically, the presence of a diffuse area indicated an abscess, a circumscribed area indicated a granuloma, and a sclerotic bony outline was a sign of a cyst; however, all attempts to correlate the radiographic appearance of an area with its histopathologic features failed.[10,29,39] As a result, a proper and accurate diagnosis can be made only when a tissue specimen has been examined microscopically (Fig. 5–6).

A chronic abscess should also be differentiated from periapical osteofibrosis, also known as cementoma or ossifying fibroma, which is associated with a vital tooth and requires no endodontic treatment.

Bacteriology. The microorganisms most commonly recovered from a pulpless tooth with a chronic abscess are alpha-hemolytic streptococci of low virulence. When special culture media are used, however, obligate anaerobes are generally found. Obligate anaerobic organisms were isolated from 18 of 19 intact teeth only when an area of periapical pathosis was present radiographically.[37] Most of these teeth contained more than 1 strain, and some had as many as 8 strains of obligate anaerobes.

Histopathology. As the infective process extends to the periapical tissues or as toxic products diffuse through the apical foramen, some of the periodontal fibers at the root apex are detached or lost, followed by destruction of the apical periodontal ligament. The apical cementum may also become affected. Lymphocytes and plasma cells are generally found toward the periphery of the abscessed area, with variable numbers of polymorphonuclear leukocytes at the center. Mononuclear cells may also be present. Fibroblasts may start to form a capsule at the periphery.

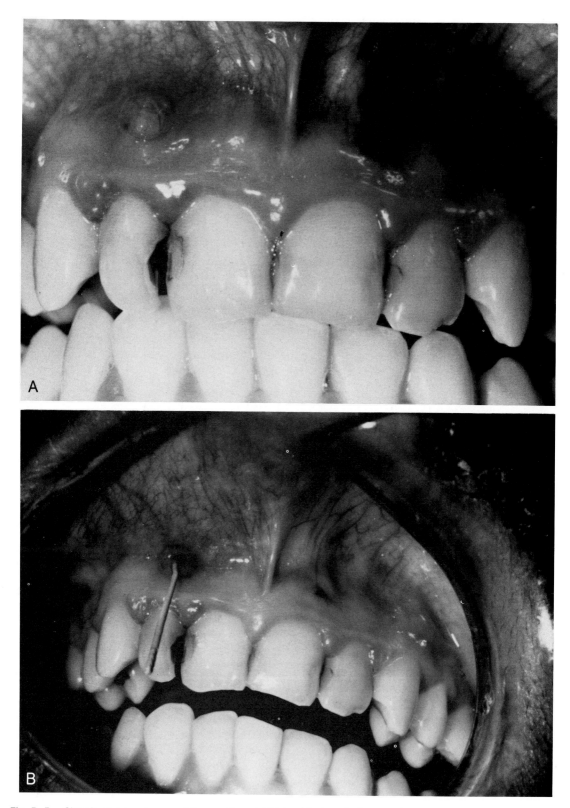

Fig. 5–5. Chronic alveolar abscess of the maxillary right lateral incisor. *A,* An extensive carious lesion is present in the mesial surface of the tooth, with an epulis in the mucosa that indicates the presence of a sinus tract. *B,* A gutta-percha cone was threaded through the stoma (foramen) of the epulis to trace the origin of the sinus tract.

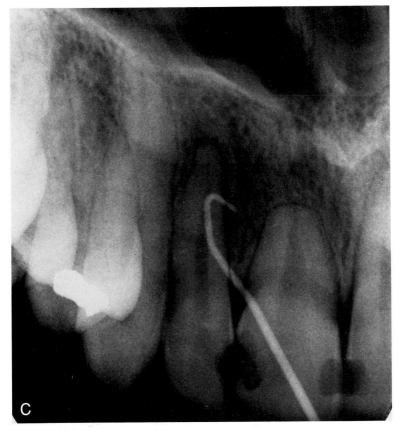

Fig. 5–5 (Continued).   *C,* Radiographic location of the origin of the sinus tract, a rarefied area of bone mesiolaterally to the root.

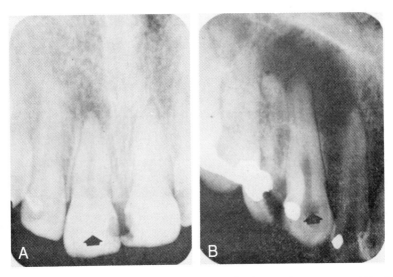

Fig. 5–6.   *A,* Chronic alveolar abscess of an upper incisor. *B,* Chronic abscess of an upper cuspid tooth. Note the diffuse area of rarefaction in the incisor and the formation of a more circumscribed area in the cuspid. The diagnosis in both cases was confirmed by biopsy.

The root canal itself may appear to be empty, or cellular debris may be present (Fig. 5–7). Bacteria were found infrequently on microscopic examination of 230 periapical tissue specimens removed during root resection.[7]

The suppurative material from the interior of the abscess is discharged on the mucosa or gingiva. The drainage may or may not be continuous. When the drainage is intermittent, the discharge is preceded by swelling of the area due to closure of the sinus opening. When pressure from the contained pus is sufficient to rupture the thin wall of soft tissue, the suppurative material is discharged into the mouth through a small opening or stoma (foramen) (see Fig. 5–5). The opening may heal and may close again, only to be reopened when pressure from the contained pus overcomes the resistance of the undermined layer of soft tissue. This small elevation of the mucosa is often referred to as a "gumboil" by the layman and is frequently observed in conjunction with infection of the deciduous and permanent teeth. Although the sinus opening is usually opposite the root apex on the labial or buccal mucosa, it may be far removed from the affected tooth.

A sinus tract may develop on the surface of the face in a patient with a chronic alveolar abscess, particularly in a young person.

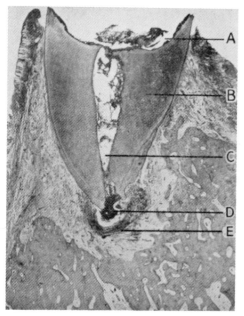

Fig. 5–7. Chronic alveolar abscess. A, Detritus; B, dentin; C, suppurative matter in the root canal; D, abscess; E, wall of the abscess. (Courtesy of the Department of Histopathology, School of Dental Medicine, University of Pennsylvania, Philadelphia.)

When a sinus tract associated with lower anterior teeth opens into the face, it generally opens near the symphysis of the jaw, whereas a sinus tract associated with posterior teeth, chiefly the first molar, generally opens along the inferior border of the mandible in the region of the affected tooth (Fig. 5–8). In rare cases, the purulent material encounters least resistance along the root and passes by way of a sinus tract into the gingival sulcus, where it exits creating the impression of a pocket of periodontal origin.

A misconception exists that the sinus tract is lined with epithelium. Such tracts are generally lined with granulation tissue. In addition to granulation tissue, acute and chronic inflammatory cells may be seen. This cellular makeup accounts for the complete disappearance of the sinus tract often observed within a few days of thorough cleansing and medicating of the root canal. Grossman has observed histologically the tissue adjacent to the tract, as well as the sinus tract itself, in a number of cases; no evidence of an epithelial lining of the tract was seen. The several tracts examined did show evidence of erosion, acute and chronic cellular infiltration, and granulation tissue. On the other hand, in a study of 13 experimentally induced sinus tracts in monkeys, 6 tracts were partially lined and 4 tracts were completely lined with epithelium.[41] Another study, in human patients, found 1 of 10 sinus tracts lined with epithelium.[16] The sinus tract ultimately heals by granulation following the elimination of the infection in the root canal. It was once thought that a sinus tract required special treatment. If a sinus tract is present, it will close up and disappear without any special treatment as soon as the root canal has been cleaned and shaped and an antiseptic has been sealed in to reduce the bacterial flora. In rare cases when a sinus tract does not heal while the tooth is under endodontic treatment, the tract should be curetted with a small spoon excavator.

Treatment. Treatment consists of elimination of infection in the root canal. Once this end is accomplished and the root canal is filled, repair of the periradicular tissues generally takes place. When the area of rarefaction is small, treatment is similar to that of a tooth with a necrotic pulp. Actually, a chronic abscess may be seen as a periapical extension of infection from a necrotic pulp. The difference is one of degree only.

Prognosis. The prognosis for the tooth

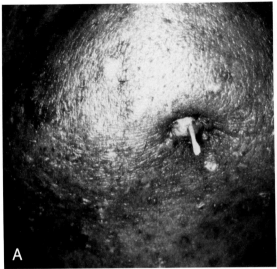

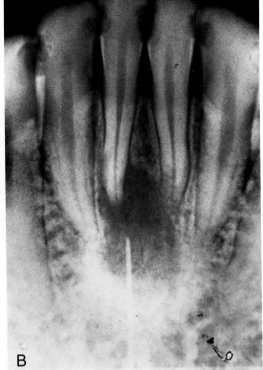

Fig. 5–8. *A,* Sinus tract opening on the chin of a patient from a chronic alveolar abscess of the mandibular right central incisor. *B,* Radiographic view of the sinus tract, as traced by a gutta-percha point.

depends on proper cleaning, shaping, and obturating of the root canals. In addition, other factors, such as the periodontal status, restorative needs, and functional potential, help to determine the prognosis.

Granuloma

Definition. A dental granuloma is a growth of granulomatous tissue continuous with the periodontal ligament resulting from death of the pulp and the diffusion of bacteria and bacterial toxins from the root canal into the surrounding periradicular tissues through the apical and lateral foramina. A dental granuloma is misnamed because its tissue is principally chronic inflammatory in composition, and it is not a tumor. In compliance with common usage, the term "granuloma" is used here. A granuloma contains "granulomatous" tissue, that is, granulation tissue and chronic inflammatory cells infiltrating its fibrous connective tissue stroma. For this reason, the term "granulomatous," rather than granulation, tissue is used in referring to a granuloma.

A granuloma may be seen as a chronic, low-grade defensive reaction of the alveolar bone to irritation from the root canal. A condition for the development of a granuloma is continued mild irritation. Like a chronic abscess, a granuloma is a further sequela of infection from a necrotic pulp. The granulomatous tissue may vary in diameter from a fraction of a millimeter to a centimeter or even larger. It consists of an outer, fibrous capsule, which is continuous with the periodontal ligament, and an inner or central portion made up of looser connective tissue and blood vessels and characterized by the presence of lymphocytes, plasma cells, and mononuclear and polymorphonuclear leukocytes in varying numbers.[23] Mast cells have been demonstrated in granulomas. Lying within the periodontal ligament near the cemental border may be clusters of epithelial cells called cell rests of Malassez. They are derived from Hertwig's sheath and represent the remains of the enamel organ.

Cause. The cause of the development of a granuloma is death of the pulp, followed by a mild infection or irritation of the periapical tissue that stimulates a productive cellular reaction. A granuloma develops only some time after the pulp has died. In some cases, a granuloma is preceded by a chronic alveolar abscess. Experimental evidence has shown that a granuloma is a cell-mediated response to pulpal bacterial products.[35]

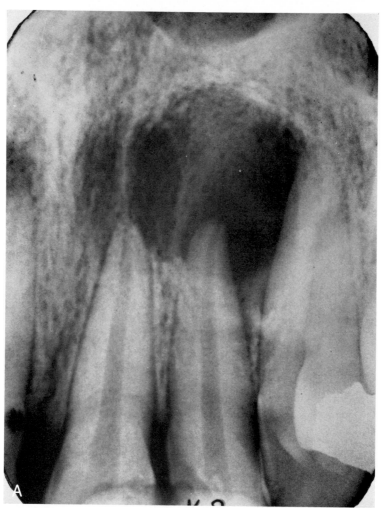

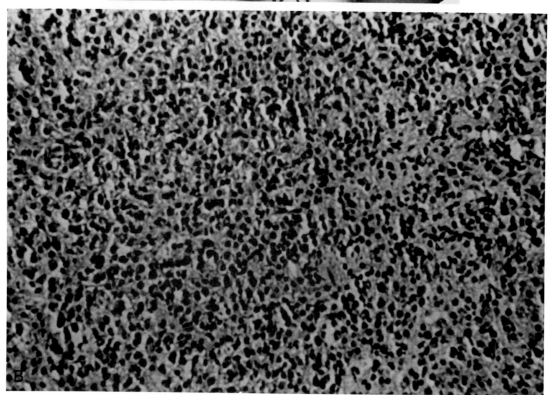

Fig. 5–9.

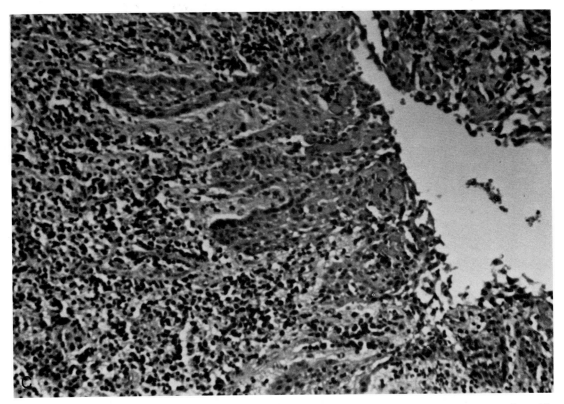

Fig. 5—9. *A,* Lobulated area of radiolucency on periradicular areas of the central and lateral left maxillary incisors. The radiolucent area in the central incisor is a granuloma, and that in the lateral incisor is a cyst. The diagnosis was confirmed by biopsy. Note the similarity in size and density of both radiolucent borders. *B,* Histopathologic section of a granuloma from the radiolucent area of the left central maxillary incisor, showing an area of chronic inflammatory infiltrate. *C,* Section of the epithelial-lined cystic wall from the lesion of the left lateral maxillary incisor. (Courtesy of G.M. McWalter, San Antonio, Texas.)

Symptoms. A granuloma may not produce any subjective reaction, except in rare cases when it breaks down and undergoes suppuration. Usually, a granuloma is asymptomatic.

Diagnosis. The presence of a granuloma, which is symptomless, is generally discovered by routine radiographic examination. The area of rarefaction is well defined, with lack of continuity of the lamina dura. An exact diagnosis can be made only by microscopic examination, however. The involved tooth is generally not tender to percussion, and it is not loose. The mucosa over the root apex may or may not be tender to palpation. A sinus tract may be present. The tooth does not respond to thermal or electric pulp tests. The patient may give a history of pulpalgia that subsided.

Differential Diagnosis. A granuloma cannot be differentiated from other periradicular diseases unless the tissue is examined microscopically (Fig. 5—9). Fortunately, the peri-

radicular diseases are all treated alike, usually endodontically, and do not have to be differentiated, only recognized. Thus, a necrotic pulp and a periapical area of rarefaction on a radiograph are usually sufficient evidence of the presence of periradicular disease. The granuloma must be differentiated from the osteolytic stage of periapical osteofibrosis, the so-called "cementoma," in which the tooth is vital (Fig. 5—10).

Bacteriology. The periapical tissue is sterile in most cases, even though microorganisms may be present in the root canal. Bacteriologic examination of the periradicular tissues has shown that bacteria, although found in the apical area of the root canal, are seldom present in the periradicular area.[7,14,21]

Histopathology. Granulomatous tissue replaces the alveolar bone and periodontal ligament. It consists of a rich vascular network, fibroblasts derived from the periodontal ligament, and a moderate infiltration of

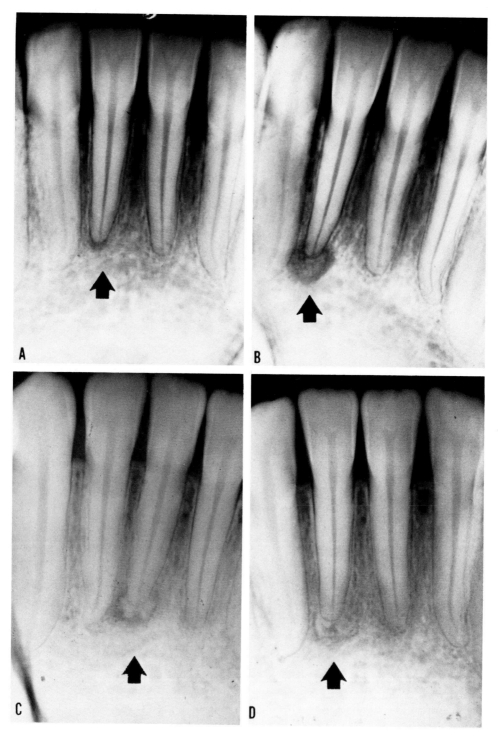

Fig. 5–10. Periapical osteofibrosis (cementoma) observed in a single patient over a 22-year period. *A,* Radiograph taken on presentation of the patient for endodontic treatment. All test results were within the normal range. The early fibrous or osteolytic stage of cementoma resembles inflammatory lesions. *B,* Radiograph taken 5 years later. In this intermediate stage of cementoma, note the mixed radiopaque and radiolucent lesion. *C,* Radiograph taken 12 years later. In this mature stage of cementoma, note the radiopaque lesion with the radiolucent halo separating it from alveolar bone. *D,* Radiograph taken 22 years later. The lesion is almost indistinct.

lymphocytes and plasma cells. Macrophages and foreign-body giant cells may also be present. As the inflammatory reaction continues, because of irritation from bacteria or their products, the exudate accumulates at the expense of the surrounding alveolar bone. This process is followed by clearing of the dead osseous tissue by macrophages or foreign-body giant cells while, at the periphery, fibroblasts actively build a fibrous wall. The outer surface of this wall of granulation tissue is continuous with the periodontal ligament. Some granulomas may have foam cells, macrophages containing lipid material, and cholesterol. The alveolar bone at the periphery of the granuloma may show resorption, and osteoclasts may be present. Young granulomas have greater cellular activity and are less dense than older granulomas, which contain more fibrous tissue and become solid. The incidence of epithelium derived from cell rests of Malassez is high in granulomas.[26,42] The root surface may show external root resorption due to cementoclastic activity or hypercementosis due to cementoblast activity[4,31] (Figs. 5–9 and 5–11).

Treatment. Root canal therapy may suffice for the treatment of a granuloma. Removal of the cause of inflammation is usually followed by resorption of the granulomatous tissue and repair with trabeculated bone.

Prognosis. The prognosis for long-term retention of the tooth is excellent.

Radicular Cyst

Definition. A cyst is a closed cavity or sac internally lined with epithelium, the center of which is filled with fluid or semisolid material (Fig. 5–12). Cysts of the jaws are divided into odontogenic, nonodontogenic, and nonepithelial. Odontogenic cysts arise from odontogenic epithelium and are classified as follicular, arising from the enamel organ or follicle, and radicular, arising from the cell rests of Malassez. Nonodontogenic cysts are classified as either fissural, arising from epithelial remnants entrapped in the fusion of the facial processes, or nasopalatine, arising from the remnants of nasopalatine duct. Pseudocysts or nonepithelial cysts are bony cavities that are not lined with epithelium and, therefore, are not truly cysts. They are divided into traumatic cysts, idiopathic bone cavities, and aneurysmal bone cysts. The reader is referred to textbooks of oral pathology for more detailed discussion.

A radicular or alveolar cyst is a slowly

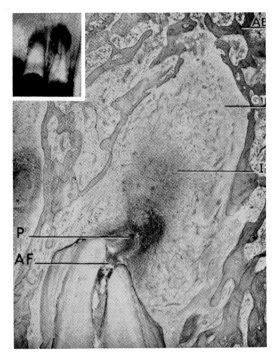

Fig. 5–11. Mesiodistal section through the apex of an upper first bicuspid with granuloma. Inset, radiograph of the specimen. Large areas of bone destruction are apparent around the root ends of both upper bicuspids. AF, Apical foramen; P, tissue breakdown and pus formation at the foramen; I, dense cellular infiltration next to the foramen; GT, granulomatous tissue; AB, alveolar bone. (From Kronfeld, R.: Histopathology of the Teeth. Philadelphia, Lea & Febiger, 1939.)

growing epithelial sac at the apex of a tooth that lines a pathologic cavity in the alveolar bone. The lumen of the cyst is filled with a low-concentration of proteinaceous fluid. The incidence of cysts reported by different authors depends on the criteria used for defining a cyst and on whether serial sections are examined. The incidence of cysts is shown in Table 5–2.

About 75% of all cysts occur in the maxilla, and about 25% occur in the mandible.[8] The distribution in the maxilla is as follows: incisors, 62%; cuspids 7%; premolars, 20%; and molars, 11%. In the mandible, the distribution is: incisors, 16%; cuspids, 2%; premolars, 34%; and molars 48%.

Cause. A radicular cyst presupposes physical, chemical, or bacterial injury resulting in death of the pulp, followed by stimulation of the epithelial rests of Malassez, which are normally present in the periodontal ligament.

Symptoms. No symptoms are associated with the development of a cyst, except those

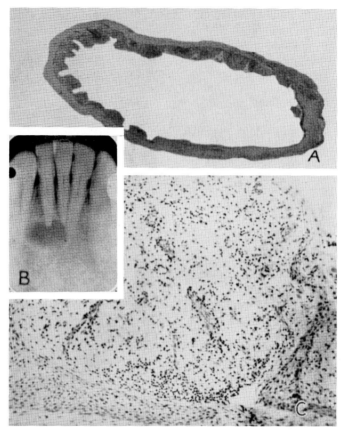

Fig. 5–12. *A,* Cyst wall. The fluid content of the cyst has been lost during preparation of the section, and the epithelial lining has been thrown into folds. The outer, light gray layer is the connective tissue capsule. *B,* Radiograph showing the cyst around the lower incisor. Note the divergence of the roots from the pressure of the cystic fluid. *C,* High-power detail of a section of the cyst lining. (Courtesy of the Department of Histopathology, School of Dental Medicine, University of Pennsylvania, Philadelphia.)

incidental to necrosis of the pulp. A cyst may become large enough, however, to become obvious as a swelling.

The pressure of the cyst may be sufficient to cause movement of the affected teeth, owing to accumulation of cystic fluid (Fig. 5–12). In such cases, the root apices of the involved teeth become spread apart, so the crowns are forced out of alignment. The teeth may also become mobile. If left untreated, a cyst may continue to grow at the expense of the maxilla or the mandible.

Diagnosis. The pulp of a tooth with a radicular cyst does not react to electrical or thermal stimuli, and results of other clinical tests are negative, except the radiograph. The

Table 5–2.   Incidence of Periradicular Cysts and Granulomas

Authors	Cases	Cysts	Granulomas	Other Disorders
Baumann and Rossman[1]	121	32(26%)	89(74%)	—
Bhaskar[6]	2,400*	1,025(42%)*	1,150(48%)*	225(10%)*
Block et al.[7]	230	14(6.1%)	202(93.9%)	—
Grossman and Ether[15]	503	85(17%)	316(63%)	102(20%)
Lalonde and Luebke[18]	800	350(43%)	361(45%)	89(12%)
Patterson et al.[27]	510	70(14%)	420(84%)	10(2%)
Priebe et al.[29]	101	55(54%)	46(46%)	—
Sommer and Kerr[34]	170	11(7%)	143(84%)	16(9%)
Wais[42]	50	13(26%)	32(64%)	5(10%)

*Approximately

patient may report a previous history of pain. Usually, on radiographic examination, one sees loss of continuity of the lamina dura with an area of rarefaction. The radiolucent area is generally round in outline, except where it approximates adjacent teeth, in which case it may be flattened and may have an oval shape. The radiolucent area may be larger than a granuloma and may include more than one tooth (see Figs. 5–9 and 5–12). Neither the size nor the shape of the rarefied area is a definitive indication of a cyst.

Clinical studies, using injection of a contrast medium into the periapical tissue through the root canal to define size and shape radiographically and then removal of the tissue for histologic study, showed no correlation between the shape and size and the histologic findings.[11] Radiographic examination alone is not sufficient for a diagnosis. Other areas of periapical rarefaction that are not the result of pulp death may resemble radicular cysts radiographically. Some of these areas are globulomaxillary cysts, lateral periodontal cysts, incisive canal cysts, aneurysmal bone cysts, traumatic bone cysts, and fibrous dysplasia. By means of a polyacrylamide gel, granulomas may be differentiated from cysts by the intense albumin pattern of cysts, as compared to that of granulomas. In two studies, specimens from the periapical area were aspirated through the root canal and, by a modified Davis technique, were placed in polyacrylamide gel and examined by electrophoresis; this method resulted in the identification of eight out of nine cysts, as confirmed by histologic examination.[25,26] The reliability of this experimental diagnostic method is yet to be confirmed.

Differential Diagnosis. The radiographic picture of a small root cyst cannot be differentiated from that of a granuloma (see Fig. 5–9). Although a positive differentiation between a cyst and granuloma cannot be made from radiographs alone, certain points may suggest the presence of a cyst. A cyst is usually larger than a granuloma and may cause the roots of adjacent teeth to spread apart because of continuous pressure from accumulation of cystic fluid (see Fig. 5–12). One should differentiate a radicular cyst from a normal bone cavity, such as the incisive foramen. A normal cavity appears dissociated from the root apex on radiographs taken at different angles, whereas a cyst remains attached to the root apex regardless

of the angle at which the radiograph is taken. A radicular cyst must also be differentiated from a globulomaxillary cyst, which is a fissural cyst that develops in the upper jaw between the roots of lateral and cuspid teeth. A globulomaxillary cyst is not the result of death of the pulp and may be marsupialized and later enucleated without involving pulp vitality of the adjacent teeth. A radicular cyst should also be differentiated from a traumatic bone cyst, also called a hemorrhagic or extravasation cyst, which is a hollow cavity lined not by epithelium, but by fibrous connective tissue. A method for treatment of a traumatic bone cyst is aspiration of fluid through a small surgical cavity in the bone, enlargement of the opening for irrigation and aspiration until blood fills the wound, and closure of the mucoperiosteum with sutures.[30] Extravasation cysts of the maxilla are rare, and diagnosis can only be made at operation.[28]

Bacteriology. A cyst may or may not be infected. Like a granuloma, a cyst represents a defensive reaction of tissue to a mild irritant. Actinomyces organisms have been isolated from a periapical cyst.[12]

Histopathology. Radicular cysts consist of a cavity lined with stratified squamous epithelium derived from epithelial cell rests of Malassez present in the periodontal ligament (see Figs. 5–9 and 5–12). A theory of cyst formation is that periradicular inflammatory changes cause the epithelium to proliferate. As the epithelium grows into a mass of cells, the center loses the source of nutrition from the peripheral tissues. These changes produce necrosis in the center; a cavity is formed, and a cyst is created. Another theory of cyst formation is that an abscess cavity is formed in the connective tissue and is lined with proliferating epithelial tissue. Evidence supports a theory that the cavity formation and the destruction of the epithelial lining of radicular cysts are mediated by immunologic reactions. Immunologically competent cells are present in the epithelial lining, and immunoglobulins are present in the cyst fluid. The epithelial cell rests of Malassez can become recognized as antigen and may produce an immunologic reaction, which in turn causes lysis of the cystic wall.[40]

Cyst growth can be explained by three possible mechanisms. The first theorizes that the shedding of epithelial cells into the cystic cavity increases the osmotic pressure. This increase produces filtration of edema and tissue fluids into the cystic cavity, with a resulting increase in pressure against the granulomatous tissue and bone. Pressure against the bone produces resorption and cyst growth. In the second theory, granulomatous tissue may proliferate and may exert pressure that results in resorption of bone and growth of the cyst. The third possibility is that the epithelium may invade the connective tissue and may cause the cyst to grow.[4]

Microscopically, because a cyst is derived from a granuloma with strands of epithelium, the lesion is a granuloma with a cavity lined with stratified squamous epithelium. The cyst is surrounded by connective tissue that is infiltrated by lymphocytes, plasma cells, and polymorphonuclear neutrophils (see Figs. 5–9 and 5–12). The cystic cavity contains debris and eosinophilic material. The connective tissue may have cholesterol clefts, macrophages, and giant cells.[4]

Treatment. Surgical enucleation of radicular cysts is not necessary in all cases. Cysts are present in about 42% or less of the areas of rarefaction at the apex of teeth.[6] Resolution of these areas of rarefaction occurs following root canal therapy in 80 to 98% of cases.[17] A percentage of these healed areas may be cysts. The success and failure studies give ample evidence that some radicular cysts heal after endodontic treatment.

The mechanism of resolution is not known. Several hypotheses have been published. The first suggests that the introduction of an endodontic instrument beyond the apex into the cystic area produces an acute inflammatory response that may destroy the epithelial lining of the cyst and may cause resolution.[5] This hypothesis is rejected because healing usually occurs from the periphery to the center of the lesion. The second hypothesis suggests that the introduction of the instrument into the cyst punctures the wall of the cyst and drains it. Drainage reduces the pressure of the cyst on the walls of the osseous cavity and stimulates fibroplasia and repair from the periphery of the lesion.[3] The first two hypotheses may explain the healing of "bay" cysts, lesions in which the cyst lumen communicates with the apical foramen.[33] They do not explain the resolution of cysts that do not connect with the apical foramen, however. The following hypotheses may explain the resolution of pathologic areas not connected with the apical foramen. When the inflammatory process has subsided, drainage is established and fibroplasia starts, producing collagen. The pressure of the proliferating collagen reduces the blood supply to the epithelium by compressing the vascular network of the granulomatous tissue. The collagen entraps the epithelial lining and causes it to degenerate. Macrophages remove the degenerating epithelial tissue.[3] The most modern hypothesis and most feasible is that: "if periapical lesions are inflammatory responses to the antigen content of the root canal system, and the epithelial proliferation is a response to these irritating materials, then when the source of irritation is removed, the immune system gradually destroys and removes the proliferating epithelial cells."[40]

The treatment of choice is root canal therapy alone, followed by periodic observation. Surgical treatment is indicated if a lesion fails to resolve or if symptoms develop.

When a cyst is large, removal by curettage may endanger the vitality of an adjacent tooth or teeth because of interruption of the blood supply during curettage. Root canal treatment of the affected tooth, together with surgical exteriorization to collapse the cyst, may be attempted. This surgical procedure involves evacuation of the cyst contents by inserting a rubber dam or gauze drain over a period of several weeks and changing it weekly. When the cyst is reduced in size, curettage is done in the usual manner without endangering the adjacent teeth. This procedure is sometimes referred to as marsupialization of the lesion.

Prognosis. The prognosis depends on the particular tooth, the extent of bone destroyed, and the accessibility for treatment.

CHRONIC PERIRADICULAR DISEASE WITH AREA OF CONDENSATION

The only disorder in this category is condensing osteitis.

Condensing Osteitis

Definition. Condensing osteitis is the response to a low-grade, chronic inflammation of the periradicular area as a result of a mild irritation through the root canal.

Cause. Condensing osteitis is a mild irritation from pulpal disease that stimulates osteoblastic activity in the alveolar bone.

Symptoms. This disorder is usually asymptomatic. It is discovered during routine radiographic examination.

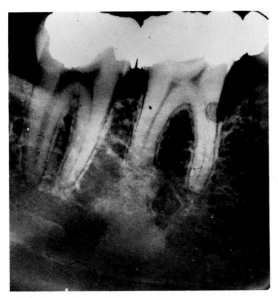

Fig. 5–13. Area of condensing osteitis surrounding the distal root of a mandibular molar. The radiopaque area has a reduced trabecular pattern.

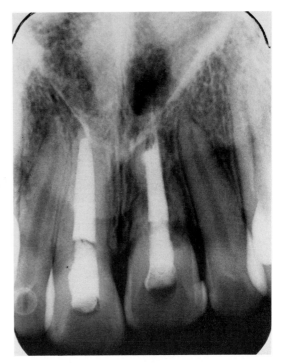

Fig. 5–15. External root resorption of the type called replacement resorption or ankylosis. The tooth had been replanted 6 years previously. As seen in the radiograph, the tooth is in infraocclusion, the root is being resorbed by alveolar bone, and the lamina dura is absent from the areas of root resorption. (Courtesy of Dr. M.L. Canales, San Antonio, Texas.)

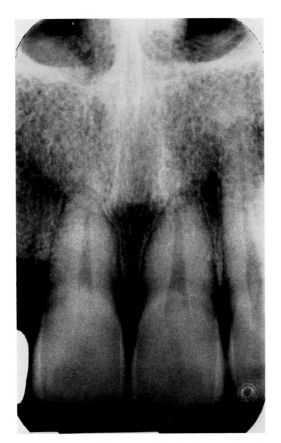

Fig. 5–14. External root resorption due to excessive orthodontic forces. Note the blunting of the roots.

Diagnosis. The diagnosis is made from radiographs. Condensing osteitis appears in radiographs as a localized area of radiopacity surrounding the affected root. It is an area of dense bone with reduced trabecular pattern (Fig. 5–13). The mandibular posterior teeth are most frequently affected. Results of vitality tests may be in the "normal" range.

Histopathology. Microscopically, condensing osteitis appears as an area of dense bone with trabecular borders lined with osteoblasts. Chronic inflammatory cells, plasma cells, and lymphocytes are seen in the scant bone marrow.

Treatment. Endodontic treatment is indicated.

Prognosis. The prognosis for long-term retention of the tooth is excellent if root canal therapy is performed and if the tooth is restored satisfactorily. Lesions of condensing osteitis may persist after endodontic treatment.

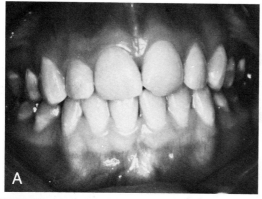

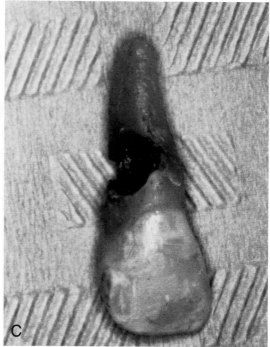

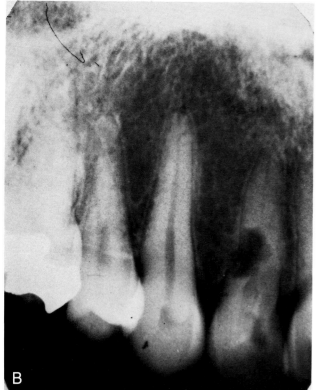

Fig. 5–16. Idiopathic root resorption discovered during routine radiographic examination. *A,* Clinically, no evidence of a resorptive process was present. The radiograph *(B)* and the extracted tooth *(C)* show an area of concave resorption. This resorptive process is called inflammatory resorption, owing to the presence of granulomatous tissue in the defect.

OTHER PERIRADICULAR LESIONS

These disorders include external root resorption and nonendodontic periradicular diseases.

External Root Resorption

Definition. External resorption is a lytic process occurring in the cementum or cementum and dentin of the roots of teeth.

Cause. Although unknown, the suspected cause of external resorption is periradicular inflammation due to trauma, excessive forces (Fig. 5–14), granuloma, cyst, central jaw tumors, replantation of teeth (Fig. 5–15), bleaching of teeth, impaction of teeth, and systemic diseases. If no cause is evident, the disorder is called idiopathic resorption (Fig. 5–16).

Histopathology. External resorption, regardless of cause, is the result of osteoclastic activity on the root surface of the involved tooth. Microscopically, it varies from small areas of cementum resorption replaced by connective tissue or repaired by new cementum, to large areas of resorption replaced by osseous tissue, to "scooped-out" areas of resorption replaced by inflammatory or neoplastic tissues (Fig. 5–16).

Symptoms. Throughout its development, external root resorption is asymptomatic. When the root is completely resorbed, the tooth may become mobile. If the external root resorption extends into the crown, it will give the appearance of "pink tooth" seen in internal resorption. Root resorption of the type called replacement resorption or ankylosis, in which the root is gradually replaced by bone, renders the tooth immobile, in infraocclusion, and with a high percussion sound (see Fig. 5–15).

Diagnosis. External resorption is usually diagnosed by radiographs. Small areas of surface resorption of cementum that cannot be seen radiographically can only be detected histologically. Radiographically, external resorption appears as concave or ragged areas on the root surface (see Fig. 5–16) or blunting of the apex (see Fig. 5–14). Areas of replacement resorption or ankylosis have a resorbed root with no periodontal ligament space and with bone replacing the defects (see Fig. 5–15). Areas of inflammatory resorption caused by the pressure of a growing granuloma, cyst, or tumor have an area of root resorption adjacent to the area of radiolucency. Cysts, usually because of their slow

growth, exert pressure on the roots of teeth and move the roots instead of causing resorption. On the other hand, neoplastic tumors cause rapid root resorption.

Differential Diagnosis. External resorption needs to be differentiated from internal resorption. In external resorption, the radiograph shows a blunting of the apex, a ragged area, a "scooped-out" area on the side of the root, or, if the area is superimposed on the root canal, the root canal clearly traverses the area of resorption. In internal resorption, one sees a root canal with a well-demarcated, enlarged "ballooning" area of resorption. It is sometimes difficult to determine whether the resorption is internal or external, that is, whether internal resorption has perforated the root surface or external resorption has penetrated the pulpal cavity. Several radiographs taken at different angles may help to resolve the question. When bone adjacent to the area of resorption is involved and the resorbed area is externally concave and when

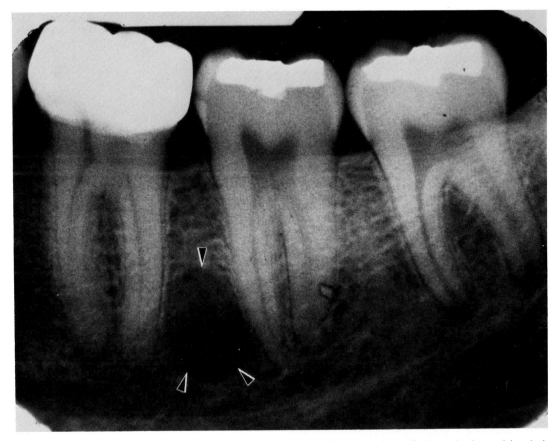

Fig. 5–17. Radiolucent area between the root of the first and that of the second mandibular molar (arrows) is a lesion of systemic origin diagnosed as multiple neurofibromatosis or von Recklinghausen's disease.

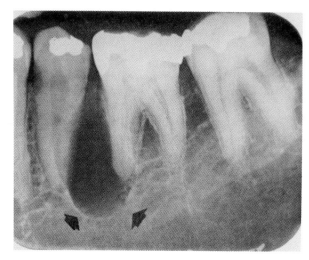

Fig. 5–18. Periodontal cyst. The teeth adjacent to the cyst are vital.

the root canal is intact, as seen in the radiograph, external resorption is present.

Treatment. Internal resorption ceases when the pulp is removed or becomes necrotic. Root canal therapy is the treatment of choice. The treatment of external resorption varies with the etiologic factor. If the external resorption is caused by extension of pulpal disease into the supporting tissues, root canal therapy will usually stop the resorptive process. External resorption produced by excessive forces from orthodontic appliances can be stopped by reducing those forces (see Fig. 5–14). In patients with external resorption

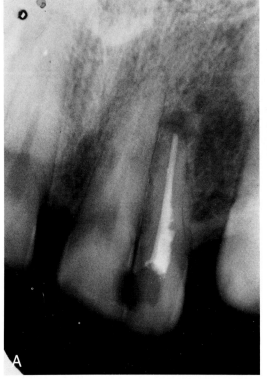

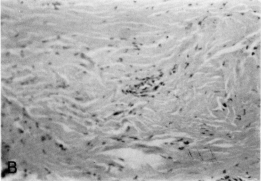

Fig. 5–19. A, Radiograph of an apical scar, showing an area of periapical radiolucency, a blunt apex due to periapical operation, lamina dura present around the apical third of the root, and an obturated root canal. The patient had undergone a surgical procedure in the past, without postoperative symptoms. B, Microscopic examination of the lesion shows dense collagen bundles or healing fibrous tissue.

due to replantation of teeth, preparation of the root canal and obturation with calcium hydroxide paste may stop the resorptive process.

Prognosis. The prognosis of a tooth with external resorption is guarded. If the etiologic factor is known and it is removed, the resorptive process will stop, but it may leave a weak tooth unable to sustain functional forces. In some cases, regardless of treatment, the tooth is lost.

Diseases of the Periradicular Tissues of Nonendodontic Origin

Periradicular lesions not only arise as extensions of pulpal diseases, but they may also originate in the remnants of odontogenic epithelium. Such lesions may be manifestations of systemic diseases, such as multiple neurofibromatosis (Fig. 5–17), or they may have other causes, such as periodontal diseases (Fig. 5–18). Some of these periradicular lesions, radiographically and clinically, resemble the sequelae of pulpal diseases in the periradicular area and should be differentiated from them to avoid errors in treatment. One of the major diagnostic differences is that, in lesions of endodontic origin, the pulp of the tooth is nonvital or is irreversibly diseased, whereas in most lesions of nonendodontic origin, the pulp is vital. Lesions of nonendodontic origin with vital pulps include periapical cemental dysplasia or cementoma, cementoblastoma, odontogenic cysts, fissural cysts, and central giant cell granuloma. Metastatic malignant tumors or ameloblastomas are aggressive lesions that produce excessive bone loss, mobility of teeth, extensive root resorption, and loss of pulp vitality. These lesions can be differentiated from endodontic lesions by their aggressiveness.

Another apical radiolucency may be confused with a lesion of endodontic origin. This lesion, the apical scar, may be differentiated from a lesion of pulpal origin by a thorough history. The tooth, which is completely asymptomatic, has undergone endodontic therapy or periradicular surgical procedures in the past. The radiograph shows a circumscribed radiolucency with an intact lamina dura and a well-obturated root canal. Microscopic examination shows a lesion of dense collagen bundles or healing by fibrous tissue (Fig. 5–19). No therapeutic intervention is necessary.

The reader is advised to consult a textbook on oral pathology for a more complete discussion of the periradicular diseases of nonendodontic origin.

BIBLIOGRAPHY

1. Baumann, E., and Rossman, S.: Oral Surg., 9:1330, 1956.
2. Bence, R., et al.: Oral Surg., 49:82, 1980.
3. Bender, I.B.: Oral Surg., 34:469, 1972.
4. Bhaskar, S.N.: Synopsis of Oral Pathology, 6th Ed. St. Louis, C.V. Mosby, 1981.
5. Bhaskar, S.N.: Oral Surg., 34:458, 1972.
6. Bhaskar, S.N.: Oral Surg., 21:657, 1966.
7. Block, R.M., et al.: Oral Surg., 42:656, 1976.
8. Browne, W.G.: Oral Surg., 14:1103, 1961.
9. Brynolf, I.: Svensk Tandlaek. Tidskr., 63:415, 1970.
10. Brynolf, I.: Odontol. Revy, 18(Suppl. 11):458, 1967.
11. Cunningham, C.J., and Penick, E.C.: Oral Surg., 26:95, 1968.
12. Fergus, H.S., and Savord, E.G.: Oral Surg., 49:390, 1980.
13. Grossman, L.I.: J. Dent. Res., 41:495, 1962.
14. Grossman, L.I.: J. Dent. Res., 38:101, 1959.
15. Grossman, L.I., and Ether, S.S.: Rev. Bras. Odontol., 22:124, 1963.
16. Harrison, J.W., and Larson, W.J.: Oral Surg., 42:511, 1976.
17. Ingle, J.I., and Taintor, J.F.: Endodontics, 3rd Ed. Philadelphia, Lea & Febiger, 1985.
18. Lalonde, E.R., and Luebke, R.G.: Oral Surg., 25:861, 1968.
19. Langeland, K., et al.: J. Endod., 3:8, 1977.
20. McConnell, G.: J. Am. Dent. Assoc., 8:390, 1921.
21. Malooley, J., et al.: Oral Surg., 47:545, 1979.
22. Mata, E., et al.: Oral Surg., 60:201, 1985.
23. Mathiesen, A.: Scand. J. Dent. Res., 81:218, 1973.
24. Matusow, R.J.: Oral Surg., 48:70, 1979.
25. Morse, D., et al.: J. Endod., 1:158, 1975.
26. Morse, D., et al.: Oral Surg., 35:249, 1973.
27. Patterson, S.S., et al.: J. Am. Dent. Assoc., 68:192, 1964.
28. Peters, R.A., and Wussow, G.C.: Oral Surg., 26:742, 1968.
29. Priebe, W.A., et al.: Oral Surg., 7:979, 1954.
30. Sapone, J., and Hansen, L.J.: Oral Surg., 38:127, 1974.
31. Shafer, W.G., Hine, M.K., and Levy, B.M.: A Textbook of Oral Pathology, 4th Ed. Philadelphia, W.B. Saunders, 1983.
32. Shear, M.: Oral Surg., 16:1465, 1963.
33. Simon, J.H.: J. Endod., 6:845, 1980.
34. Sommer, R., and Kerr, D.: Quoted in Clinical Endodontics. Philadelphia, W.B. Saunders, 1961, p. 445.
35. Stern, M.H., et al.: J. Dent. Res., 150:130, 1979.
36. Strindberg, L.Z.: Acta Odontol. Scand., 14:100, 1956.
37. Sundqvist, G.: Bacteriologic studies of necrotic dental pulps. In Umea University Odontological Dissertations. Umea, Sweden, 1976, p. 5.
38. Suzuki, A.: Shikwa Gakuho, 60:37, 1960.
39. Toller, P.: Br. Dent. J., 129:317, 1970.
40. Torabinejed, M.: Int. J. Oral Surg., 12:14, 1983.
41. Valderhaug, J.: Int. J. Oral Surg., 3:7, 1974.
42. Wais, F.T.: Oral Surg., 11:650, 1958.
43. Walton, R.E.: Dent. Clin. North Am., 4:783, 1984.

6 Pulpotomy and Apexification

PULPOTOMY

Pulpotomy is the surgical removal of the coronal pulp.

Objectives

Pulpotomy has as its objective the preservation of vitality of the radicular pulp and the relief of pain in patients with acute pulpalgia.

Rationale

When the coronal pulp is exposed by trauma, operative procedures, or caries, ingress of bacteria produces inflammatory changes in the tissue. Through the surgical excision of the coronal pulp, the infected and inflamed area is removed, leaving vital, uninfected pulpal tissue in the root canal. The remaining pulp may undergo repair while completing apexogenesis, that is, root-end development and calcification. In addition, removal of the inflamed portion of the pulp affords temporary, rapid relief of pulpalgia.

A dressing is placed over the pulp stump to protect it and to promote healing. The two most commonly used dressings contain either calcium hydroxide or formocresol. These dressings are discussed later in the chapter. Under either dressings, an area of necrosis is formed on the surface of the pulp stump (Figs. 6–1 and 6–3).

Under calcium-hydroxide dressings, beyond the layer of induced necrosis, undifferentiated mesenchymal cells in the cell-rich zone proliferate, differentiate into odontoblasts, and move subjacent to the area of necrosis. These newly differentiated odontoblasts form a one-cell layer that produces reparative dentin, to form a "bridge" to cover and protect the pulp[12,48] (Fig. 6–2). Another theory proposes that new odontoblasts develop from fibroblasts rather than from undifferentiated mesenchymal cells.[4,6,48]

The severity of the inflammatory process dictates the quality and quantity of reparative dentin produced in the dentinal bridge. Severe inflammation produces limited reparative dentin devoid of dentinal tubules. Mild inflammation produces reparative dentin with varying numbers of dentinal tubules.[25] Although the term "bridge" implies a solid barrier and a seal between the surface of the new reparative dentin and the pulp, communications exist in the form of openings.[31] Experiments have shown that the formation of reparative dentin bridges is reduced in the presence of an inflammatory process. Therefore, in the presence of severe inflammation of the pulp, pulpotomy procedures to preserve pulp vitality are contraindicated.[35]

In contrast to calcium hydroxide, formocresol does not stimulate the pulp to form a calcific bridge. Formocresol produces an area of necrosis in the pulp adjacent to it. The effect of the fixative diminishes as it progresses apically through the layers of pulp. Usually, the apical third of the pulp is unaffected and retains its vitality for an extended time (Fig. 6–3). Pulpotomy is a safe and useful operation for maintaining the vitality of the radicular pulp. The operation should be limited to teeth with uninfected pulps in children and young adults in whom reparative ability is possible. Cases for pulpotomy should be chosen carefully, to ensure success.

Pulpotomies are classified according to the mode of action of the dressing material used: (1) material that promotes healing of the pulp, that is, calcium hydroxide; and (2) material that sanitizes and fixes pulp tissue, that is, formocresol.

Calcium-Hydroxide Pulpotomy

The materials usually used to promote healing of the pulp are calcium hydroxide and zinc oxide and eugenol. Calcium hydroxide is used because of its predictability in bridge formation and maintenance of vitality of the residual pulp. In contrast, zinc oxide-eugenol cement causes a persistent chronic inflammatory response when applied directly to the pulp, with less likelihood of dentin bridge formation. Calcium hy-

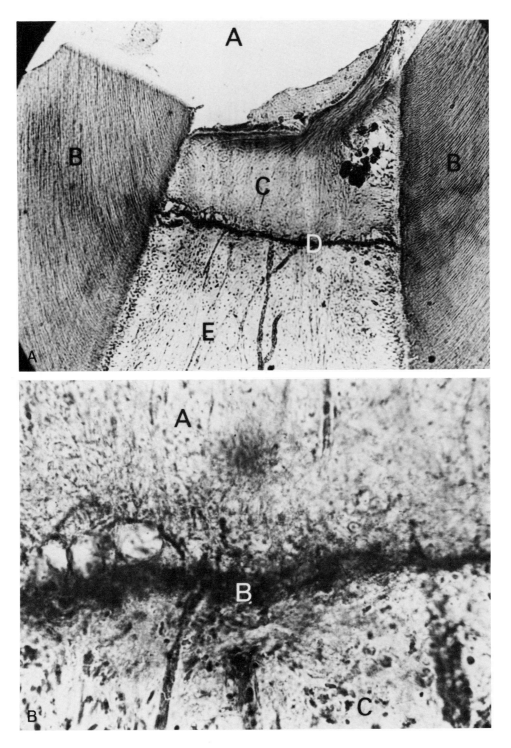

Fig. 6–1. *A,* Twenty-four hours after exposure of the pulp to calcium hydroxide: A, Site of exposure; B, dentin walls; C, necrotic area; D, line of demarcation and calcium proteinate precipitate; E, pulp. *B,* High magnification of the line of demarcation: A, Necrotic area; B, line of demarcation and calcium proteinate precipitate; C, vital pulp tissue. (From Glass, R.L. and Zander, H.A.: J. Dent. Res., *28:*97, 1949.)

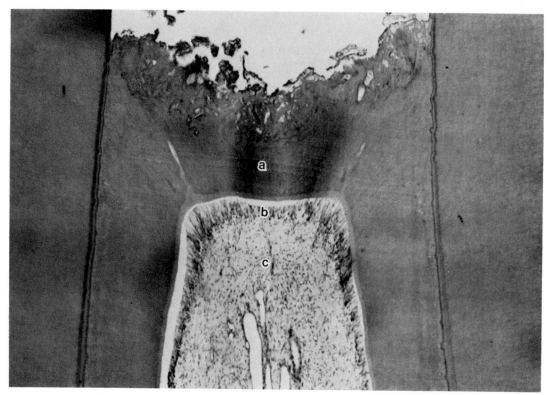

Fig. 6–2. Thirty days after pulpotomy with calcium hydroxide powder in dog's pulp. Note the complete bridge formation (a) covering the pulp stump, new odontoblast formation (b), and vital, uninflamed pulp (c). (From Holland, R., et al.: The healing process of dog's dental pulp after pulpotomy and pulp covering with calcium hydroxide in powder or paste form. Acta Odontol. Pediatr., 2:47, 1981.)

droxide, introduced by Hermann in 1930,[22] is available as a dry powder, a paste mixed with sterile water, or a commercially prepared paste such as Pulpdent, Dycal, or Life. Calcium-hydroxide powder can be used alone or with a radiopaque material, such as barium sulfate, to render the mixture more visible in radiographs.

Of a number of agents studied experimentally by Hunter, calcium hydroxide, magnesium hydroxide, and zinc oxide-eugenol were the only ones that produced dentinal bridging; Hunter conjectured that both calcium and magnesium anions stimulate bridging because of their high pH, and "the cation appears to be unimportant so long as it remains bland."[26]

The histologic reactions to three proprietary preparations intended for pulpotomy, namely, Pulpdent, Dycal, and Hydrex, have been studied.[40] Of these, Hydrex was irritating and caused inflammation and necrosis of the pulp.[24,40,46,47] The undesirable reaction was due to the catalyst.[47] Pulpdent and Dycal were clinically and histologically satisfac-

tory. Regardless of the preparation used, the result will be satisfactory if the teeth to be treated are carefully chosen and if the technique of treatment is aseptically performed.

Indications

Pulpotomy is indicated in pulpally involved children's permanent teeth in which the root apex is not completely formed. In such cases, pulp extirpation and obturation are contraindicated because of the immature root and wide-open foramen, and extraction is not justified because of the effect on the eruption of adjacent teeth and the development of the dental arches. The open foramen contraindicates root canal therapy, which should be postponed until the foramen matures. The pulpotomy procedure permits the completion of apexogenesis, the physiologic maturation of the root. Even if only the apical 3 or 4 mm of the pulp tissue are still vital, the root apex can complete development.

Pulpotomy should be undertaken only in teeth with healthy, hyperemic, or slightly inflamed pulps, such as a child's permanent

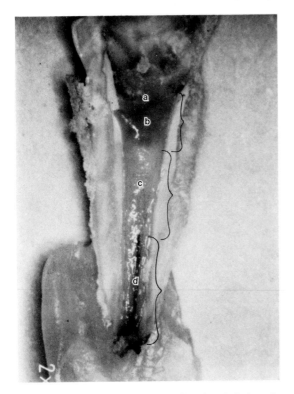

Fig. 6–3. Formocresol pulpotomy in a female baboon by means of a pledget of cotton saturated with formocresol for 5 min against the pulp stump. Macroscopically, after 30 days, one sees evidence of an area of necrosis (a), and area of fixation (b), an area of transition (c), and an area of vital pulp (d). Note the increased vascularity in the area of the vital pulp. (From García-Godoy, F.: J. Pedod., 5:102, 1981.)

anterior tooth with a wide-open apex that is fractured during sports or an automobile accident, or a child's posterior tooth with wide-open apices that has a small, asymptomatic carious exposure. Although pulpotomy may be attempted in selected cases of chronic hyperplastic pulpitis, where only the coronal pulp is involved, in teeth of young, healthy persons, the procedure is still questionable because of the restorability of the tooth. Pulpotomy is contraindicated in patients with irreversible pulpitis. Contraindications to pulp capping and pulpotomy are abnormal sensitivity to heat and cold, chronic pulpalgia, tenderness to percussion or palpation because of pulpal disease, periradicular radiographic changes resulting from extension of pulpal disease into the periapical tissues, and marked constriction of the pulp chamber or root canals (calcification).[2]

Technique

A diagnostic radiograph should be examined to determine the approach to the pulp chamber, to evaluate the shape and size of the root canals, and to ascertain the condition of the periradicular tissues. The tooth should be tested for vitality, and the result should be recorded. The tooth is anesthetized with a local anesthetic, using either infiltration or conduction methods. The rubber dam is applied, and the field of operation is disinfected with a suitable antiseptic. An aseptic technique is used throughout the entire procedure (Figs. 6–4 to 6–6). On removal of carious tooth structure, access is gained to the pulp chamber along a straight line, using the area of exposure as a starting point and removing the roof of the pulp chamber entirely with a sterile bur. Bleeding may be controlled with a moist pledget of sterile cotton. The coronal portion of the pulp is removed with a sharp, sterile, large spoon excavator or periodontal curette. A long-shank spoon excavator is preferable to a bur for removing the soft pulp tissue because it allows more accurate control in severing coronal from radicular pulp tissue. In anterior teeth, however, in which the pulp chamber is small and indistinct from the root canal, it may be necessary to use a bur to remove the coronal portion of the pulp. In posterior teeth, the bulbous portion of the pulp contained in the pulp chamber down to the orifices of the root canals should be removed; in anterior teeth, the bulbous portion up to, but not beyond, the cervical third of the root canal should be removed. As much pulp tissue as possible should be left in the root canal, to allow maturation of the entire root, rather than just of a portion of it. A partially matured root is weak and is susceptible to fracture by occlusal forces. Excavators with extra long shanks are often necessary for reaching into the pulp chambers of molar teeth to scoop out pulp remnants adhering to the pulpal floor. A sharp No. 31L endodontic excavator* is excellent for this purpose (Fig. 6–7).

Twisting of the pulp stump compresses the tissue, with consequent necrosis.[38] The pulp tissue at the entrance to the root canals and that confined within the root canals should not be disturbed.

The pulp chamber is next irrigated thoroughly with sterile water or with anesthetic

---

*Miltex, Lake Success, New York.

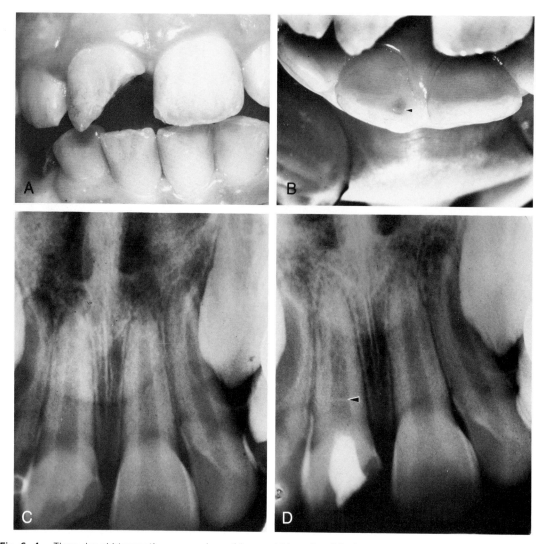

Fig. 6–4. Three-day-old traumatic exposure in an 11-year-old boy. *A* and *B*, Gross appearance. *C*, Radiograph shows an immature apex. Calcium hydroxide pulpotomy was performed to maintain vitality of the radicular pulp and to promote apexogenesis. *D*, Three-month recall radiograph shows the level of the calcific barrier (arrow) and a still-immature apex.

solution. Anesthetic solution is preferred because it is sterile, contains epinephrine, which controls hemorrhage, and is convenient to use. The pulp chamber is dried with sterile cotton and is examined for remnants of pulp tissue. Hemorrhage is controlled with large, moist, sterile cotton pledgets left in contact with the pulp stump for 2 or 3 min.

Calcium hydroxide is then applied to the amputated pulp in the form of a paste made with water or a commercial paste consisting of calcium hydroxide and methyl cellulose (Pulpdent) (Fig. 6–8). A small amount of the paste is deposited from a syringe in contact with the amputated pulp and is tamped against the pulp with a sterile pledget of cotton. Calcium hydroxide may also be applied

in the form of a quick-setting paste (Dycal). Histologic evaluation has found this preparation to be satisfactory.[51] The pulp chamber should be filled to a depth of at least 1 to 2 mm with calcium hydroxide, on which one applies a base of cement, either zinc oxide-eugenol or zinc phosphate. An intermediary is not necessary because the acidity of zinc-phosphate cement is neutralized by the calcium hydroxide. A permanent restoration is placed over the base. The rubber dam is then removed, and the occlusion is checked. A radiograph should then be taken as a record of the operation, for future comparison of apical closure, bridge formation, internal resorption, calcific degeneration, or development of periapical disease.[31,48]

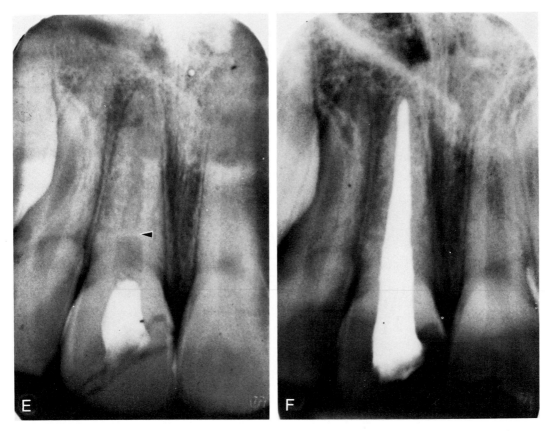

Fig. 6–4 (Continued). *E,* A broader calcific barrier (arrow) is evident, and the apical foramen appears mature in the 10-month recall radiograph. *F,* Root canal therapy was performed after removal of the calcific barrier, and the tooth was restored with a composite material. (Courtesy of Drs. L. Fox and G. Walters, San Antonio, Texas.)

The tooth should be checked with radiographs and vitality tests every 3 months. Slightly more current than normal may be necessary to elicit a response to the electric pulp test. Because teeth with a calcium-hydroxide pulpotomy may develop internal resorption or may undergo complete calcification of the root canal, endodontic therapy should be performed as soon as apexogenesis is complete. The calcific bridge is penetrated, and root canal therapy is started if the apex is mature. In the event of pain or death of the pulp, the root canal contents should be removed as soon as possible, and endodontic therapy should be started if the apex is mature. If the apex is immature, however, apexification therapy should be initiated. Apexification is discussed later in this chapter.

Histopathology

The histopathology of a large series of pulpotomies has been studied.[23] In this study, cases were divided into four groups: (1) those in which building of odontoblast cells on the surface of the wound occurred, protecting the pulp with a dentinal bridge from outside influences (Fig. 6–9); (2) those in which the surface of the pulp was covered with a hard, bony substance, with only partial building of an odontoblast layer; (3) those in which the pulp was protected with an osteoid layer traversed by many canaliculi; and (4) those few cases in which deposition of an osteoid layer on the surface of the pulp was accompanied by small areas of infection; cases in this last group were considered unsuccessful.

Prognosis

Radiographic evidence of the formation of a "bridge" is one criterion for success of a pulpotomy (see Figs. 6–4 and 6–9). Evaluation of the integrity of a bridge is impossible, however, because radiographs are bidimensional images of a tridimensional object. Although many pulps return to normal after a pulpotomy procedure, some are chronically inflamed and may eventually become ne-

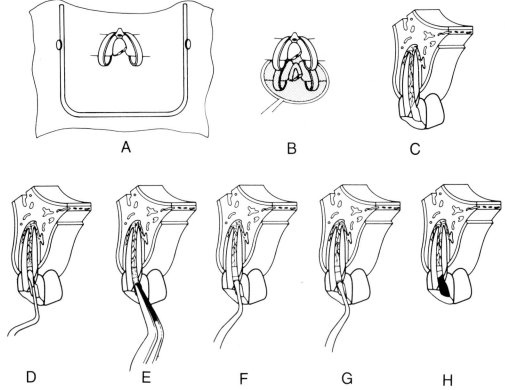

Fig. 6–5. Anterior pulpotomy. *A* and *B*, The rubber dam is applied. *C*, Access is gained into the pulp chamber. *D*, The coronal portion of the pulp is removed with a sharp spoon excavator. *E*, The pulp chamber is irrigated with sterile water and is dried with a sterile cotton pledget. *F*, Calcium hydroxide paste is applied to the pulp stump. *G*, A zinc phosphate cement base is applied. *H*, The tooth is restored by composite restoration.

crotic.[48] Therefore, pulpotomy procedures are temporary therapy, and definitive therapy should be instituted once pulpotomy has served its purpose.

Formocresol Pulpotomy

The effects of formocresol appear to be necrosis and fixation of tissue cells and microorganisms. Coagulation necrosis is produced in the tissues in the immediate vicinity of the application of formocresol, and a less-severe effect is observed in the adjacent tissue. Tissue further removed from the site of application appears vital and is little affected, if at all (see Fig. 6–3).

Indications

Formocresol pulpotomy is indicated for the treatment of pulpally involved primary teeth with clinical manifestation of inflammatory changes confined to the coronal pulp or mechanical exposure during operative procedures. It is contraindicated in a primary tooth that is abnormally sensitive to heat and cold, has chronic pulpalgia, is tender to percussion or palpation because of a pulpal dis-

order, has radiographic changes resulting from extension of pulpal disease, or has constricted pulp chamber or root canals.[2]

Formocresol pulpotomy is also used in permanent posterior teeth for the expedient treatment of pulpalgia. This procedure is used to relieve pain in an emergency. The formocresol "fixes" the contiguous pulp left in the root canal and renders it painless.

Technique

The method for primary teeth consists of removing the coronal pulp down to the root canal orifices, controlling the hemorrhage by pressure, and then applying a pledget of cotton moistened with formocresol for at least 5 min. A thick, creamy mix of zinc oxide and eugenol cement is then applied to the amputated pulp. A quick-setting cement is placed as a base, over which a stainless steel crown or amalgam restoration is made. Variations on this procedure consist of: (1) sealing a cotton pledget moistened with formocresol for 3 to 4 days; (2) using a creamy mix of cement, consisting of equal parts of for-

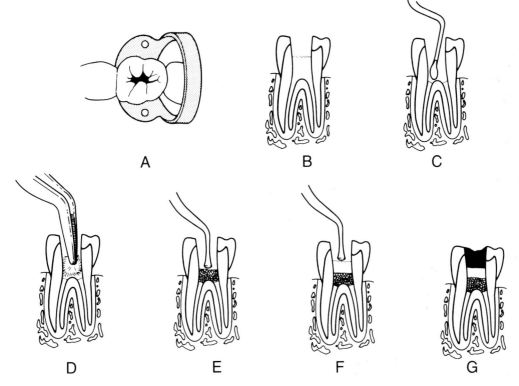

Fig. 6–6. Posterior pulpotomy. *A*, The rubber dam is applied. *B*, Access is gained into the pulp chamber. *C*, The coronal portion of the pulp is removed with a sharp spoon excavator. *D*, The pulp chamber is irrigated with sterile water and is dried with a sterile cotton pledget. *E*, Calcium hydroxide paste is applied to the pulp stump. *F*, A zinc phosphate cement base is applied. *G*, The tooth is restored by amalgam restoration.

mocresol and eugenol mixed with zinc oxide in contact with the pulp tissue; and (3) the use of glutaraldehyde as the medicament of choice in place of formocresol.

The emergency procedure for permanent posterior teeth with pulpalgia is as follows:

1. Anesthetize the tooth.
2. Remove the roof of the pulp chamber.
3. Curette and remove the coronal pulp tissue up to the canal orifices.
4. Irrigate and debride the chamber with local anesthetic solution to promote hemostasis.
5. Place a cotton pledget moistened with formocresol over the pulp stumps, and seal the access cavity with Cavit.
6. Disocclude the tooth if necessary.
7. Prescribe analgesics if needed.
8. Ask the patient to return within the next few days to complete endodontic treatment.

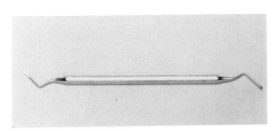

Fig. 6–7. Endodontic excavator No. 31L. Long shanks are useful for reaching into the pulp chamber to remove pulp tissue during pulpotomy.

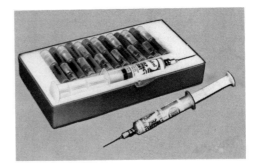

Fig. 6–8. Pulpdent syringe for applying radiopaque calcium hydroxide compound. (Courtesy of the Pulpdent Corporation, Brookline, Massachusetts.)

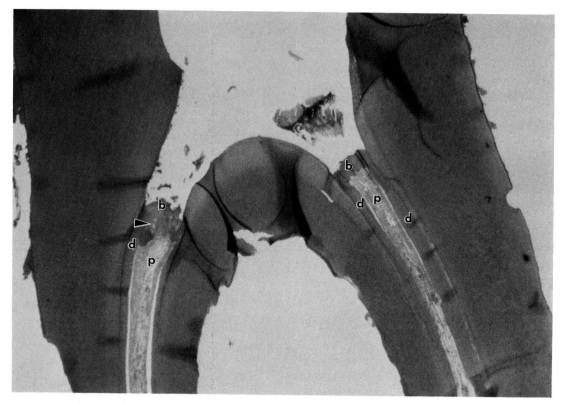

Fig. 6–9. A calcific bridge (b) of reparative dentin covering the pulp stump (p) in a primary tooth after calcium hydroxide pulpotomy. The root canal is lined by reparative dentin (d), which reduces the size of that structure. Note the defect in calcification in the bridge (arrow). (Courtesy of M.C. Russo, Araçatuba, Brazil.)

Histology

Three distinct zones develop in pulp tissue in the area subjacent to formocresol application: (1) a zone of fixation or necrosis; (2) a zone of diminished cellular and fiber definition; and (3) a zone of inflammation contiguous with the vital pulp apically[5] (see Fig. 6–3). Some recent studies have advocated the use of glutaraldehyde, rather than formocresol, as the fixative agent for pulpotomies in primary teeth.[42,43,57] Because of its high degree of cross linkage, glutaraldehyde does not penetrate the periradicular areas, whereas formocresol, which has a high degree of penetrability and the potential to cause antigenic alteration of pulp tissue, increases the probability of a periradicular immunologic reaction.[3,49] Clinical studies have also shown a high success rate for glutaraldehyde pulpotomy procedures.[16,29] Histologically, multilayer zones of pulpal necrosis and fixation are absent in glutaraldehyde pulpotomies. Only a fixed tissue zone is contiguous with the vital radicular pulp tissue. It is likely that glutaraldehyde will replace formocresol as the drug of choice in primary-teeth pulpotomies.

Prognosis

Formocresol pulpotomy in both primary and permanent teeth is a temporary procedure. In primary teeth, it is performed to maintain the integrity of the dental arch until the eruption of the permanent successor. In permanent posterior teeth, it is an emergency procedure to relieve pain until definitive endodontic treatment can be performed.

APEXIFICATION

Apexification is a method to induce development of the root apex of an immature, pulpless tooth by formation of osteocementum or other bone-like tissue. It differs from apexogenesis, the physiologic process of root development.

Objective

The aim of apexification is to induce either closure of the open apical third of the root canal or the formation of an apical "calcific barrier" against which obturation can be achieved.

Rationale

Although apexification had been attempted in the past, the technique was given impetus by the description of 3 cases of apexification by Frank in 1966.[15] This report was followed by a series of experimental procedures by others, to elucidate some factors in apexification. The technique of treatment in the first 3 cases was the usual cleaning and irrigation of the root canal, followed by sealing with a paste composed of camphorated chlorophenol and calcium hydroxide. Radiographic examination was made 3 and 6 months after the procedure, and when evidence of a root apex cap or barrier appeared, the root canals were obturated. Actual root growth does not occur as a result of apexification, but radiographic evidence of a calcified mass at the root apex gives that impression.

In discussing apexification, it has been speculated that "the residual undamaged pulp tissue, if there is any, and the odontoblastic layer associated with the pulp tissue resume their matrix formation and subsequent calcification, guided by the reactivated sheath of Hertwig. The fact that the sheath of Hertwig and the pulp tissue were once damaged may explain why some of the apical formations appear atypical".[62]

From all experimental studies reported, it appears that disinfection of the root canal is indispensable to apical closure. Infection prevents further root-end development.[3,9,11,13,15,20,21,54,56] Normal linear growth of the root does not occur in the absence of a vital pulp.[53] If apexification is successful, a hard substance, in configurations histologically described variously as bone, dentin, osteodentin, or cementum, will develop against which dense obturation of the root canal can be done[10,13,21,62] (Fig. 6–10). Although several materials have been used, such as collagen-calcium phosphate gel or tricalcium phosphate, none are as effective in promoting a calcific barrier as calcium hydroxide.[28,36,37,43]

Technique

In apexification procedures, every effort should be made to preserve any vital apical pulp tissue that will help the closure of the immature apex. The tooth is anesthetized, the rubber dam is applied, access is gained to the pulp chamber and root canal, and irrigation is performed with sterile water or saline solution, to prevent further irritation to the periapical tissues from sodium hypochlorite. The actual length of the tooth is determined by radiograph when a file whose stop is set to a measured length has been inserted to the apparent length of the tooth, as determined from the preoperative radiograph. The measured difference between the file tip and the root tip in the radiograph is used to adjust the apparent length to the actual length.

The working length should be at least 2 mm short of the length of the tooth, to prevent injury to the apical tissues and the thin walls at the apical third of the root (Fig. 6–10). Circumferential enlargement is effected by lateral pressure against the walls with a large file. The instrument should follow the natural shape and contour of the root canal, which is usually not entirely round. In some cases, the walls are thin and fragile so care must be used to prevent a perforation or a fractured wall. The purpose of cleaning and shaping is to remove any necrotic pulpal tissue and to prepare the root canal for a calcium-hydroxide dressing.

After thorough cleaning, shaping, and irrigation with sterile water or saline solution, the root canal is dried with blunt absorbent points; one must take care not to injure the apical tissues. Calcium hydroxide is mixed with sterile water or anesthetic solution to a thick consistency on a sterile glass slab. Because calcium hydroxide has antimicrobial properties, additional antimicrobial agents, especially those that are irritating to the periapical tissues, are unnecessary.[1,59] Barium sulfate can be added to the paste (1 part barium sulfate to 10 parts calcium hydroxide) to increase radiopacity of the mixture. The paste is picked up in an amalgam carrier and is ejected into the pulp chamber. The amalgam carrier should have plastic tips and should be used only for this purpose. By means of a thick, blunt finger plugger, the paste is forced into the root canal. Finally, the tip of the amalgam carrier is pressed into a mound of calcium hydroxide, to pack the powder well into the carrier. The dry pledget of calcium hydroxide is then ejected into the pulp chamber and is forced against the paste ahead of it. The dry paste is forced into the root canal with a blunt finger plugger until the entire root canal is filled with calcium-hydroxide paste. The calcium-hydroxide

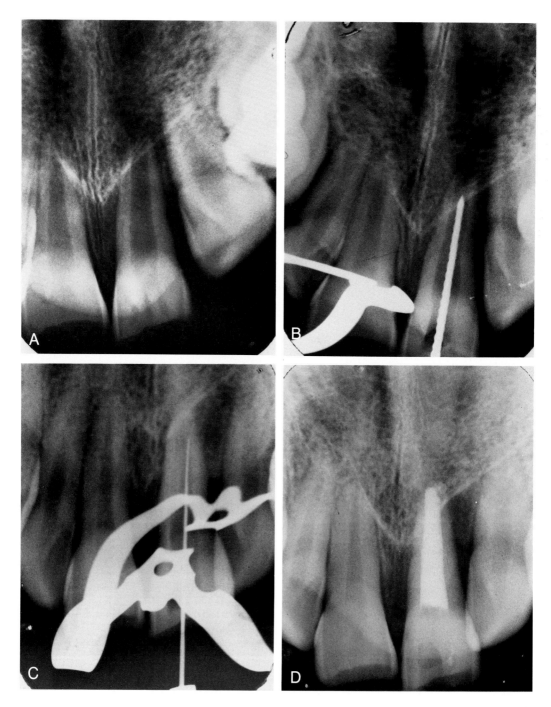

Fig. 6—10. A traumatic accident fractured the incisal ledges of a maxillary central incisor and caused necrosis of the pulp of a maxillary left central incisor in a 9-year-old boy. *A,* Note the diffuse area of rarefaction and the loss of lamina dura in the periapical area, the immature apex, and the cessation of dentinogenesis in the root canal and the pulp chamber denoting pulp necrosis. *B,* The root canal was cleaned and shaped 2 mm short of the apex and was packed with calcium hydroxide. *C,* Apical closure occurred in 6 months, as determined by radiographs and sounding of the calcific barrier with a small file. *D,* The root canal was obturated, the teeth were restored with composite material. Note the calcific barrier and the size of the root canal of the left central incisor, as compared to the normal development of the right central incisor.

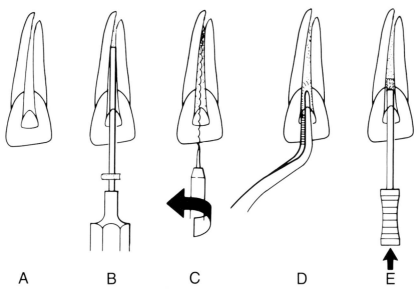

Fig. 6–11. Apexification. *A*, The root canal is cleaned and shaped. *B*, Radiopaque calcium hydroxide paste is delivered into the root canal by means of a syringe. *C*, The paste is gently carried into the periapical area by means of a lentulo spiral. *D*, A cotton pledget is introduced into the root canal. *E*, With the cotton pledget and a blunt-finger plugger, the calcium hydroxide is condensed apically.

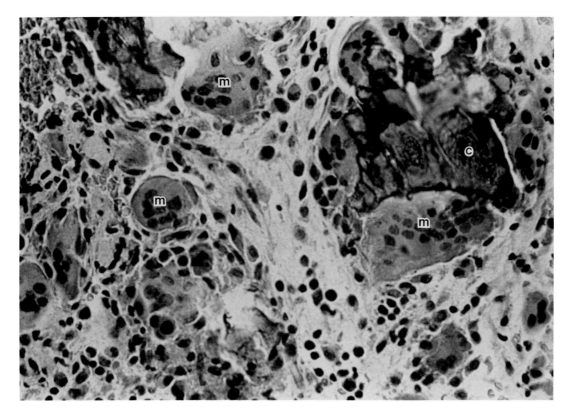

Fig. 6–12. Particle of calcium hydroxide (c) being phagocytized by multinucleated giant cells (m). (Courtesy of E.S. Senia, San Antonio, Texas.)

mixture must be in contact with the periapical tissues to be effective. Excess calcium hydroxide is removed from the pulp chamber and around the cavity margins. Zinc-phosphate cement is condensed into the access cavity, and the access cavity is sealed with composite.

An alternate method is the use of a radiopaque paste of calcium hydroxide in a methyl cellulose base (Pulpdent) available in a syringe (see Fig. 6–8). A rubber stop is placed on the needle to the working length. The needle is introduced, and the calcium-hydroxide paste is delivered into the root canal (Fig. 6–11). With a rotating lentulo spiral, the paste is gently carried to the periapical area. A cotton pledget is introduced with the help of a blunt finger plugger, and the paste is condensed. Excess calcium hydroxide in the periradicular tissues will be removed by multinucleated giant cells (Fig. 6–12). The cotton pledget and the excess calcium hydroxide are removed, and the access cavity is sealed as previously described.

The patient should be recalled for radiography in 3 months, to determine whether a calcific barrier has developed at or near the root apex; such a barrier denotes that apexification has occurred (see Fig. 6–10). If not, a fresh supply of calcium-hydroxide paste is applied to the root canal, and the patient is recalled every 3 months until one sees radiographic evidence of an apical barrier denoting apexification. The old calcium-hydroxide paste is removed with the help of large files and copious irrigation with sterile water. Sterile water is used to prevent irritation to the periapical tissues. One should try not to let the instrument harm the periapical tissues when removing the paste. Although apexification is usually complete in 6 months, or 2 years at most, in one reported case, 4 years of treatment were required for complete apexification.[41] The root canal is obturated after completion of apexification (see Fig. 6–10). Thermoplasticized gutta-percha technique is our method of choice for obturation.

Prognosis

The prognosis for a tooth that has undergone apexification is guarded. The root is underdeveloped, and the tooth is fragile and is subject to fracture from minimal trauma.

BIBLIOGRAPHY

1. Anthony, D.R., et al.: Oral Surg., *54*:560, 1982.
2. Berk, H., and Krakow, A.A.: Oral Surg., *34*:944, 1972.
3. Block, R.M., et al.: Oral Surg., *45*:282, 1978.
4. Brindsen, G.I.: Northwest. Univ. Bull., *56*:4, 1955.
5. Camp, J.H.: *In* Pathways of the Pulp, 3rd Ed. Edited by H. Cohen and R.C. Burns. St. Louis, C.V. Mosby, 1984.
6. Cooke, C., and Rowbotham, C.E.: Br. Dent.J., *100*:174, 1956.
7. Coviello, J., and Brilliant, J.D.: J. Endod., *5*:1, 1979.
8. Cvek, M.: J. Endod.,*4*:232, 1978.
9. Cvek, M.: Odontol. Revy, *23*:27, 1972, and Transactions of the Fifth International Conference on Endodontics. Philadelphia, University of Pennsylvania, p. 30, 1973.
10. Cvek, M., and Sundström, E.: Odontol. Revy, *25*:379, 1974.
11. Das, S.: J. Am. Dent. Assoc., *100*:880, 1980.
12. Diamond, R.D., and Stanley, H.: Personal communication.
13. Dylewski, J.J.: Oral Surg., *32*:82, 1971.
14. Englander, H.R., et al.: J. Dent. Child., *23*:48, 1956.
15. Frank, A.L.: J. Am. Dent. Assoc., *88*:87, 1966.
16. Garcia-Godoy, F.: Acta Odontol. Pediatr., *4*:41, 1983.
17. Goldberg, F., et al.: J. Endod., *10*:318, 1984.
18. Gordon, T., et al.: J. Endod., *11*:156, 1985.
19. Hallett, G.E.M., and Porteus, J.R.: Br. Dent. J., *115*:279, 1963.
20. Ham, J.W., et al.: Oral Surg., *33*:438, 1972.
21. Heithersay, G.S.: Oral Surg., *29*:620, 1970, and J. Br. Endodont. Soc., *8*:74, 1975.
22. Hermann, B.W.: Zahnaerztl. Rdsch., *39*:890, 1930.
23. Hess, W.: Zahnaerztl. Rdsch., *47*:149, 1938.
24. Hirschfeld, Z., et al.: Oral Surg., *34*:364, 1972.
25. Horsted, P., et al.: Oral Surg., *52*:531, 1981.
26. Hunter, H.A.: J. Dent. Res., *34*:697, 1955.
27. Kakehashi, S., et al.: Oral Surg., *20*:340, 1965.
28. Koenigs, F.J., et al.: J. Endod., *1*:263, 1975.
29. Kopel, H.M., et al.: J. Dent. Child., *47*:425, 1980.
30. Krakow, A., et al.: Oral Surg., *43*:735, 1977.
31. Langeland, K., et al.: Oral Surg., *32*:943, 1971.
32. Law, D.B.: J. Dent. Child., *23*:40, 1956.
33. Low, M., and Krasnow, F.: N.Y. State Dent. J., *6*:59, 1950.
34. Mills, J.S.: Austr. Dent. J., *57*:241, 1953.
35. Mjör, IA.: Reaction Patterns in Human Teeth. Boca Raton, FL, CRC Press, 1983.
36. Nevins, A.J., et al.: Oral Surg., *49*:360, 1980.
37. Nevins, A.J., et al.: J. Endod., *2*:159, 1976.
38. Nyborg, H.: Odontol. Revy, *11*:247, 1960.
39. Nyborg, H., and Halling, A.: Odontol. Tidsskr., *71*:277, 1963.
40. Phaneuf, R.A., et al.: J. Dent. Child., *35*:61, 1968.
41. Piekoff, M.D., and Trott, J.R.: J. Endod., *2*:182, 1976.
42. Ranly, D.M.: Pediatr. Dent., *6*:83, 1984.
43. Roberts, S.C., and Brilliant, J.D.: J. Endod., *1*:263, 1975.
44. Sawyer, H.P., and Amaral, W.J.: U.S. Armed Forces Med. J., *5*:155, 1954.
45. Sciaky, I., and Pisanti, S.: J. Dent. Res., *30*:1128, 1960, and *43*:641, 1964.
46. Sekine, N., et al.: Bull. Tokyo Dent. Coll., *12*:149, 1973.
47. Sela, J., et al.: Oral Surg., *35*:118, 1973.
48. Seltzer, S., and Bender, I.B.: The Dental Pulp, 3rd Ed. Philadelphia, J.B. Lippincott, 1984.

49. S'Gravenmade, E.J.: J. Endod., *1*:233, 1975.

50. Shubick, J., et al.: J. Endod., *4*:242, 1978.

51. Stanley, H.R., and Lundy, T.: Oral Surg., *34*:818, 1972.

52. Stark, M.M., et al.: J. Oral Ther. Pharmacol., *1*:290, 1964.

53. Steiner, J.C., and Van Hassel, J.H.: Oral Surg., *31*:409, 1971.

54. Stewart, G.G.: J. Am. Dent. Assoc., *90*:793, 1975.

55. Strange, E.M.: J. Dent. Child., *20*:38, 1953.

56. Torneck, C.D., and Smith, J.: Oral Surg., *30*:258, 1970.

57. Van Velzen, S.K.T.: Ned. Tijdschr. Tand., *82*:23, 1975.

58. Via, W.F.: J. Am. Dent. Assoc., *50*:34, 1955.

59. Weber, R.T.: Dent. Clin. North Am., *28*:669, 1984.

60. Zander, H.A.: J. Dent. Res., *18*:373, 1939.

61. Zander, H.A., and Law, D.B., J. Am. Dent. Assoc., *29*:737, 1942.

62. Zeldow, L.L.: N.Y. State Dent. J., *33*:327, 1967.

7 Rationale of Endodontic Treatment

REACTIONS OF THE PULP AND PERIRADICULAR TISSUES

Injury to the calcified structure of teeth and to the supporting tissues by noxious stimuli may cause changes in the pulp and the periradicular tissues. Noxious stimuli can be physical, chemical, or bacterial and can produce changes in the pulp and periradicular tissues that are either reversible or irreversible, depending on duration, intensity, and pathogenicity of the stimulus and the host's ability to resist the stimulus and to repair tissue damage. Based on these premises, we can generalize that mild-to-moderate noxious stimuli to the pulp may produce sclerosis of the dentinal tubules, formation of reparative dentin, or reversible inflammation. Irreversible inflammatory changes caused by severe injury can lead to necrosis of the pulp and subsequent pathologic changes in the periradicular tissues.

The inflammatory response of the connective tissue of the dental pulp is modified because of its milieu. Because the pulp is encased in hard tissues with limited portals of entry, it is an organ of terminal and limited circulation with no efficient collateral circulation and with limited space to expand during the inflammatory reaction. A clear concept of the fundamentals of inflammation is necessary for the understanding of the diseases of the pulp and their extension to the periradicular tissues.

Inflammation

Inflammation is the local physiologic reaction of the body to noxious stimuli or irritants. Any irritant, whether of traumatic, chemical, or bacterial origin, produces a sequence of basic physiologic and morphologic reactions in vascular, lymphatic, and connective tissues. Host-resistance factors and intensity, duration, and virulence of the irritant modify the ultimate character, extent, and severity of the tissue changes and, to some degree, the clinical manifestations.

The object of inflammation is to remove or to destroy the irritant and to repair damage to the tissue. Inflammation brings to the area phagocytic cells to digest bacteria or cellular debris, antibodies to recognize, attack, and destroy foreign matter, edema or fluid to dilute and neutralize the irritant, and fibrin to limit the spread of inflammation.

Repair of the tissues depends on the severity of injury and host resistance. The injurious agent may cause reversible or irreversible changes to the tissues. Irreversible damage leads to tissue necrosis, whereas reversible damage leads to repair. Repair, or the return of the tissue to normal structure and function, begins as the tissue becomes involved in the inflammatory process. Removal of the irritant, exudate, and cellular debris and return of the vascular bed to normal enhance the reparative process. Fibroblasts from adjacent connective tissue and capillary buds from adjacent blood vessels proliferate in the area. The result is the production of new collagen fibers, matrix, and a rich supply of blood vessels to the area of injury. This reparative tissue, which contains new blood vessels, fibroblasts, collagen fibers, and inflammatory cells, is called granulation tissue. The inflammatory process resolves when repair has been completed.

Symptoms

Inflammation produces the following symptoms: (1) pain, from the action of cytotoxic agents released from humoral, cellular, and microbial elements on the nerve endings; (2) swelling, produced by filtration of macromolecules and fluids into the affected tissues; (3 and 4) redness and heat, produced by vasodilatation of the vessels and the rushing of blood to the affected tissues; and (5) disturbance of function, resulting from changes in the affected tissues. In an inflamed pulp, as in any other inflamed organ of the body, these symptoms also occur, but only pain and disturbance of function are recognized clinically because of the encasement of the pulp by unyielding tissues. In acute inflammation involving the periapical tissues, all symptoms of inflammation may be recognized clinically.

In the dental pulp and periradicular tissues, inflammation may be either acute or chronic. These two stages can be recognized only at the histologic level and depend on the preponderant type of cells in the lesion. The main cell of an acute inflammatory lesion is the polymorphonuclear neutrophil. In chronic inflammation lymphocytes, plasma cells, monocytes, and macrophages are predominant. As a rule, no definite demarcation exists between acute and chronic inflammation. Lesions usually have both types of cells, with either acute or chronic cells predominating.

Polymorphonuclear Neutrophils

The polymorphonuclear neutrophils morphologically consist of a nucleus with three or more connected lobules and cytoplasm containing lysosomal and specific granules. They are present during the acute or early stages of inflammation, and although their main function is to phagocytize bacteria, they may also phagocytize and lyse fibrin and cellular debris. They are attracted to the area of inflammation by chemotactic factors produced by bacteria or by complement, and they are the first cells to migrate from the vessels. Serum factors of complement and immunoglobulins called opsonins bind bacteria to the surfaces of the polymorphonuclear neutrophils. In the binding sites, the bacteria are encapsulated in vacuoles that move into the cytoplasm of the polymorphonuclear neutrophils and come in contact with the lysosomal granules, which degranulate and release lysosomal enzymes inside the vacuoles for lysis of the bacteria. The polymorphonuclear neutrophils have a narrow range of life; they are destroyed in the inflammatory site when the tissue fluids fall to a pH of 6.5. This tissue change is due to the increased production of lactic acid during phagocytosis and the release of this product into the tissues during the death of the polymorphonuclear neutrophils. Destruction of the polymorphonuclear neutrophils also causes the release of the proteolytic enzymes, pepsin and cathepsin, with resulting tissue lysis. Polymorphonuclear neutrophils, with the products of cellular lysis and debris, are the principal constituents of pus.

Macrophages

Macrophages are derived from circulating monocytes. Immature monocytes in extravascular areas, such as areas of inflammation, differentiate into macrophages. Macrophages are phagocytic cells that ingest cellular debris, microorganisms, and particulate matter. The macrophages secrete certain mediators of inflammation, such as lysosomal enzymes, complement proteins, and prostaglandins.

Macrophages enhance the immunologic reaction by ingesting, processing, and degrading antigen before it is presented to the lymphocytes. Their capacity to remove debris from the area facilitates repair. Macrophages are mononucleated cells that, in periods of great activity, may fuse with other macrophages to produce a multinucleated giant cell.

Lymphocytes

The small lymphocytes appear in the chronic stage of the inflammatory reaction. These lymphocytes are intimately related to the immunologic system of the organism. Small lymphocytes have a large, spherical or slightly indented nucleus surrounded by a thin band of cytoplasm containing small granules. Two types of small lymphocytes, B cells and T cells, are known. Both are derived from the pluripotential hemopoietic stem cells. Stem cells are carried by the blood to the thymus, where they become immunologically competent T cells. B cells, in contrast, are believed to become immunocompetent in the bone marrow (Fig. 7–1).

T cells have a long life span and are the most common cell of the lymphocytic series in the blood. They are responsible for cell-mediated immunity and for the immunosurveillance of the human organism. They recirculate through the lymphoid tissues and organs of the body, except the thymus, and are found in the paracortical areas of the lymph nodes. When T cells are stimulated by an antigen, a foreign substance, they develop into sensitized T lymphocytes. These T lymphocytes have various immunologic manifestations, as follows: memory T cells, which speed the immunologic reaction in subsequent encounters with the same antigen; helper or suppressor T cells, which stimulate or suppress the development of effector T or B cells; and effector T cells, which may produce cell-mediated immune reactions, such as delayed hypersensitivity. The sensitized T lymphocytes also release chemical

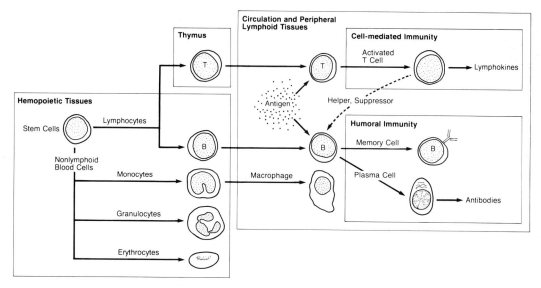

Fig. 7—1. Differentiation of lymphocytes. (Modified from Cooper, M.D., and Lawton, A.R., III: The development of the immune system. *In* Readings from *Scientific American:* Immunology. San Francisco, W.H. Freeman, 1955.)

mediators called lymphokines. Lymphokines may activate macrophages, polymorphonuclear leukocytes, and nonsensitized T cells, or they may produce interferon, which inhibits viral replication as needed by the immune response.

B cells have a shorter life span than T cells. They are found in the blood in lesser numbers than T cells and in the cortical areas of the lymph nodes. When activated by an antigen, B cells become larger cells called plasmablasts, which divide to form plasma cells and memory B cells. The memory B cells speed the immunologic reaction in subsequent encounters with the same antigen. The plasma cells are large, oval or round cells with eccentric nuclei containing chromatin arranged in cartwheel form. The plasma cells produce immunoglobulins. Immunoglobulins are called antibodies when the antigen that triggers its production is known.

The immunoglobulins, of which the five major classes are IgM, IgG, IgA, IgD, and IgE, are involved in different defense reactions. These reactions include the neutralization of bacterial toxins by antitoxins; the coating of bacteria by antibodies, or opsonization, to facilitate phagocytosis; the lysis of bacteria by complement activation; the agglutination of bacteria; and the combining of the antibody with viruses to prevent their entry into the cells. The B cells are responsible for the humoral immunity of the human organism.

Eosinophils, Basophils, and Mast Cells

Other cells found in the pulp and periradicular tissue during the inflammatory response are eosinophilic leukocytes, basophilic leukocytes, and mast cells. The eosinophils are found in allergic and parasitic reactions. During the immune response, they are involved in phagocytosis of the antigen-antibody complexes and in the detoxification of histamine. Basophils and mast cells are considered similar cells; basophils are found in the hemopoietic system, and the mast cells are found in tissue. They both contain granules that, when stimulated by tissue injury or antigen, degranulate and release chemical mediators, such as histamine, a vasodilator, and heparin, an anticoagulant, which can initiate an inflammatory or allergic response.

Vascular Changes

Injury, regardless of the cause or intensity, causes two fundamental vascular changes, vasodilatation and increased capillary permeability, which, in turn, lead to a series of interrelated physiologic and morphologic changes characteristic of the inflammatory response. A brief vasoconstriction is followed by vasodilatation of the arterioles caused by the relaxation of the arteriolar and capillary sphincters. This process is followed by the opening of dormant capillary beds that increases the blood supply to the affected area. Proteolytic enzymes released from injured cells, bacterial toxins, and traumatic mechanical forces are some of the injurious agents that may release histamine from mast cells to start the vasodilatation of the vessels.

This vasodilatation is accompanied by an increased rate of blood flow through the vessels, a reduction in vascular reactivity, and a decrease in flow resistance. These changes increase intravascular pressure, blood flow, and permeability of capillaries. Histamine enhances the permeability reaction by contracting the endothelial cells of the venules and producing intracellular gaps. This process favors the filtration of plasma and macromolecules from the venules. The blood plasma escaping through the vessel walls is usually less viscous and contains less protein than blood plasma remaining in the blood vessels. In inflammation, the blood plasma that leaks into the tissues contains plasma proteins such as albumins, fibrinogen, and immunoglobulins and is called inflammatory exudate. Blood plasma containing macromolecules brings the chemical mediators and cells of inflammation into the inflammatory site to start the inflammatory reaction; this plasma also dilutes bacterial toxins, thereby reducing the potential of tissue damage, and helps to form fibrin to contain the inflammatory reaction.

Hageman factor or factor XII of the blood-clotting system is released into the tissues in the inflammatory exudate. This factor is activated by collagen, by damaged basement membrane of blood vessels, or by an antigen-antibody complex and reacts with prekallikrein of the plasma or tissues to produce kinins. The kinins, such as bradykinin, produce dilatation and permeability of blood vessels. The Hageman factor also activates the fibrinolytic and blood-coagulating systems. Fibrinogen in the inflammatory exudate is acted on by the Hageman factor to produce fibrin, which confines the inflammatory reaction to a limited area. Plasminogen from the plasma found in the inflammatory exudate is activated to plasmin. Plasmin may activate the complement system. Moreover, it digests fibrin and thereby aids in the removal of blood clots or fibrin plugs, or it may activate the kinin system. The inactive serum proteins of complement are also released from the blood in the inflammatory exudate. Immunoglobulins activate the complement cascade and produce anaphylatoxin, which acts on mast cells and causes the release of histamine. Complement activation also results in the release of a chemotactic factor, which aids in leukocytosis and lysis of bacteria.

The fluid leaked from the vessels into the tissues accumulates, producing edema. The subsequent increase in tissue pressure causes the venules to collapse and reduces both the venous drainage from the area and the blood flow. The stasis of blood in the venules due to increased viscosity of blood from loss of fluid and the increased pressure resistance of the venules cause the leukocytes to migrate from the center of the blood vessels to the periphery. This process is called margination of leukocytes. After margination, the leukocytes adhere to the vessel walls. This adherence is termed pavementation of leukocytes. The next step in the inflammatory reaction is the emigration of the leukocytes. The leukocytes are attracted by complement to the site of inflammation and migrate through the vessel walls by ameboid movement. This migration process is called chemotaxis. The polymorphonuclear neutrophils migrate first, followed by the monocytes and lymphocytes. Complement, prostaglandins, kallikrein, and bacterial products all may produce chemotaxis.

The presence of complement, kallikrein, and bacterial products in the inflammatory site has been previously discussed. Prostaglandins, mediators of inflammation, produce vasodilatation, vascular permeability, and pain. They are derived from the cell-membrane phospholipids. Phospholipase, a lysosomal enzyme produced by polymorphonuclear leukocytes, reacts with the cell-membrane phospholipids to produce arachidonic acid, which, in turn, produces prostaglandins, thromboxanes, and leukotrienes. Thromboxanes and leukotrienes are mediators of inflammation about which little is known. The polymorphonuclear neutrophils also produce lysosomal enzymes, which give rise to chemotactic substances that attract more leukocytes to the area of inflammation.

The vascular response continues with the aggregation of red blood cells in the vessels. This aggregation increases the resistance of the blood to flow. This resistance, along with the increase in blood viscosity produced by the loss of plasma, causes metabolic changes, such as a decrease in the oxygen concentration, an increase in carbon dioxide levels, and a lower pH in the inflammatory site. These changes are detrimental to the metabolism of the pulpal tissue, as elsewhere in the body, because they prevent the removal of waste products. The aforementioned changes may spread inflammation to the adjacent tissues; this vicious cycle of inflammation may lead to total necrosis of the pulp (Fig. 7–2). The foregoing discussion of the pathophysiologic features of pulpal disorders is based on Syngcuk Kim's hypothetic model.[24]

The migration of monocytes and lymphocytes renders the inflammatory site capable of an immunologic reaction. As the inflammatory reaction progresses, macrophages necessary to process the antigen, plasma cells derived from B lymphocytes and synthesizers of immunoglobulin, and lymphocyte mediators of the immune response are found in the inflammatory site. Extravascular immunoglobulins found in inflamed pulp tissues, as well as those in plasma cells, are predominantly IgG, although IgA, IgE and IgM containing plasma cells are present. The presence of these immunoglobulins indicates that the pulp possesses the mechanism for immunologic reactions, which in themselves contribute to pulpal and periradicular disorders.

The recovery of the pulp may be explained by some unique vascular responses. Arteriovenous anastomoses and "U-turn" loops open in the pulpal vasculature to reduce the flow to the area of inflammation and thereby decrease the vascular pressure. The increased tissue pressure plays a role in the recovery of the pulp by allowing return of macromolecules and fluids to the venules. These two changes return vascular pressure and tissue pressure to normal and stimulate the repair process.[24]

Periradicular Manifestations

If the inflammatory response overwhelms the pulp, with resulting partial or total necrosis, the root canal will serve as a pathway to the periradicular area for the noxious products of tissue necrosis and antigenic agents. The inflammatory and immunologic responses in the periradicular area occur as in the pulp. On reaching the periradicular area, these noxious products produce bone resorption and granulation tissue in place of

PATHOPHYSIOLOGY OF PULPAL DISORDER

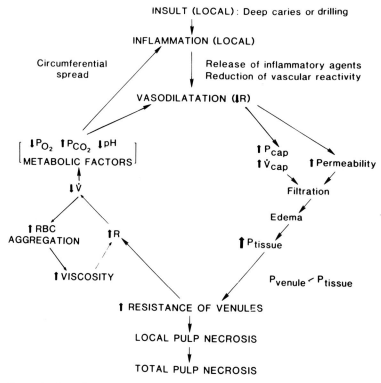

Fig. 7–2. Hypothetic mechanism of the pathophysiology of pulpal disorder. (From Kim, S.: J. Endod., 11:465, 1985.)

normal periradicular tissues. The periradicular pathologic tissues contain polymorphonuclear neutrophils, lymphocytes, plasma cells, macrophages, and mast cells, along with immunoglobulins IgG, IgA, IgM, IgE and complement. In the presence of inflammatory cells, immunoglobulins, and complement in the periradicular tissues, anaphylactic, cytotoxic, antigen-antibody complex, and delayed hypersensitivity reactions may occur. Recent reports indicate that some endodontic flare-ups are mediated by IgE reactions and that bone resorption is mediated by a lymphokine called osteoclastic-activating factor. These findings point to the important role that immunologic reactions play in the physiology and pathology of the periradicular tissues.

Tissue Changes Following Inflammation

Tissue changes following inflammation are either degenerative or proliferative.

Degenerative Changes

Degenerative changes in the pulp may be fibrous, resorptive, or calcific. If the degeneration continues, necrosis will result, especially if thrombosis of the blood vessels occurs, or if leukotoxin is released as a result of damage to the tissue cells. Another form of degeneration is suppuration. When the polymorphonuclear cells are injured, they release proteolytic enzymes, with resulting liquefaction of the dead tissue. This process is suppuration or formation of pus. Three requisites are necessary for suppuration: (1) necrosis of tissue cells; (2) a sufficient number of polymorphonuclear leukocytes; and (3) digestion of the dead material by proteolytic enzymes. If the reaction is not great enough, because the irritant is weak, an exudation consisting chiefly of serum, lymph, and fibrin (serous exudate) will result.

All dead cells, particularly polymorphonuclear cells, liberate proteolytic enzymes. In this way, an abscess is formed because the enzymes digest not only the leukocytes, but also the adjacent dead tissue. Microorganisms are not necessary for development of an abscess. For example, a sterile abscess may result from chemical or physical irritation in the absence of microorganisms.

Proliferative Changes

Proliferative changes are produced by irritants mild enough to act as stimulants. Within the same area, a substance may be both an irritant and a stimulant, such as calcium hydroxide and its effect on adjacent tissue. In the center of the inflammatory area, the irritant may be strong enough to produce degeneration or destruction, whereas at the periphery, the irritant may be mild enough to stimulate proliferation. Generally, if the tissue is in apposition, as in the case of an incision for root resection, fibroblastic repair will take place. When a gap is present between the tissue parts, repair is made with granulation tissue. Granulation tissue is resistant to infection. The principal cells of repair are the fibroblasts, which lay down cellular fibrous tissue. In some cases, collagen fibers may be substituted; dense acellular tissue is then formed. In either case, fibrous repair is the result. Destroyed bone is not always replaced by new bone, but it may be replaced by fibrous tissue. The process of repair is discussed again in Chapter 14 with regard to repair following root canal treatment.

ENDODONTIC IMPLICATIONS

The reaction of the periradicular tissues to noxious products of tissue necrosis, bacterial products, and antigenic agents from the root canal has been described by Fish, who established experimental foci of infection in the jaws of guinea pigs by drilling openings in

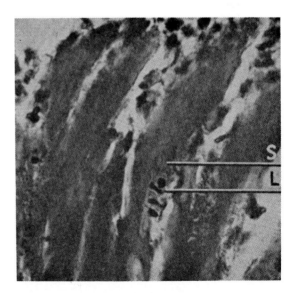

Fig. 7–3. Photomicrograph of zone of infection, showing staphylococci (S) in clefts of bone caused by bur; polymorphonuclear leukocytes (L) seek out the microorganisms. (From E.W. Fish: J. Am. Dent. Assoc.)

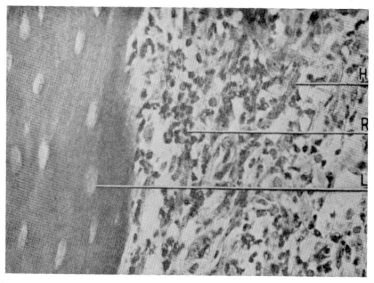

Fig. 7–4. Photomicrograph of zone of contamination. The osteocytes have died in the bone lacunae (L), and none of the normal cells (fibroblasts and osteoblasts) are left in the soft tissues infiltrated by round cells (R) and a few phagocytic macrophages (H). (From E.W. Fish: J. Am. Dent. Assoc.)

the bone and packing in wool fibers saturated with a broth culture of microorganisms.[20] Four well-defined zones of reaction were found: (1) zone of infection; (2) zone of contamination; (3) zone of irritation; and (4) zone of stimulation.

Zone of Infection

This zone is characterized by polymorphonuclear leukocytes. In Fish's study, infection was present in the center of the lesion, and microorganisms were found only in that area. The only microorganisms not disposed of by polymorphonuclear leukocytes were found in haversian canals or in fissures in the bone matrix made by the bur[20] (Fig. 7–3).

Zone of Contamination

This zone is characterized by round cell infiltration. Around the central zone, Fish observed cellular destruction, not from bacteria themselves, but from toxins discharged

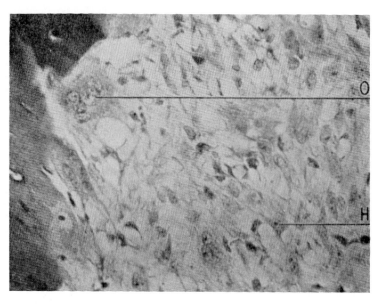

Fig. 7–5. Photomicrograph of zone of irritation, showing osteoclasts (O) digesting matrix, and numerous macrophages (H) digesting intracellular collagen fibers. (From E.W. Fish: J. Am. Dent. Assoc.)

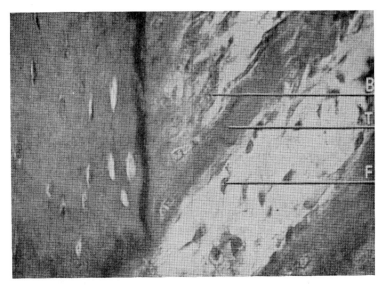

Fig. 7–6. Photomicrograph of zone of stimulation. The bone cells are alive in the lacunae. New bone trabeculae (T) are laid down by young osteoblasts (B), and young fibroblasts (F) are building new collagen fibers. (From E.W. Fish: J. Am. Dent. Assoc.)

from the central zone.[20] Whether the toxins were tissue-breakdown products or exotoxins was not established. In this area, bone cells had died and had undergone autolysis, so the lacunae appeared empty. Lymphocytes were prevalent everywhere (Fig. 7–4).

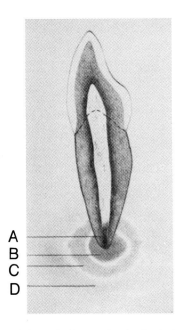

A
B
C
D

Fig. 7–7. Schematic diagram showing bacteria in the root canal and the zones of infection (A), contamination (B), irritation (C), and stimulation (D).

Zone of Irritation

This zone is characterized by macrophages and osteoclasts. Fish found evidence of irritation further from the central lesion as the toxins became more diluted.[20] In this area, also distinguished by small, round cells, normal bone cells and osteoclasts could just about survive. The collagen framework was digested by phagocytic cells, the macrophages, while osteoclasts attacked the bone tissue. "The interesting result of their activity is that they open up a gap in the bone all around the center of the lesion; as trees are felled to isolate a forest fire. The space thus obtained becomes filled with polymorphonuclear leukocytes and, until that has taken place, the danger of widespread necrosis remains."[20] In this area, the histologic picture is one of much activity preparatory to repair (Fig. 7–5).

Zone of Stimulation

This zone is characterized by fibroblasts and osteoblasts. At the periphery, Fish noted that the toxin was mild enough to be a stimulant.[20] In response to this stimulation, collagen fibers were laid down by the fibroblasts, which acted both as a wall of defense around the zone of irritation and as a scaffolding on which the osteoblasts built new bone. This new bone was built in irregular fashion (Fig. 7–6).

By analogy, we can apply the knowledge gained in Fish's experiment to understand

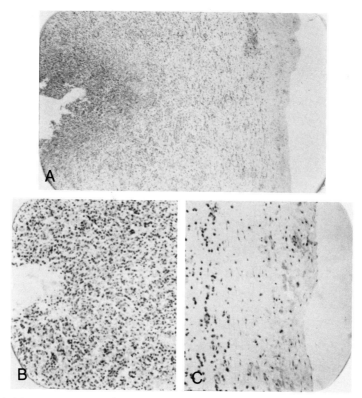

Fig. 7–8. *A,* At the left is a necrotic area surrounded by dense leukocytic infiltrations. As the distance from the necrotic area is increased, the polymorphonuclear cells become decreased in number until at the periphery (the right-hand side of the figure), collagen fibers are being laid down and repair is in evidence. *B* and *C,* Higher magnifications of the left and right areas of *A.* (Courtesy of the Department of Histopathology, School of Dental Medicine, University of Pennsylvania, Philadelphia.)

better the reaction of the periradicular tissues to a pulpless tooth. The root canal is the seat of infection (Fig. 7–7). The microorganisms in the root canal are rarely motile and do not move from the root canal to the periradicular tissues; however, they can multiply sufficiently to grow out of the root canal, or the metabolic products of these microorganisms or the toxic products of tissue necrosis may be diffused to the periradicular tissues. As the microorganisms gain access to the periradicular area, they are destroyed by the polymorphonuclear leukocytes. When the microorganisms are sufficiently virulent, or when enough are present, they overwhelm the defensive mechanism, and a periradicular lesion results. When they are of low virulence and numbers, however, a stalemate occurs. The polymorphonuclear leukocytes destroy the microorganisms as rapidly as they gain access to the periradicular tissues. The result is a chronic abscess. The toxic products of the microorganisms and the necrotic pulp in the root canal are irritating and destructive to the periradicular tissue and,

together with the proteolytic enzymes released by the dead polymorphonuclear leukocytes, help to produce pus.

At the periphery of the destroyed area of osseous tissue, toxic bacterial products may be diluted enough to act as a stimulant. The toxic products from the root canal are diffused from the apical foramen and destroy bone in the immediate vicinity of the root apex; further away, the toxins are so diluted that they act as a stimulant and form a granuloma. Fibroblasts then build fibrous tissue, and osteoblasts delimit the area with a wall of sclerotic bone (Fig. 7–8). If, in addition, the epithelial rests of Malassez are stimulated, a cyst will form.

Microorganisms are usually transients in periradicular tissue, even when an area of rarefaction is present radiographically.[21,25] These transient invaders are destroyed by the polymorphonuclear leukocytes in the manner already described. Although this phenomenon explains the development of radiolucent areas as a result of infection of the pulp, it does not altogether explain the development of such areas following trauma. The pulp may be sterile, but a radiolucent area develops nevertheless because of tissue-breakdown products of the pulp that irritate the periradicular tissues.

When the root canal has been treated, the reservoir of bacteria or noxious products has been eliminated, and the root canal has been thoroughly obturated, the destroyed periapical bone will undergo repair.

BIBLIOGRAPHY

1. Barnes, C.W., and Langeland, K.: J. Dent. Res., 45:1111, 1966.
2. Bergenholtz, G.: J. Endod., 7:100, 1981.
3. Bergenholtz, G., and Lindhe, J.: Scand. J. Dent. Res., 83:153, 1975.
4. Bergenholtz, G., and Warfringe, J.: Scand. J. Dent. Res., 90:354, 1982.
5. Bergenholtz, G., et al.: Scand. J. Dent. Res., 85:396, 1977.
6. Beveridge, E.E., and Brown, A.C.: Oral Surg., 19:655, 1965.
7. Bhaskar, S.N.: Synopsis of Oral Pathology, 6th Ed. St. Louis, C.V. Mosby, 1981.
8. Björlin, G., et al.: Oral Surg., 39:488, 1975.
9. Block, R.M., et al.: Oral Surg., 48:168, 1979.
10. Block, R.M., et al.: Oral Surg., 47:372, 1979.
11. Block, R.M., et al.: J. Endod., 4:178, 1978.
12. Block, R.M., et al.: J. Endod., 4:110, 1978.
13. Block, R.M., et al.: J. Endod., 4:53, 1978.
14. Block, R.M., et al.: J. Endod., 3:424, 1977.
15. Block, R.M., et al.: J. Endod., 3:309, 1977.
16. Burnet, F.M.: Readings from Scientific American: Immunology. San Francisco, W.H. Freeman, 1955.
17. Cymerman, J.J., et al.: J. Endod., 10:9, 1984.
18. Dahlen, G., and Bergenholtz, G.: J. Dent. Res., 59:1033, 1980.
19. Dood, E.E.: Atlas of Histology. New York, McGraw-Hill, 1979.
20. Fish, E.W.: J. Am. Dent. Assoc., 26:691, 1939.
21. Grossman, L.I.: J. Dent. Res., 38:101, 1959.
22. Hood, L.E., et al.: Immunology. Menlo Park, CA, Benjamin/Cummings Publishing, 1984.
23. Houck, J.C.: Ann. N.Y. Acad. Sci.,105:765, 1963.
24. Kim, S.: J. Endod., 11:465, 1985.
25. Korzen, D.H., et al.: Oral Surg., 37:783, 1974.
26. Mathiesen, A.: Scand. J. Dent. Res., 81:218, 1973.
27. Miller, G.S., et al.: Oral Surg., 46:559, 1978.
28. Moist, R.R., and Yanof, H.M.: J. Dent. Res., 44:570, 1965.
29. Morse, D.D.: Oral Surg., 58:327, 1984.
30. Naidorf, I.J.: J. Endod., 3:223, 1977.
31. Naidorf, I.J.: J. Endod., 1:15, 1975.
32. Nilsen, R., et al.: Oral Surg., 58:160, 1984.
33. Okada, H., et al.: Arch. Oral Biol., 12:1017, 1967.
34. Orban, B.: J. Dent. Res., 19:537, 1940.
35. Perrini, N., and Fonzi, L.: J. Endod., 11:197, 1985.
36. Pitts, D.L., et al.: J. Endod., 8:10, 1982.
37. Pulver, N.H., et al.: Arch. Oral Biol., 23:435, 1978.
38. Pulver, N.H., et al.: Arch. Oral Biol., 22:103, 1977.
39. Roitt, I.M., and Lehner, T.: Immunology of Oral Diseases. Oxford, Blackwell Scientific Publications, 1980.
40. Ryan, G.B., and Majno, G.: Inflammation. Kalamazoo, MI, Upjohn, 1977.
41. Schonfeld, S.E., et al.: Oral Surg., 53:82, 1982.
42. Synderman, R., et al.: J. Dent. Res., 50:304, 1971.
43. Stern, M.H.: J. Dent. Res., 61:1408, 1982.
44. Stoughton, R.B.: Arch. Dermatol., 93:601, 1966.
45. Taintor, J.F., et al.: Oral Surg., 51:442, 1981.
46. Tonder, J.: Acta Odontol. Scand., 41:247, 1983.
47. Torabinejad, M.: J. Endod., 6:766, 1980.
48. Torabinejad, M.: J. Endod., 6:733, 1980.
49. Torabinejad, M., and Kettering, J.D.: J. Endod., 11:122, 1985.
50. Torabinejad, M., and Kettering, J.D.: Oral Surg., 48:256, 1979.
51. Torabinejad, M., et al.: J. Endod., 11:479, 1985.
52. Torabinejad, M., et al.: J. Endod., 5:196, 1979.
53. Torneck, C.D.: J. Can. Dent. Assoc., 44:510, 1978.
54. Trowbridge, H., and Daniels, T.: Oral Surg., 43:902, 1977.
55. Trowbridge, H.O., and Emling, R.C.: Inflammation: A Review of the Process, 2nd Ed. Bristol, PA, Comsource/Distribution Systems, 1983.
56. Van Hassel, H.J.: Inflammation. Atlanta, American Association of Endodontists, 1978.
57. Van Hassel, H.J.: Oral Surg., 32:126, 1971.
58. Walton, R.E., and Langeland, K.: J. Endod., 4:167, 1978.
59. Wesselink, P.R., et al.: Oral Surg., 45:789, 1978.
60. Wynn, W., et. al.: J. Dent. Res., 42:1169, 1963.
61. Zachrisson, B.U.: Arch. Oral Biol., 16:555, 1971.
62. Zmener, O.: Oral Surg., 58:330, 1984.

8 Selection of Cases for Treatment

Proper selection of cases avoids pitfalls during endodontic treatment and helps to ensure success. Not every tooth is a suitable candidate for endodontic treatment. Errors in case selection, some of which could have been avoided, constituted 22% of failures reported in a study by Ingle and Beveridge.[13]

In most instances, case selection is dictated by what we see in the radiograph. What cannot be seen on the radiograph is often encountered during operation in the root canal. An examination of the radiograph may disclose the following problems: a large periapical lesion; a supernumerary root or root canal; a dilacerated, bayonet, curved, or other misshapen root apex; a pathologically resorbed root tip; a flaring, everted, wide apical foramen in a young tooth; a partial or completely calcified root canal; an obstruction in a canal; a pulp stone occupying almost the entire pulp chamber and root canal; internal or external resorption; subgingival fracture or fracture of a root; subgingival decay of a crown; dens in dente; or taurodontism.

The selection of cases for endodontic treatment has been discussed by a number of authors, among them Bender,[2] Grossman and associates,[8] Healey,[9] Luebke and associates,[15] Luks,[16] Maurice,[17] Siskin,[21] and Strindberg.[22]

Four factors enter into the decision to do or not to do root canal treatment: (1) accessibility of the apical foramen through the root canal; (2) restorability of the involved tooth; (3) strategic value of the involved tooth; and (4) general resistance of the patient.

Many more root canals are treated today than before because of a greater interest in endodontics by the practitioner not only to save endodontically involved teeth, but also to use them as abutments for bridges or partial dentures. Unfortunately, a general practitioner's best effort may not be good enough because of a mistaken diagnosis, such as when treating a curved canal not capable of being instrumented or filled to the apex, with

a resulting persistence of the area of rarefaction. On the other hand, certain kinds of cases formerly thought to contraindicate endodontic treatment, such as a sinus tract discharging into the gingival sulcus, are treated successfully today because of advances in both endodontal and periodontal therapy. To depend on root canal treatment alone for all endodontic cases is bound to meet with a certain degree of failure, unless such treatment is combined with other endodontic procedures, such as apexification to induce the formation of a calcific barrier in root perforation or periapical curettage to remove chronic inflammatory tissue. On the other hand, resection is not indicated simply because an area of rarefaction is present.

LOCAL CONTRAINDICATIONS

Endodontic treatment may be done when it is not contraindicated by the patient's health, provided the entire extent of the root canal can be instrumented, disinfected, and obturated satisfactorily (Fig. 8–1). It is simpler to enumerate the contraindications to root canal treatment, because they are few in number, than to list the indications for treatment. In the following cases, additional procedures, such as periradicular surgery, should be considered in addition to root canal treatment to enhance the potential for tissue repair.

1. When there is extensive destruction of the periapical tissues involving more than one-third of the length of the root. The statement "more than one-third of the length of the root" is arbitrary, and in some cases, an area of rarefaction of this extent or greater undergoes repair. These cases are exceptional, however, and our observation has been that the greater the amount of bone destroyed, the less will be the likelihood of repair. In a 4-year follow-up study of 529 teeth, Strindberg found that: (1) the rate of success was lower in cases with areas of rar-

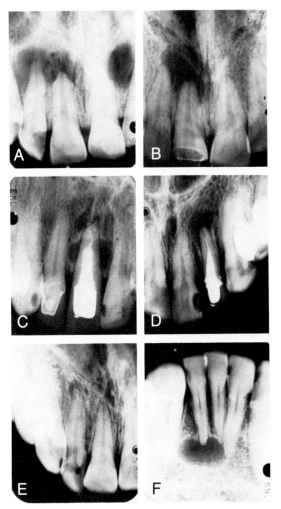

Fig. 8–1. Examples of anterior teeth which are not considered amenable to endodontic treatment alone and which could require root resection/curettage in addition. *A,* Resorption of root and large area of rarefaction. *B,* Large area of rarefaction. *C,* Combined periodontal and endodontal lesion and poorly filled canal. *D,* Poorly filled canal. *E,* Broken instrument and area of rarefaction offering poor prognosis. *F,* Cyst.

efaction than in those of vital pulp extirpation; and (2) the incidence of success decreased with an increase in the size of the area of rarefaction.[22] In an evaluation of 800 endodontally treated teeth, Eggink found that the larger the initial periapical lesion, the less likely were the chances of repair.[3] Such has also been our experience in evaluating 432 cases in which the rate of success was lower when areas of rarefaction were present; some cases had undergone progressive rather than complete repair at the time of the evaluation.[8] Holland and colleagues have cited 17 studies showing that the presence of a

periapical lesion reduces the probability of success following endodontic treatment.[10] Hörting-Hansen's experience has been that periapical lesions less than 10 mm in diameter are more likely to show evidence of repair than those over 10 mm.[11] Kerekes and Tronstad made a 3- to 5-year follow-up study of 501 roots, 50% of which were necrotic or had areas of rarefaction, and found that those with areas of rarefaction were less successful than those without rarefied areas.[14] In a study of 299 root fillings followed from 2 to 30 years, Nelson found that the presence of an area of rarefaction reduced the success rate, and early diagnosis and treatment increased the success rate.[18] Tay and coworkers also found that the larger the size of the periapical rarefaction, the less successful the result.[23]

Frank, however, stated that large lesions heal as readily as small, but no statistical data confirm this finding.[4] In young people, repair of a large area of rarefaction occurs more readily than in older persons. Even when the rate of repair is low, healing is still possible without surgical treatment. The involved tooth, whenever it is practical to do so, should be treated nonsurgically and monitored until repair occurs or surgery becomes necessary

2. When the root canal of a pulpless tooth with a radiolucent area is obstructed by a curved root, a tortuous canal, secondary dentin, a pulp stone that cannot be removed or bypassed, a calcified or partially calcified canal, a malformed tooth, or a broken instrument, for example. In such cases, when it is impossible to instrument the root canal or to fill it apically for at least 3 to 4 mm, the prognosis is poor. Instrumentation, disinfection, and obturation of the coronal and middle thirds of the canal are less important, provided the apical third of the root is properly cleaned, disinfected, and obturated. The best example of this situation is in preparing the canal for the reception of a post-type or dowel crown during which the middle and coronal thirds of the root canal are left open to ingress of saliva for hours, at times, without undesirable effect. The apical third of the root canal is critical and therefore must be disinfected and obturated so microorganisms can no longer reach the periapical tissues and continue their destruction. If this procedure cannot be done because of blockage of the apical portion of the canal, repair of the damaged bone is not likely to occur because microorganisms can still reach the periapical structures through the apical foramen. An example is in teeth with areas of rarefaction in which a reamer or file had been accidentally broken in the root canal. According to an evaluation made by Grossman, repair of periapical bone in such cases occurred in only 47% of teeth, as against 84% in which no area of rarefaction had been present originally.[6] In such cases, complete endodontic treatment of the patent portion of the root canal and surgically place a retrograde apical filling, such as amalgam, to seal the remainder of the untreated, inaccessible root canal.

3. *When there is incomplete development of the root apex with death of the pulp.* In such cases, the root canal is difficult, if not impossible, to fill satisfactorily not only because of divergence of the canal as the apex is approached, but also because of persistent moist seepage. Apexification should be attempted and when an apical stop of hard cementoid tissue has developed, the root canal should be obturated. When apexification has not been successful, however, the root canal must be filled from the apical end after smoothing the root apex. When the walls of the canal are parallel, a rolled gutta-percha cone may be prepared for filling the canal, if seepage can be controlled by suitable irrigation, and the tooth may be kept under observation afterward.

4. *When there is accidental or pathologic perforation of the root surface.* Perforation of the root surface may occur accidentally by misdirection of the bur while attempting to reach the pulp chamber or by a hand-operated or engine-driven reamer or file. Perforation of the root surface may also be the result of internal or external resorption. In cases of resorption, an effort should be made to induce repair by means of calcium hydroxide, or the perforated area must be walled off by amalgam; otherwise, hemorrhage will continue into the root canal, and it will not be possible to disinfect and fill the canal properly. An external surgical approach is necessary to wall off the perforation in some cases.

5. *When there is persistent excessive periapical exudate that cannot be controlled prior to filling the root canal, or when negative cultures cannot be obtained.* Such cases are rare today. If seepage cannot be controlled in severely infected upper anterior teeth of young people by the usual irrigating solutions or by sealing in an iodine solution or calcium hydroxide paste, then periapical surgery is indicated.

6. *In cases of retreatment, when a foreign body, such as a fragment of gutta-percha or of root canal filling material, lies in the periapical tissues of radiolucent teeth.* The presence of a foreign body increases the difficulty of eliminating infection by intracanal treatment alone. Periapical curettage should be done in addition to canal filling, to clear the periapical structures of the foreign body.

7. *When an acute infection in a previously treated and filled pulpless tooth has occurred, treatment or resection is indicated after the acute symptoms are controlled.* In some cases, the administration of an antibiotic controls the acute stage of the infection; in others, incision and drainage are necessary to relieve pain. Retreatment should be considered when the acute symptoms have subsided if the canal filling can be removed. Otherwise, resection with a retrograde amalgam filling should be done, to ensure a proper apical seal.

8. *When the root apex has been fractured and the pulp has died.* Root fracture alone is not a reason for endodontic treatment, and resection is contraindicated if the pulp is vital and the tooth can be stabilized. When the fracture is in the apical third and the pulp has died, endodontic treatment should be carried out. When the apical fragment cannot be lined up with the main canal, complete the endodontic treatment to the fractured segment. The untreated apical root tip and the treated root segment are monitored radiographically. If an area of rarefaction develops, the root fragment should be removed by root resection.

In addition, special consideration should be given to certain cases, such as a combined *periodontal-endodontal lesion* in which an acutely infected pulpless tooth communicates with the gingival sulcus through a sinus tract that cannot be eliminated. Although it is possible to eliminate infection in the root canal in such cases by simultaneous periodontal treatment, and although the gingival sulcus area heals once the endodontic treatment is completed, consideration should be given to the extent of the periodontal lesion prior to endodontic treatment. If destruction of the periodontal attachment is considerable, repair of the periodontal fibers may not occur even after endodontic treatment.

Another special case is when alveolar resorption is extensive, involving at least half the root surface. When the periodontal involvement is severe and the tooth is mobile, or when the crown-root ratio is unfavorable, an effort should be made to improve the periodontal status in conjunction with endodontic therapy. If class III mobility is present, extraction of the tooth will be preferable to root canal treatment because the prognosis from a periodontal standpoint is poor even though the endodontic treatment may be successful. In some cases, however, the tooth may be firm despite radiographic evidence of considerable bone resorption. In such cases, endodontic treatment is not contraindicated.

In another special case, damage to the crown is so extensive that endodontic treatment cannot be carried out under aseptic conditions. In our opinion, if the crown of the tooth can be restored, and if a rubber dam can be applied, routine endodontic treatment may then be done. A stainless steel band will need to be applied in some cases, and in others, a gingivectomy will have to be done. Root canal treatment should not be attempted unless the crown can be restored properly.

In all cases, an effort should be made to determine whether the tooth is strategic. This determination is especially important if the patient is already wearing a partial denture, or if a partial denture is planned for the patient, particularly if an area of rarefaction is present or if the crown is in poor condition. Extraction of the tooth in such cases may make for a better design of denture, may save time, and may not only be more economical, but also more satisfactory in the long run. On the other hand, salvaging a tooth by endodontic treatment may mean the difference between a bridge and a partial or full denture.

When more than one focus of infection are present in the oral cavity, each focus should be considered as an individual unit of the same problem and treated coordinately. Examples are as follows: (1) when two adjacent untreated pulpless teeth are present; (2) when periapical rarefaction and periodontal disease of the same tooth are coexistent; and (3) when periapical rarefaction of the maxillary posterior teeth and sinus involvement are coexistent. Unless coordinate treatment of the foregoing conditions is carried out, the prognosis for endodontic treatment is less favorable.

SYSTEMIC CONDITIONS

At one time, the treatment of pulpless teeth was questioned. Instead, teeth were extracted. This rationale was based on the focal-infection theory, which stated that microorganisms from a localized area of infection, such as an abscess, escape into the blood and lymph channels and establish themselves elsewhere in the body. Ergo, the removal of such chronic foci of infection would be followed by abatement of the disease and its symptoms. After acceptance of the focal-infection theory for more than three decades, even its most ardent advocates began to question its validity, and, in its fourth decade the theory was laid to rest.

In deciding whether to retain or to extract a pulpless tooth, it should be remembered that: (1) pulpless teeth generally are not the cause or contributing cause of systemic disease; (2) in patients with severe systemic disease, such as active diabetes, syphilis, tuberculosis, a severe anemia, infected pulpless teeth with areas of rarefaction may not respond as readily to treatment; repair of periapical tissue may be delayed or may not occur as the potential for repair is reduced; and (3) on the other hand, in certain cases, extraction is contraindicated because of an existing systemic condition of the patient, such as leukemia or radiation necrosis.

A concise medical history, including careful questioning, should be obtained whenever possible. The questions should be designed to throw light on the existence of a suspected systemic disease. Under certain circumstances, the patient's physician should be consulted.

When a patient has a history of rheumatic fever with valvular heart damage, physicians generally prefer that endodontic treatment be done rather than extraction. Cardiovascular-renal diseases, hypertension, and arteriosclerosis are on the increase, and we should premedicate and treat such patients with empathy and care. Special consideration should also be given to those who have had an open heart operation or valve defect replaced by plastic substitutes. In all cases where the patient is at risk, endodontic treatment, especially instrumentation of the root canal, should be done after the administration of antibiotic premedication, as follows: 2 g penicillin V 1 hour before the operation, and 1 g 6 hours after the operation; or 1 g erythromycin 1 hour before the operation and 500 mg 6 hours after the operation, as recommended by the American Heart Association. In addition, Bender and associates have recommended oral rinsing and application of an antiseptic to the gingiva before applying the rubber-dam clamp, to preclude the possibility of a transient bacteremia resulting from injury to the gingiva from the clamp.[1]

It is the consensus among a large number of physicians that pulpless teeth probably play no role in the origin of rheumatoid arthritis, rheumatic fever, peptic ulcer, gall-bladder disease, ulcerative colitis, regional ileitis, and other diseases formerly associated with dental foci of infection.

Bender and colleagues are of the opinion that "in the presence of blood dyscrasias, hemophilia, hyperthyroidism, Paget's disease, and many other systemic disorders patients would fare best if endodontic procedures were performed rather than exodontic procedures. We know of no systemic disorder that negates endodontic treatment."[2]

In patients with acute or chronic leukemia, hemophilia, purpura hemorrhagica, rheumatic heart disease, radium necrosis, or other severe illness, endodontic treatment is preferable to extraction.

PULPLESS TEETH AS ABUTMENTS

Many dentists believe that pulpless teeth may be used satisfactorily for bridge abutments. From an analysis of many case histories, Tylman found that pulpless teeth are satisfactory bridge abutments,[25] and in an in vitro study, Trabert and associates found no difference in impact fractures between untreated and endodontally treated teeth.[24]

Pulpless posterior teeth that are to be used as abutments for bridges or for partial dentures should have complete occlusal coverage. When the crown of an anterior tooth is weak and is undermined by the presence of mesial or distal fillings, it may be strengthened by cementing an Endopost (Kerr) or KG Endowel (Star) in the root canal and extending it into the crown. These prefabricated posts are of the same diameter and taper as standardized root canal instruments, as suggested by Gerstein and Burnell.[5] When a crown is to be made for a broken-down posterior tooth, a cast core deriving its support from an Endopost or a KG Endowel casting should be made.

The following types of teeth may be retained and used for fixed-bridge abutments or as abutments for removable bridges or dentures: (1) any vital tooth requiring pulp extirpation; (2) any pulpless tooth without an area of rarefaction; (3) any pulpless tooth with an area of rarefaction requiring root resection, provided sufficient alveolar support will remain; (4) any pulpless tooth with an area of rarefaction considered to be of strategic importance to the retention of the denture, and the potential for repair is good; and (5) any previously treated pulpless tooth with no periapical involvement. When the root canal filling is inadequate, however, the canal should be retreated and refilled.

Before deciding to remove a salvageable pulpless tooth, one should consider the relation of the tooth to other teeth in the arch. One must be careful not to create an orthodontic problem or a difficult prosthetic problem by heedless removal of a tooth. Removed, but not replaced, first molars are often the cause of disturbed occlusion in the young and of "bite collapse" in the adult. Certain teeth are considered strategic teeth in the dental arch from a prosthetic standpoint. For example, any terminal second molar is difficult to replace by itself. In most cases, replacement is not done because of inherent technical difficulties. In addition, if the first molar is missing and if the second molar requires endodontic treatment, the second molar may be considered a strategic tooth because its removal presents difficulties in replacement if no other tooth is missing in the arch. The problem is similar when a second molar is already missing and the first molar is in need of endodontic treatment. Other difficult prosthetic problems are conceivable. For example, if the lateral incisor and both premolars are missing on one side and the cuspid on the same side is in need of endodontic treatment, extraction of the cuspid will present a problem from the standpoint of both fixed and removable bridgework. The replacement of a single anterior tooth, particularly mandibular, by any type of removable appliance or fixed bridgework is not usually satisfactory. Under no circumstances should endodontic treatment be dictated only by the strategic need for the tooth, however.

PULPLESS TEETH AND ORTHODONTIC TREATMENT

Will pulpless teeth respond to orthodontic treatment as well as vital teeth? This question has been answered by Huettner and Young on the basis of experimental work in monkeys,[12] and by clinical observation in humans. Whether a vital or a pulpless tooth was stimulated to movement by the orthodontic appliance, the histologic picture was the same. Clinical observation in many cases compels one to conclude that no difference exists in the degree of tooth movement regardless of whether the tooth moved is vital or pulpless. In fact, Peskin and Graber surgically repositioned teeth for orthodontic reasons and found that the pulps remained vital if the apices of the teeth were luxated minimally.[20] Ohzeki and Takahashi performed maxillary anterior osteotomies in 7 dogs; they found pulpal changes from hyperemia to necrosis.[19] Cholinesterase-positive nerve fibers appeared at 6 weeks and began to be distributed throughout the tooth in bundles, indicating nerve regeneration.

It is advisable to relieve or remove any strain on the tooth by an orthodontic appliance while the tooth is under endodontic treatment, to avoid confusion as to whether the discomfort is from the appliance or from endodontic treatment. Appliances should not be placed for a week or two after endodontic treatment, to allow sufficient time for recovery because the periodontal ligament is sometimes irritated during endodontic treatment and may need a rest for recovery.

BIBLIOGRAPHY

1. Bender, I.B., et al.: J. Am. Dent. Assoc., *109*:415, 1984.
2. Bender, I.B., et al.: Oral Surg., *16*:1102, 1963.
3. Eggink, C.O.: Results of Endodontic Treatment Based on a Standardized Evaluation. Utrecht, Schotemus en Jens, 1964, p. 208; and Int. Endod. J., *15*:79, 1982.
4. Frank, A.L.: J. Am. Dent. Assoc., *96*:202, 1978.
5. Gerstein, H., and Burnell, S.C.: J. Am. Dent. Assoc., *68*:787, 1964.
6. Grossman, L.I.: J. Br. Endod. Soc., *2*:35, 1968.
7. Grossman, L.I.: J. Can. Dent. Assoc., *18*:181, 1952.
8. Grossman, L.I., et al.: Oral Surg., *17*:368, 1964.
9. Healey, H.J.: J. Am. Dent. Assoc., *55*:434, 1956.
10. Holland, R., et al.: Oral Surg., *55*:191, 1983.
11. Hörting-Hansen, E.: Studies of Implantation of an Organic Bone in Cystic Jaw Lesions. Copenhagen, Munksgaard, 1970.
12. Huettner, R.J., and Young, R.W.: Oral Surg., *8*:189, 1955.
13. Ingle, J.I., and Beveridge, E.E.: Endodontics, 2nd Ed. Philadelphia, Lea & Febiger, 1976, p. 48.
14. Kerekes, K., and Tronstad, L.: J. Endod., *5*:83, 1979.
15. Luebke, R.G., et al.: Oral Surg., *18*:97, 1964.
16. Luks, S.: N.Y. State Dent. J., *23*:31, 1957.
17. Maurice, C.G.: Dent. Clin. North Am., *Nov.*:761, 1957.
18. Nelson, F.A.: Int. Endod. J., *15*:168, 1982.
19. Ohzeki, H., and Takahashi, S.: Bull. Tokyo Dent. Coll., *21*:21, 1980.
20. Peskin, S., and Graber, T.M.: J. Am. Dent. Assoc., *80*:1320, 1970.
21. Siskin, M.: J. Am. Dent. Assoc., *66*:648, 1963.
22. Strindberg, L.Z.: Acta Odontol. Scand., *14 (Suppl. 21)*:100, 1956.
23. Tay, W.M., et al.: J. Br. Endod. Soc., *11*:3, 1978.
24. Trabert, K.C., et al.: J. Endod., *4*:341, 1978.
25. Tylman, S.: Theory and Practice of Crown and Bridge Prosthodontics. St. Louis, C.V. Mosby, 1970, p. 68.

9 Principles of Endodontic Treatment

The basic principles underlying the treatment of teeth with endodontic problems are those underlying surgery in general. An aseptic technique, debridement of the wound, drainage, and gentle treatment of the tissues with both instruments and drugs—all are cardinal principles of surgery. Specifically, pain must be controlled, if present. During treatment, all pulp tissue must be removed, the root canal enlarged and irrigated, the canal surface rendered sterile as determined by bacteriologic examination, and the root canal well obturated to prevent the possibility of reinfection.

APPLICATION OF RUBBER DAM

To maintain a safe and aseptic operating technique, application of the rubber dam is imperative. It is the only sure safeguard against bacterial contamination from saliva and accidental swallowing of root canal instruments. All endodontic operations should be performed under the rubber dam. In some cases, it is first necessary to supply a missing wall with amalgam or to cement a stainless steel band to prevent the rubber-dam clamp from slipping off the tooth. In other cases, a gingivectomy may need to be done, with removal of about 2 mm gingival tissue to provide enough tooth structure for application of a rubber-dam clamp. Gingivectomy may be necessary in any event for restoration of the crown of the tooth.

Treatment of posterior teeth should not be attempted under cotton rolls or napkins. The risk of losing a reamer or file down the patient's trachea or esophagus is too great to warrant this practice.

In a survey of the use of the rubber dam in endodontic treatment by general practitioners, Going and Sawinski found that 36% of dentists never, or seldom, used the rubber dam.[6] Their survey emphasizes the need for more general use of the rubber dam by the dentist, especially in view of the more than threefold increase in ingestion or aspiration of instruments during endodontic treatment in the last decade. To risk operating without a rubber dam is to risk one's professional reputation. A variety of objects used in endodontic practice may be swallowed accidentally if the rubber dam is not applied (Fig. 9–1). Root canal instruments swallowed during endodontic treatment have been reported by Christen,[3] Goultchin and Heling,[7] Govila,[8] Hanzely,[13] Heling,[15] Israel and Laban,[18] Kitamura,[19] and Taintor and Biesterfeld.[30]

If an instrument is swallowed or aspirated during endodontic treatment without a rubber dam, one is likely to be confronted with a lawsuit. Grossman has stated that: "in the eyes of the court, when an endodontic instrument escapes from the dentist's fingers and is ingested or aspirated, expert opinion is unnecessary to justify claims of negligence. In most other liability cases against a professional practitioner, the plaintiff is required to produce expert testimony to convince a jury of negligence, but when an endodontic instrument is swallowed or aspirated, a jury is competent enough from 'common knowledge' to pass on the question of negligence without expert testimony. Even if the accident was caused by the patient's moving, the patient will usually deny having moved."[9]

In many cases, the rubber dam can be applied in less than 2 min and often within 1 min. Heise timed the application of the rubber dam in 302 cases and found that it took an average of 1 min 48 sec.[14] Only the tooth to be operated on should be isolated. This limitation consumes less operating time and lessens the possibility of contamination from adjacent teeth and saliva.

Most anterior teeth may be clamped satisfactorily with an Ivory No. 9 or No. 9 ON clamp (Fig. 9–2). When the tooth is small, as in the case of upper lateral incisors or lower anterior teeth, the HF* No. 211 clamp or its equivalent may be used. In posterior teeth,

---

*All SSW clamps are manufactured by Hu-Friedy, Chicago, IL, under their own label.

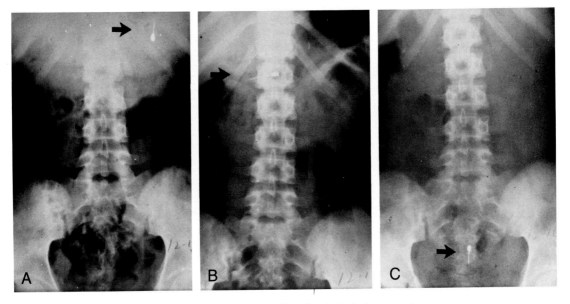

Fig. 9–1. *A* to *C*, Radiographic views of the trail of a swallowed endodontic instrument.

the HF or Ivory No. 27 clamp (wingless) may be used on all premolars and the HF No. 26 clamp or its equivalent on all molars. Figure 9–3 shows a tray for holding rubber-dam clamps.

In tapering, young upper anterior teeth that have not completely erupted, an HF No. 27 (premolar) clamp can often be applied to advantage (Fig. 9–4). Moreover, if a No. 27 clamp slips toward the cervix and pinches the gingiva when applied on a lower premolar, a No. 9 clamp may at times be substituted for it. When two adjacent anterior teeth are to be treated, one clamp may be applied to one tooth while the other is simply ligated, so both teeth may be treated simultaneously. One may also use two No. 27 HF clamps, one facing mesially, the other distally. Three adjacent anterior teeth can be

treated simultaneously by applying the Ivory No. 9 ON clamp over only one tooth and by tucking the rubber dam under the gingiva of the adjacent teeth. The handling of similar unusual clinical situations is left to the ingenuity of the operator (Figs. 9–5 to 9–7).

In summary, only four clamps are needed for applying the rubber dam to most teeth: (1) Ivory No. 9, for upper central incisors and all cuspids; (2) HF No. 211, for upper lateral and all lower incisors; (3) HF No. 27, for all premolars; and (4) HF No. 26, for all molars.

A proximal cavity in an involved anterior tooth may be disregarded from the standpoint of applying the rubber dam, provided a filling is inserted to prevent contamination of the root canal, because the approach will be made lingually. When a proximal cavity is present in an involved posterior tooth, the

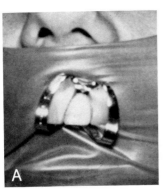
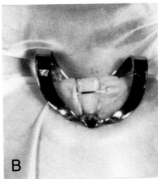
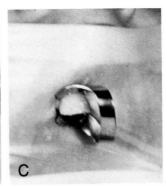

Fig. 9–2. *A*, Ivory No. 9 clamp on an upper central incisor. *B*, HF No. 211 clamp on a lower incisor under orthodontic treatment. *C*, HF No. 27 clamp on a partially erupted central tooth of a child.

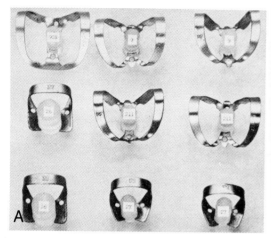
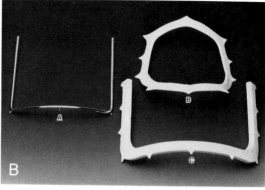

Fig. 9–3. *A.* Plastic tray for holding rubber-dam clamps. The tray is easily made from sheet plastic and plastic rods that are cemented to the tray with plastic cement. Such trays are also available commercially. Hu-Friedy (Chicago, IL) manufactures all the old SSW clamps shown above. *B.* Rubber dam frame holders. A. Stainless steel (Young); B. Plastic (Nygaard-Ostby); C. Plastic. (A,B, Courtesy of Union Broach, York, Pa.; C, Courtesy of Hygenic Corp., Akron, Ohio.)

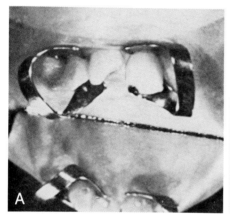
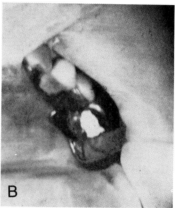

Fig. 9–4. *A,* Two upper central and a lateral incisor simultaneously under endodontic treatment, with two HF No. 27 clamps to keep the rubber dam in place. *B,* Entire bridge under the rubber dam. First, one punches a large hole in the dam and uses an HF No. 26 clamp, and then one ligates the entire bridge to prevent leakage.

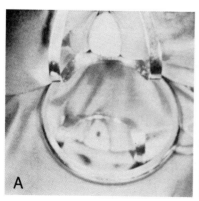
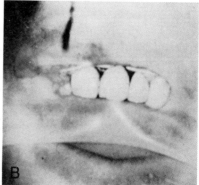

Fig. 9–5. *A,* Rubber dam applied over a porcelain jacket crown that serves as an abutment for a bridge. *B,* An entire ceramic bridge under the rubber dam; dental floss is used to keep the dam in place.

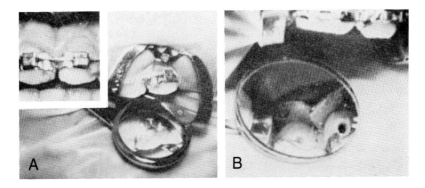

Fig. 9–6. *A,* Rubber dam applied despite the presence of an orthodontic appliance. The inset shows the orthodontic appliance before the application of the rubber dam. *B,* Two teeth under orthodontic treatment placed under the rubber dam. Note that the orthodontic bands do not interfere with the preparation of access cavities, nor does the endodontic operation interfere with the orthodontic treatment.

adjacent tooth must also be isolated under the rubber dam. If the cavity is mesioocclusal, the involved tooth may be clamped, and the tooth immediately anterior to it may be ligated. If the cavity is distoocclusal, the tooth distal to the involved tooth may be clamped, and the involved tooth may be ligated. In some posterior teeth, it may be necessary to ligate the clamped tooth as well, to bring the distal fold of rubber dam down into the interproximal space and thereby to prevent leakage around the clamp.

When gingivitis is present, it is desirable to remove gross accumulations of calculus before applying the rubber dam and to apply a suitable antiseptic to the gingiva. The contact points should be tested with dental floss to determine the presence of a sharp edge of a restoration or a cavity, which may tear the rubber dam, and to determine whether inter-

proximal clearance is sufficient to permit application of the rubber dam. Slight separation of the teeth or smoothing of the tooth surface may be necessary, especially if a temporary filling is present.

The holes in the rubber dam should be punched approximately over the center of the incisal or occlusal surfaces of the teeth to be engaged. In addition, guide holes should be punched along the upper border of the rubber dam for ready identification of the upper surface while adjusting the dam, particularly over a posterior tooth.

When a clamp is used on an anterior tooth, the rubber dam should first be slipped over the tooth. One should stretch the dam over the tooth between the thumb and index finger of the left hand while the clamp is adjusted with the right hand. In posterior teeth, the clamp is preferably inserted half-

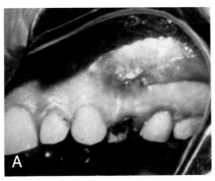
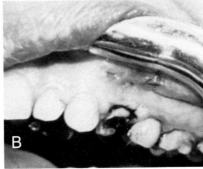

Fig. 9–7. *A,* Gingiva had overgrown the edge of a cavity of a premolar. *B,* After gingivectomy, a rubber-dam clamp an be applied for retention of the rubber dam.

way into the previously punched hole in the rubber dam, and the arms of the clamp are then spread apart with clamp forceps. The rubber dam is held in the left hand and is kept from obstructing the view while the clamp is slipped over the tooth with the right hand. The forceps are then disengaged from the clamp, and the rubber dam is slipped under the anterior arms of the clamp. If a wing clamp is used, the wing of the clamp is inserted into the hole of the rubber dam, the clamp is applied to the tooth, the clamp forceps are removed, and the rubber dam is slipped under the arms of the clamp.

The type of rubber-dam holder one uses is a matter of individual preference, but whichever one chooses, it should not interfere with the endodontic operation. Some operators prefer one that lies flat against the patient's face because it permits easy access to the operating field around the tooth. Others prefer the "frame" type of holders made of stainless steel (Young) or plastic (Nygaard-Ostby, Brave) because they can be applied quickly and effectively. The plastic frames, contoured facially, have the additional advantage of being radiolucent and do not have to be removed when taking working radiographs of the tooth during treatment.

To facilitate slipping the rubber dam over the tooth, especially if the contact point is tight, the surface of the rubber dam adjacent to the hole should be wiped with liquid soap, or a wet finger may be rubbed on a cake of soap and applied to the rubber dam around the punched hole. Petrolatum or cocoa butter should not be used for this purpose because these substances soften and weaken the rubber dam, and leakage may result.

In upper or lower anterior teeth, when little is left of the crown as a result of caries, or when the crown has been broken off by traumatic injury, generally enough root surface is still exposed on which to attach a cervical clamp when the rubber dam has been pulled taut over the exposed crown or root surface. Although access to the pulp chamber may be obtained in such cases before applying the rubber dam, all other endodontic procedures should be done only after the rubber dam has been applied. In partially erupted anterior teeth, in which the rubber-dam clamp may slip off, or when one of the surfaces is completely broken away, a narrow orthodontic band may be fitted and cemented in place, over which the rubber dam can then be attached.

In badly broken down posterior teeth, it may be necessary to build up the crown of the tooth with a stainless steel band and to contour and cement the band in place before endodontic treatment is begun (Fig. 9–8). An aluminum or stainless steel crown may be cemented instead of a band. A core of gutta-percha is first placed in the pulp chamber to keep cement out of the root canals. The band is cemented with zinc-phosphate cement, and the excess cement and core of gutta-percha, lying within the approach to the root canal, are then removed. The band should remain in place until the endodontic operation is completed. In some cases where the crown is badly broken down, gingivectomy may be necessary before a rubber-dam clamp can be applied. In other cases, it may also be necessary to cement a band after a gingivectomy has been done to ensure against leakage of the medicament (Fig. 9–9). When one of the abutments of a fixed bridge is to be treated, it is often possible to slip the rubber dam completely over the bridge, if the hole in the rubber dam is large enough, without leakage of saliva into the field of operation. In most cases, it is more feasible to slip the rubber dam over the abutment tooth only, where it is kept in place with a suitable clamp.

STERILIZATION OF INSTRUMENTS

Once the rubber dam has been applied, the teeth and dam should be thoroughly swabbed with a large pellet of cotton soaked in a quick-evaporating, nonstaining antiseptic. Ray has recommended 2% benzalkonium chloride in 50% isopropyl alcohol,[25] while Möller prefers swabbing with hydrogen peroxide followed by tincture of iodine,[21] and Baumgartner found povidone-iodine no more effective than 99% isopropyl alcohol for this purpose.[21] Burs for opening into the pulp chamber should be autoclaved, dry heat sterilized, or sterilized by being dipped in alcohol and flamed 2 or 3 times, before use in the pulp cavity. Sanderson has shown that 3 parts ethyl alcohol and 1 part formalin, when ignited, will destroy even spore formers.[27] This finding has been confirmed by Bartels and Rice.[1] Figure 9–10 shows a typical selection of endodontic instruments.

Instruments should first be cleansed of debris regardless of the method used to sterilize them. They should be wiped clean by squeezing the instrument blade with a 2 × 2 gauze

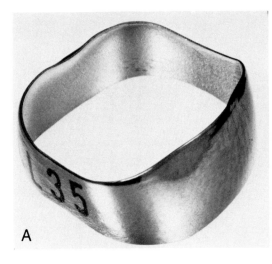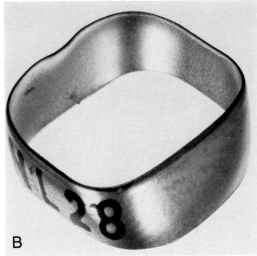

Fig. 9–8. *A and B,* Contoured stainless-steel bands by Unitek are available for all shapes and sizes of premolar and molar teeth.

or cotton roll, moistened with hydrogen peroxide or alcohol, while withdrawing the instrument, using a counter-clockwise rotary motion before subjecting them to sterilization. Segall found an alcohol sponge effective for cleansing instruments of debris.[29] Hubbard and associates have shown that simply plunging a file into a dry sponge removes some of the microorganisms, and a saline gauze wipe removes almost 98% of microorganisms.[17]

Cold sterilization of instruments, that is, sterilization by cold chemical solutions, is not recommended for two reasons: (1) the process is not effective against all varieties of microbial life; (2) the length of time necessary to destroy microorganisms against which these solutions are effective, namely, a minimum of 20 min, is too long. Quaternary-ammonium compounds are effective against vegetative organisms; ethyl alcohol and isopropyl alcohol are effective against vegetative bacteria and tubercle bacilli; alcohol-formalin solutions are effective against vegetative bacteria, tubercle bacilli, and spores; orthophenylphenol and benzyl-parachlorophenol are effective against vegetative bacteria, tubercle bacilli, certain fungi, and viruses, but not spores. The manufacturer of a cold-sterilizing solution (Sporicidin) consisting of phenol (7.05%), sodium tetraborate (2.35%), glutaraldehyde (2.0%), and sodium phenate (1.2%) claims that the solution disinfects cleaned instruments in 10 min at room temperature; kills aerobic spore formers including Bacillus subtilis in 3 hours, and achieves sterilization in 6.75 hours.

Absorbent points, broaches, files, and

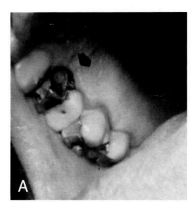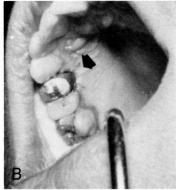

Fig. 9–9. *A,* Fracture of the lingual cusp of an upper premolar; gingivectomy has just been done, to expose the fracture line. *B,* Immediate cementing of a copper band makes it possible to treat the tooth under aseptic conditions after application of the rubber dam.

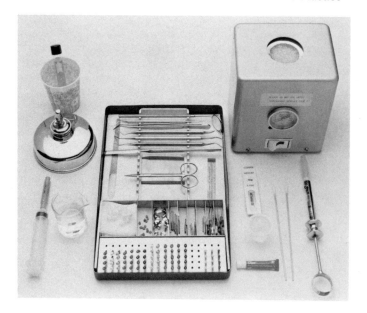

Fig. 9–10. Arrangement of instruments before beginning endodontic treatment. From left to right: dappen dishes (one for alcohol, one for absorbent points), mirror, cotton pliers, explorer, excavator, plastic instruments, dappen dishes containing irrigating solutions, irrigating syringes, and scissors for cutting absorbent points and gutta-percha cones.

other root canal instruments should be sterilized immediately before use in a *hot-salt sterilizer* (Figs. 9–11 and 9–12). This type of sterilizer is indispensable for endodontic work. The apparatus itself is compact as well as efficient. It consists essentially of a metal cup in which table salt is kept at a temperature of between 425° F (218° C) and 475° F (246° C), although a slightly higher temperature is not critical and does not impair the temper of root canal instruments. A suitable thermometer should be inserted in the salt at all times, if one is not incorporated into

the unit, so the temperature can be checked at a glance. At this temperature, root canal instruments such as broaches, files, and reamers may be sterilized in 5 sec and absorbent points and cotton pellets in 10 sec. The need for a thermometer to monitor the temperature of the sterilizer is imperative; the desired temperature may not be attained because of malfunction of the thermostat. The hot-salt sterilizer has superseded the molten-metal sterilizer and the glass-bead sterilizer because the metal or the small glass beads occasionally clung to a wet instrument, escaped

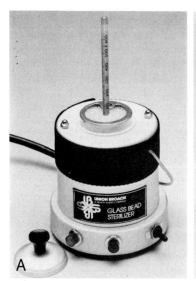
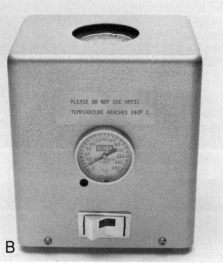

Fig. 9–11. *A,* Electric glass-bead sterilizer, which can be converted to a hot-salt sterilizer. Note the thermometer stuck in the salt. The temperature of the salt should be between 425 and 475° F. (Courtesy of Union Broach Co., Long Island City, New York.) *B,* Electric glass-bead sterilizer. (Courtesy of Pulpdent Corporation America, Brookline, Massachusetts.)

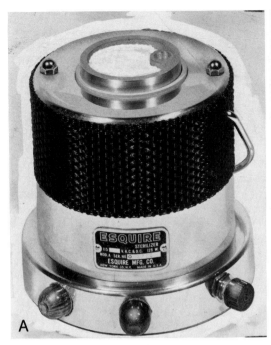
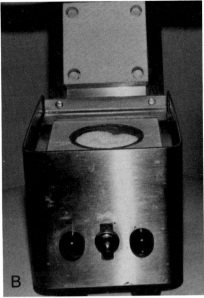

Fig. 9–12. *A,* Glass-bead or hot-salt sterilizer. The temperature should be adjusted to the maximum, and only the smallest of glass beads (about the size of grains of sand) or table salt should be used in these sterilizers. (Courtesy of Esquire Manufacturing Co., New York, New York.) *B,* Thermostatically controlled sterilizer, which can be converted from a glass-bead to a hot-salt sterilizer. (Courtesy of Buffalo Dental Manufacturing Co., Brooklyn, New York.)

detection, and then clogged the root canal as the instrument was inserted. The advantage of the hot-salt sterilizer lies in the use of ordinary table salt, which is readily available for replacement, instead of metal or beads, and eliminates the risk of clogging the canal.[10,22] The salt, the usual commercial table salt, contains a small amount (1%) of sodium silicoaluminate, magnesium carbonate, or sodium carbonate, so it pours more readily and will not become fused under heat. Pure sodium chloride should not be used without the previously mentioned additives because high heat may cause fusion of the granules, nor should the salt contain dextrose as an additive because it may coalesce the granules of salt at high heat. Any salt accidentally carried into the root canal can easily be irrigated from the canal with the usual irrigating solutions. The salt should be changed weekly, or more often, depending on the degree of humidity.

Glass beads may be effectively substituted for the salt in a hot-salt sterilizer, provided the beads are less than 1 mm in diameter. Larger beads are not so effective in transferring heat to endodontic instruments, according to tests carried out by Oliet,[22] because of the large air spaces between the beads that reduce the efficiency of the sterilizer. The glass-bead sterilizer is operated at approximately the same temperature as the hot-salt sterilizer, namely, between 218 and 246° C (425 to 475° F). Comparable tests also carried out by Oliet showed that a slightly higher temperature is reached with salt than with glass beads at the same temperature setting of the thermostat, probably because the salt granules are smaller than glass beads, the air space between granules thus is reduced, and the conductivity of heat by the salt is higher.[22] The hottest part of the salt bath in the sterilizer is along its outer rim, starting at the bottom layer of salt; the temperature is lowest in the center of the surface layer of salt. To sterilize an instrument properly, one should immerse it at least a quarter-inch below the salt's surface and in the peripheral area of the sterilizer. This finding has been confirmed by Engelhardt,[4] Koehler and Hefferren,[20] and by Windeler and Walter.[32]

Root canal instruments are immersed in the hot-salt or glass-bead sterilizer for 5 sec, whereas absorbent points and cotton pellets require immersion for 10 sec to sterilize them. Absorbent points are preferably immersed butt end first in the hot-salt sterilizer to avoid bending them. Several absorbent points may be submerged and sterilized at one time and then left on the surface of the hot salt until ready for use. Root canal instruments should not be placed in the hot salt and left there much longer than the usual 5 sec because the instrument may become too hot to handle.

Hooks and colleagues have found that exposure of infected endodontic instruments for 3 sec to a laser beam is sufficient to destroy microorganisms, including spores.[16]

A device for keeping reamers and files together according to size is available. This device consists of a plastic case containing sponge rubber, which is saturated with a cold disinfectant solution, and a lid with perforations identified by numbers arranged serially, corresponding to the sizes of the instruments. The apparatus holds both short-handle and long-handle reamers and files and has additional perforations for instruments that have been used and cleaned of debris. The apparatus is intended to maintain sterility of instruments that have already been sterilized in the hot-salt sterilizer, not to be a primary means of sterilization (Fig. 9–13).

Dappen dishes may be sterilized just before use by swabbing thoroughly with tincture of thimerosal (merthiolate) followed by alcohol. Such swabbing should be done under pressure with the intent of physically removing debris and microorganisms attached to the glass surface.

Long-handle instruments, tips of cotton pliers, blades of scissors, and other implements used in the course of an endodontic operation may be sterilized by dipping the working point in alcohol and flaming twice. Isopropyl alcohol (90%) may be used for this purpose, but alcohol-formalin (3:1) is preferable. It is assumed, of course, that such instruments were sterile when placed on the tray at the beginning of the operation and that they had become contaminated only from use in the cavity, pulp chamber, or root canal of the tooth undergoing operation. This method of sterilization, which Grossman and Appleton have found effective by bacteriologic tests,[11] is not intended as a means of primary sterilization, but as an auxiliary method of sterilization during the course of an endodontic operation.

Bulky instruments such as cotton pliers and cement spatulas may be sterilized quickly by passing the working blade(s) through a flame several times. The temper of the blade remains unaffected even after numerous passes through the flame. Trebitsch found that both spore-bearing and nonsporulating microorganisms were destroyed on cotton pliers when held in a flame for 2 sec.[31]

Root canal and other instruments may be sterilized by autoclaving, but this process subjects carbon steel instruments to rusting. Sterilization is accomplished when the instruments are kept at 15 lb pressure at 120° C (248° F) for at least 15 min. The objection to using autoclaved instruments over resterilized instruments is that although one begins the endodontic operation with sterile instruments, they soon become contaminated.

A dry-heat autoclave or a dry-heat oven may also be used for sterilization of root canal instruments, but this operation is time consuming because it requires an elapsed time of 2 hours for sterilization at a temperature of 320° F, 1 hour at 340° F,[26] or 30 min at 380° F.[22]

The slab for mixing root canal cement may be sterilized by swabbing the surface with stainless tincture of thimerosal, followed by a double swabbing with alcohol. The swabbing is done by discharging a dropperful of the thimerosal or alcohol on the slab and rubbing the surface with a cotton roll held in a pair of cotton pliers. The cement spatula may be sterilized in this manner also, but it is preferably flamed 3 or 4 times by passing it through the Bunsen flame.

Gutta-percha cones may be kept sterile in screw-capped vials containing alcohol. Several such vials, each containing a different size of gutta-percha cone, may be used. To sterilize a gutta-percha cone freshly removed from the manufacturer's box, one should immerse it in 5.2% sodium hypochlorite for 1 min,[28] then rinse the cone with hydrogen peroxide and dry it between 2 layers of sterile gauze. Frank and Pellieu have demonstrated that 5.2% sodium hypochlorite is 5 times more effective than Sporicidin and 7 times as effective as activated dialdehyde (Cidex) for sterilizing gutta-percha cones.[5]

Silver cones may be sterilized by slowly passing them back and forth through a Bunsen flame 3 or 4 times. The silver cone should not be held in the flame, however, because it might melt the fine tip. Silver cones may

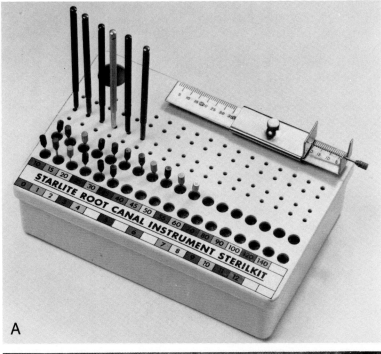

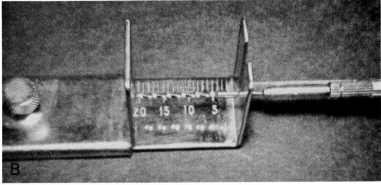

Fig. 9–13. *A,* Apparatus for holding both short- and long-handled root canal instruments. An instrument gauge is shown at the rear. The apparatus contains a rubber sponge, which may be saturated with a cold sterilizing solution for maintaining sterility of instruments after prior sterilization in a bead or salt sterilizer. *B,* Close-up view of the instrument gauge with a root canal instrument in place, to which is attached a Krueger stop. See also Figure 11–12.

also be sterilized by immersion in the hot-salt sterilizer for 5 sec.

The use of an instrument case in which root canal instruments are allegedly kept sterile by vapors of formaldehyde is not recommended. To be effective, formaldehyde gas must be in solution or must enter into solution with bacterial protoplasm. Because bacteria on root canal instruments are generally in a dry state, that is, adhering to dry instruments, formaldehyde cannot be depended on to exert a bactericidal effect.

Glassware used during endodontic treatment should be made of "Pyrex"* because it

———
*Corning Glassworks, Corning, NY.

can withstand the high temperatures needed for autoclaving or dry-heat sterilization. Plastic disposable suction tips, syringes (and needles), pipettes, and other similar products are recommended for use whenever possible.

DEBRIDEMENT

It is a principle of surgery that an infected wound must first be cleansed mechanically. It is equally true that an infected root canal must first be cleansed of debris. Devitalized tissue encourages bacterial growth, whereas healthy tissue resists such growth. Just as the surgeon rids the wound of debris initially, so too must the dentist remove all necrotic material in the root canal as soon as possible. In surgery, "cleanliness is next to godliness." The pulp chamber and root canal should preferably be carefully irrigated with sodium hypochlorite solution before one attempts instrumentation because this solution has a solvent effect on pulp tissue and also exerts an antibacterial effect. When the root canal contains pulp remnants, they may be removed by instrumentation at the first visit, provided care is taken to confine all instrumentation to the canal. In all cases, a combination of biomechanical and chemical means, namely, instrumentation and irrigation, is necessary for complete debridement and cleansing of the root canal. Provided one is careful not to force debris through the root canal or otherwise irritate the periapical tissue, complete instrumentation of the root canal in one sitting is a safe procedure if the canal is thoroughly irrigated. Dead tissue is a handicap to disinfection and repair. One should be ever mindful that: "It is not so much what you put into a root canal, but what you take out, that counts."

DRAINAGE

When gross infection and swelling are present, the surgeon generally makes an incision to provide drainage. When an acute alveolar abscess with much edema is present, drainage should be established at once, either through the root canal, or by incision, or by both. The extent and condition of the swelling govern the choice in each case. Drainage through the root canal is preferable because it allows the pent-up pus and gas to escape. To determine whether gas is generated by microorganisms in the root canal, Grossman and Demp studied the flora in 100 consecutive cases for gas-producing ability.[12] In 12% of these cases, the microorganisms isolated were gas producers.

Drainage is established by preparing a cavity lingually, in an anterior tooth, and occlusally, in a posterior tooth. The air turbine facilitates rapid entry into the root canal, whether a stone or bur is used to pierce the enamel. Pulp tissue, if present, should be removed with appropriate instruments. When drainage through the root canal is slow or access is difficult, or when the tooth is so tender that preparing a cavity to allow drainage is impractical, and a soft, fluctuant swelling is present, an incision should be made in the most dependent part of the swelling near the root apex. Care should be taken not to lance the gum before the swelling has "pointed" or "come to a head." If the tissues are lanced prematurely, no pus will escape, and the incision will only add to the pain and discomfort. If the swelling is still hard, a counterirritant, or moist heat, should be applied to the mucosa over the apex of the affected tooth to break down the tissue and to soften the contents, most effectively by means of hot mouth rinses or a proprietary poultice applied to the gum. Heat should not be applied to the outside of the face under any circumstances, lest the abscess break through the skin surface and cause a sinus tract (fistula), leaving an unsightly scar. Once the incision is made, a drain should be inserted to keep the wound open. A 1-inch length of "T-shaped" rubber-dam strip may be inserted into the wound.

CHEMOPROPHYLAXIS

If the patient has a history of rheumatic fever or heart ailment involving the heart valves, an antibiotic such as 2 g phenoxymethyl penicillin (V-Cillin, Pen-Vee-K) should be given 1 hour before the operation and then 1 g 6 hours postoperatively. Erythromycin (Erythrocin) may be substituted if the patient is allergic to penicillin. The dosage is 1 g 1 hour before treatment and 500 mg 6 hours after treatment.

IMMOBILIZATION

Immobilization is employed by the surgeon to rest an organ, to allay pain or promote healing. Immobilization reduces the potential for spreading of microorganisms. The endodontist may well follow the example of the surgeon and immobilize the affected tooth by relieving occlusal stress or by relieving contact with apposing teeth if pain is present. In fact, it may be considered good practice to relieve occlusion slightly in all endodontic cases because it lessens the possibility of traumatizing the periodontal ligament. Orban has stated that "traumatized tissue may more easily become infected and inflamed, and inflamed tissue will yield more easily to trauma."[23]

AVOIDANCE OF TRAUMA

Soft tissues should be handled gently, delicately, as by a surgeon when operating. All trauma should be avoided. Instruments should not be passed beyond the apical foramen. Ripened judgment may help to prevent this complication, but instrument stops are more certain for beginners and seasoned veterans alike. To prevent the instrument from being passed through the foramen, a mechanical stop or disc of rubber or plastic may be slipped over the instrument and adjusted short of the tooth length from apex to incisal or occlusal surface. In every instance, the radiograph should be carefully studied, and the operator should visualize the shape, length, and outline of the canal before passing a root canal instrument into the tooth. When the endodontist has inserted the instrument into the canal to the level assumed to be correct by measurement on the preoperative radiograph, a radiograph is taken to determine whether it is correct. Any adjustment in the length of the root canal instrument to compensate for the difference between the assumed and the actual length is now made, and subsequent instrumentation of the canal is carried out in conformity with the revised length. In this way, periapical trauma is minimized.

Trephination

Trephination as a means of relieving pain has been used from time to time. By trephination is meant the creation of a surgical passage in the region of the root apex, usually by a bur or special drill. The purpose of trephination is to provide a channel for the escape of pus and blood, to relieve the pressure of accumulated fluid or gas in the jawbone.

We do not use this procedure, which in itself causes surgical trauma and relies on drainage through the root canal, an antibiotic when needed, and an incision and drain when the condition of the tissues warrants it.

Prophylactic trephination is the intentional use of trephination with the object of preventing postoperative pain when root canal treatment and obturation are done in one visit. In a series of 50 cases, Peters found this procedure unjustified,[24] a result confirmed by Oliet in his study in which 264 teeth were treated endodontally in a single visit.[22a]

Trephination has been advocated in the following cases: acute alveolar abscess where drainage through the root canal is inadequate and much pain or swelling is present; teeth with large areas of rarefaction; when the root canal has been overfilled and pain or discomfort is present; and for postoperative pain following obturation of the canal by conventional means. In most cases, proper treatment of the root canal, with aseptic technique and obturation of the canal, precludes the need for trephination.

Chemical irritation may do as much damage as mechanical trauma. Irritating drugs should be confined to the root canal itself and should not be forced through the apical foramen where they may come into contact with the periradicular tissues. For example, careless irrigation of the root canal to an extent that either hydrogen peroxide or sodium-hypochlorite solution is forced through the apical foramen causes considerable pain and edema. Preference should always be given to nonirritating root canal medicaments. The dictum of Hippocrates, "whatever you do, do no harm," should be carefully observed.

BIBLIOGRAPHY

1. Bartels, H.A., and Rice, E.: J. Am. Dent. Assoc., *29*:1389, 1942.
2. Baumgartner, J.C., et al.: J. Endod., *1*:276, 1975.
3. Christen, A.G.: Oral Surg., *24*:684, 1967.
4. Engelhardt, J.P., et al.: J. Endod., *10*:465, 1984.
5. Frank, R.J., and Pellieu, G.B.: J. Endod., *9*:368, 1983.
6. Going, R.E., and Sawinski, V.J.: J. Am. Dent. Assoc., *75*:158, 1967.
7. Goultschin, J., and Heling, B.: Oral Surg., *32*:261, 1971.
8. Govila, C.P.: Oral Surg., *48*:269, 1979.
9. Grossman, L.I.: J. Am. Dent. Assoc., *82*:395, 1971.
10. Grossman, L.I.: Br. Dent. J., *100*:283, 1956, and J. Am. Dent. Assoc., *56*:144, 1958.
11. Grossman, L.I., and Appleton, J.L.T.: J. Am. Dent. Assoc., *27*:1632, 1940.
12. Grossman, L.I., and Demp, S.: J. Dent. Res., *41*:495, 1962.
13. Hanzely, B.: Fogorv. Sz., *66*:55, 1973.
14. Heise, A.L.: J. Dent. Child., *38*:52, 1971.
15. Heling, B.: Oral Surg., *43*:464, 1977.
16. Hooks, T.W., et al.: Oral Surg., *49*:263, 1980.
17. Hubbard, T.M., et al.: Oral Surg., *40*:148, 1975.
18. Israel, H.A., and Laban, S.G.: J. Endod., *10*:452, 1984.
19. Kitamura, A.: J. Am. Dent. Assoc., *89*:169, 1974.
20. Koehler, H.M., and Hefferren, J.J.: J. Dent. Res., *41*:182, 1962.
21. Möller, A.J.R.: Microbiologic Examination of Root Canal and Periapical Tissues of Teeth. Göteborg, Akademiförlaget, 1966, p. 25.
22. Oliet, S.: Oral Surg., *9*:666, 1956, and *11*:37, 1958.
22a. Oliet, S.: J. Endod., *9*:147, 1983.
23. Orban, B.: J. Period., *10*:39, 1939.
24. Peters, D.D.: J. Endod., *6*:518, 1980.
25. Ray, G.E.: Br. Dent. J., *99*:263, 1955.
26. Reddish, G.F.: Antiseptics, Disinfectants, Fungi-

cides and Sterilization. Philadelphia, Lea & Febiger, 1954, p. 703.

27. Sanderson, E.A.: J. Lab. Clin. Med., *7*:360, 1922.
28. Senia, E.S., et al.: J. Endod., *1*:136, 1975.
29. Segall, R.O., et al.: Oral Surg., *44*:786, 1977.
30. Taintor, J.F., and Biesterfeld, R.C.: J. Endod., *4*:254, 1978.
31. Trebitsch, F.: J. Dent. Res., *46*:1302, 1967.
32. Windeler, A.S., and Walter, R.G.: J. Endod., *1*:273, 1975.

10 Anatomy of the Pulp Cavity

"Of all the phases of anatomic study in the human system, one of the most complex is that of pulp cavity morphology."[1] Variations in the external morphologic features of the crowns of teeth accord with variations in the shape and size of the head. The length of the crown varies with the size and sex of the person and is generally shorter in females than in males. As the external morphology of the tooth varies from person to person, so does the internal morphology of the crown and root. Changes in pulp cavity anatomy result from age, disease, and trauma. Although morphologic variations occur, clinical experience indicates that these changes usually follow a general pattern, and thus the study of pulp cavity morphology is a feasible undertaking.

The pulp cavity is the central cavity within a tooth and is entirely enclosed by dentin except at the apical foramen (Fig. 10–1). The pulp cavity may be divided into a coronal portion, the pulp chamber, and a radicular portion, the root canal. In anterior teeth, the pulp chamber gradually merges into the root canal, and this division becomes indistinct. In multirooted teeth, the pulp cavity consists of a single pulp chamber and usually three root canals, although the number of canals can vary from one to five. The roof of the pulp chamber consists of dentin covering the pulp chamber occlusally or incisally (Fig. 10–1). A pulp horn is an accentuation of the roof the pulp chamber directly under a cusp or developmental lobe. The term refers more commonly to the prolongation of the pulp itself directly under a cusp. The floor of the pulp chamber runs parallel to the roof and consists of dentin bounding the pulp chamber near the cervix of the tooth, particularly dentin forming the furcation area. The canal orifices are openings in the floor of the pulp chamber leading into the root canals. The canal orifices are not separate structures, but are continuous with both pulp chamber and root canals. The walls of a pulp chamber derive their names from the corresponding walls of the tooth surface, such as the buccal wall of a pulp chamber. The angles of a pulp chamber derive their names from the walls forming the angle, such as the mesiobuccal angle of a pulp chamber.

The root canal is that portion of the pulp cavity from the canal orifice to the apical foramen. It may be divided for convenience into three sections, namely: coronal, middle, and apical thirds. Accessory canals, or lateral canals, are lateral branchings of the main root canal generally occurring in the apical third or furcation area of a root (Fig. 10–1). A distinction sometimes made between an accessory canal and a lateral canal is that a lateral canal is an accessory canal that branches to the lateral surface of the root and may be visible on a radiograph. The apical foramen is an aperture at or near the apex of a root through which the blood vessels and nerves of the pulp enter or leave the pulp cavity. Accessory foramina are the openings of the accessory and lateral canals in the root surface (Fig. 10–1).

ANATOMY OF THE PULP CAVITY

Much of the knowledge of the anatomy of root canals is based on the exhaustive work of Hess.[27] He made vulcanite corrosion preparations of almost 3000 permanent teeth. These preparations showed in minute detail the extensions, ramifications, and branchings as well as the shape, size, and number of root canals in the different teeth. Through the years, subsequent anatomic studies have also contributed to our knowledge of the anatomy of the pulp cavity.[1,15,25,28,54,63,77]

Root Canals

A straight root canal extending the entire length of the root is uncommon (Fig. 10–2). Either a constriction is present before the apex is reached or, as is often the case, a curvature is present. The curvature may be a gradual curvature of the entire canal, a sharp curvature of the canal near the apex,

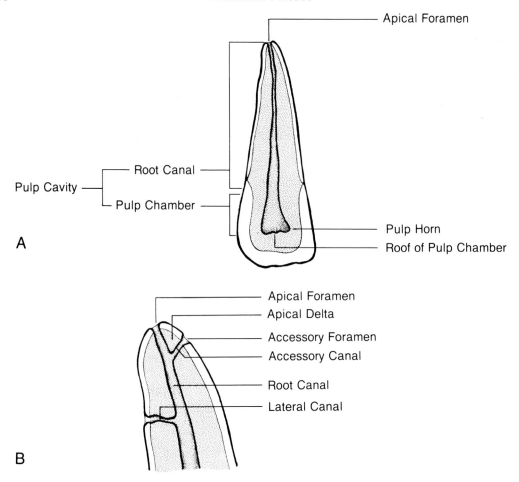

Fig. 10–1. Various views of the root canal system. *A*, Labial view of a central incisor. *B*, Apical third of a root.

or a gradual curvature of the canal with a straight apical ending. Double curvatures in the form of the letter "S" may also occur. A curvature of about 20° in a narrow root canal may be difficult or even impossible to negotiate with endodontic instruments, whereas a curvature of even 30° may be negotiated if the root canal is wide. Success in negotiating a narrow, curved canal depends on the degree of curvature, the size and constriction of the root canal, the size and flexibility of the endodontic instrument blade, and, most important, the skill of the operator.

In most cases, the number of root canals corresponds with the number of roots, but a root may have more than one canal. The mesial root of the mandibular first molar almost always has two canals, which sometimes meet in a common foramen; the distal root of the mandibular first molar occasionally has two canals; the mesiobuccal root of the maxillary first molar sometimes has two

canals; and even the pulp cavity of a mandibular anterior or premolar tooth may be bifurcated, to present two separate root canals. These variations can be classified as: one canal exiting as one canal, two canals exiting as two canals, two canals exiting as one canal, and one canal exiting as two canals (bifurcated canal)[22] (Fig. 10–3). Many other configurations occur in these roots, such as ribbon-shaped canals, and "C-shaped" canals, but those previously mentioned are the most common.

Apical Foramen

In young, incompletely developed teeth the apical foramen is funnel shaped, with the wider portion extending outward. The mouth of the funnel is filled with periodontal tissue that is later replaced by dentin and cementum. As the root develops, the apical foramen becomes narrower (see Figs. 10–1 and 10–2). The inner surface of the root apex becomes lined with cementum, which may

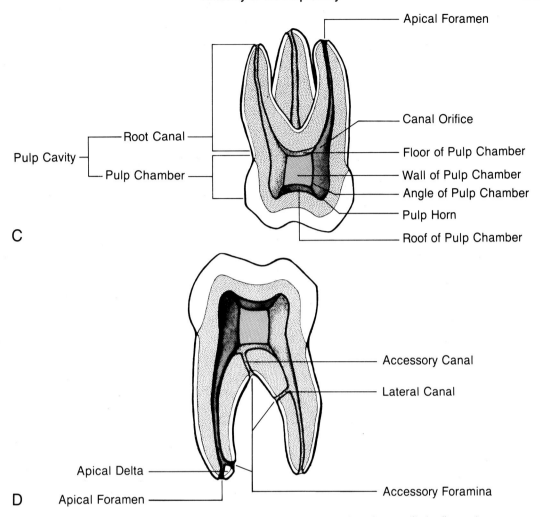

Apical Foramen

Root Canal

Pulp Cavity

Pulp Chamber

Canal Orifice

Floor of Pulp Chamber

Wall of Pulp Chamber

Angle of Pulp Chamber

Pulp Horn

Roof of Pulp Chamber

C

Accessory Canal

Lateral Canal

Apical Delta

Apical Foramen

Accessory Foramina

D

Fig. 10–1 Continued.　*C*, Buccal view of a maxillary first molar. *D*, Buccal view of a mandibular first molar.

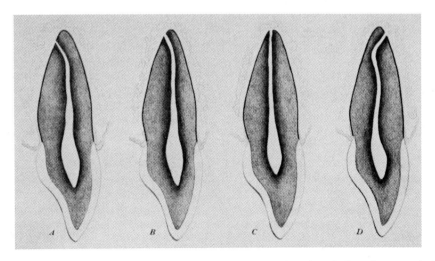

Fig. 10–2.　Various courses taken by root canals and locations of apical foramina. *A*, Curved root canal with the apical foramen distant from the root apex. *B*, Curved root canal with the foramen near the apex. *C*, Constricted root canal as the apical foramen is approached. *D*, Double curvature of the root canal with the foramen at a distance from the root apex.

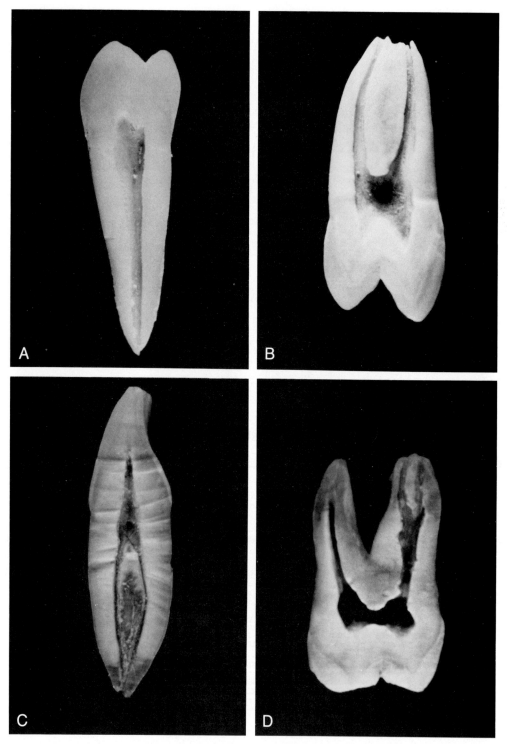

Fig. 10–3. Root canal systems. *A*, Mandibular cuspid with one canal exiting as one canal. *B*, Maxillary first premolar with two canals exiting as two canals. *C*, Mandibular incisor with two canals exiting as one canal. *D*, Mesiobuccal root of a maxillary first molar with one canal exiting as two canals.

even extend for a short distance (1 mm or so) into the root canal. The dentinocemental junction, therefore, does not necessarily occur at the extreme end of the root, but may occur within the main root canal. Consequently, it is not necessary to clean, shape, or fill root canals to their anatomic apices, but rather to the dentinocemental junction, which usually lies within the canal just short of the apex.[24] Because the location of the dentinocemental junction varies in the root canal, filling to this level is more often accomplished by accident than by intent.

The apical foramen is not always the most constricted portion of the root canal. Constrictions can and do occur before the extremity of the root is reached. Apical constrictions are found 0.5 to 1.0 mm away from the root apex.[12]

The apical foramen is not always located in the center of the root apex. It may exit on the mesial, distal, labial, or lingual surface of the root, usually slightly eccentrically (Fig. 10–4). Anatomic studies have shown that the apical foramen coincides within the anatomic apex in only 17 to 46% of cases and it is located an average of 0.4 to 0.7 mm away

from the anatomic apex. In a few cases, the apical foramen has been found as much as 2 to 3 mm away from the anatomic apex.[8,9,20,52,74] These studies have led to the recommendation that root canal obturation should end approximately 0.5 mm from the root anatomic apex as seen in the radiograph.

A knowledge of the age at which calcification of the root apex occurs is essential for endodontic practice, particularly when dealing with pulp-involved or pulpless teeth of children and young persons. As a general rule, a root apex is completely formed about 2 to 3 years after eruption of the tooth. Table 10–1 gives the approximate time in years of eruption of the teeth and calcification of the root apices. Endodontic treatment of young teeth does not affect normal eruption.[31]

Lateral Canals and Accessory Foramina

Lateral canals and accessory foramina have been found with enough regularity to prove that they are integral parts of a normal pulp cavity rather than exceptions (Figs. 10–4 and 10–5). The periodontal vessels curve around the root apex of a developing tooth and often become entrapped in Hertwig's epithelial

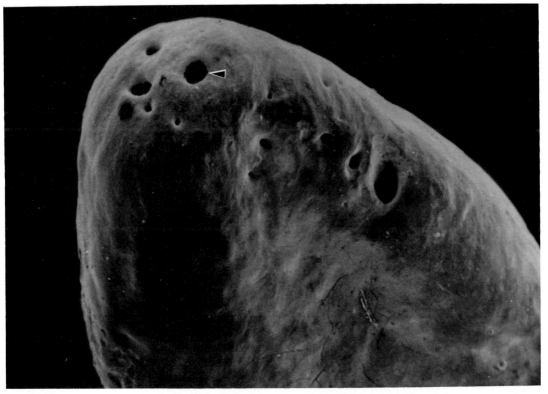

Fig. 10–4. Scanning electron micrograph of the apex of the mesial root of a maxillary first molar, showing the apical foramen (arrow) and multiple accessory foramina. (Courtesy of J. M. Brady, Washington, D.C.)

Table 10–1. Ages of Tooth Eruption and Calcification of Root Apices (in years)

	Central Incisor	Lateral Incisor	Cuspid	First Premolar	Second Premolar	First Molar	Second Molar
Eruption	6–8	7–9	10–12	9–11	11–12	5–7	12–13
Calcification	10–12	11–12	13–14	12–14	13–14	10–11	15–16

root sheath, with resulting formation of lateral canals and accessory foramina during calcification.[14] That this phenomenon frequently occurs in the apical third of the root explains the high incidence of lateral canals and accessory foramina in this region.[16] Lateral canals may occur also in the area of bifurcation or trifurcation of multirooted teeth.[68] These canals result from the entrapment of the periodontal vessels during the fusion of the parts of the diaphragm that become the floor of the pulp chamber.[14] The reported incidence of lateral canals ranges from 27.4 to 35.5%.[16,68] One researcher found lateral canals in the bifurcation or trifurcation areas of premolars and molars in 2.3% of the sample,[16] whereas another found them in 9.45%.[68]

One may well ask whether root canal therapy is justified in view of the complexity of the root canal system, because, by current methods, no one can clean and obturate all minute ramifications. Studies of a large number of serial sections of root apices showed that "many canals seen in the apical region in individual sections, both ground and decalcified, do not communicate directly with the pulp cavity. Many of them are imbedded vessels, their looping being plainly demonstrated in serial sections. Sometimes such looping arises from and terminates in the pulpal wall."[46] Moreover, "microscopic findings on extracted teeth with clinically well-filled, uninfected main canals prove that nature takes care of the remaining unfilled lateral branches and apical ramifications. All these fine canals remain vital after the pulp has been removed from the main canal and form cementum which eventually may completely obliterate the lateral canals."[34]

Much importance has been assigned to the

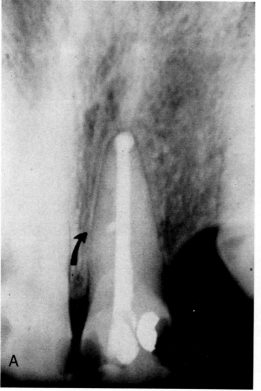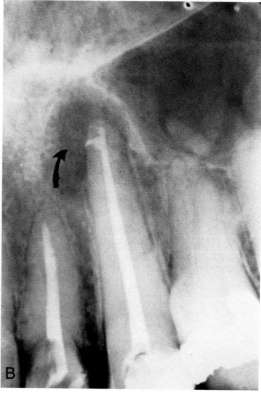

Fig. 10–5. *A*, Accessory canal filled in an upper central incisor. *B*, Accessory canal filled in an upper cuspid.

accessory foramina with regard to endodontic treatment. Such foramina are lined with cementum and in some cases lie entirely within the cementum. Pulp tissue, however, lies within a dentinal enclosure of the accessory or lateral canal. When the pulp is removed, the blood vessels lying within the accessory or lateral canals are sealed or obliterated by cementum unless injury occurs, whether mechanical, chemical, or bacterial. With increasing age, the number of accessory foramina normally diminishes because of calcification of their contained soft tissue.

Age

The size and shape of the pulp cavity are influenced by age (Fig. 10–6). In the young person, pulp horns are long, pulp chambers are large, root canals are wide, apical foramina are broad, and dentinal tubules are wide, regular, and are filled with protoplasmic fluid. With increasing age, pulp horns recede, pulp chambers become smaller in height rather than in width, and root canals become narrower from deposition of secondary and reparative dentin. Moreover, apical foramina deviate from the exact anatomic apex, and their minor diameter becomes narrower while their major diameter becomes wider from the deposition of dentin and cementum. Dentinal tubules become narrower or even obliterated by the deposition of peritubular dentin forming sclerotic dentin, and they lose their regularity and become tortuous. Reparative dentin may be devoid of dentinal tubules, and the moisture content of the dentin is reduced.

TOOTH ANATOMY AND ITS RELATION TO THE PREPARATION OF ACCESS OPENINGS

Maxillary Central Incisor

Average Tooth Length. The average length of this tooth is 21.8 mm.[54]

Pulp Chamber. The pulp chamber of the maxillary central incisor is located in the center of the crown equidistant from the dentinal walls (Figs. 10–7 and 10–8). It is broad mesiodistally, with its broadest part incisally. The pulp chamber usually follows the contours of the crown and has three pulp horns that correspond to the developmental mamelons in a young tooth. The chamber is ovoid mesiodistally. The division between root canal and pulp chamber is indistinct.

Root and Root Canal. The maxillary central incisor has one root with one root canal. The root canal is broad labiopalatally, large and simple in outline, conical in shape, and centrally located. A definite apical constriction is present in the mature root canal. In cross section, the canal is ovoid mesiodistally in the cervical third, ovoid to almost

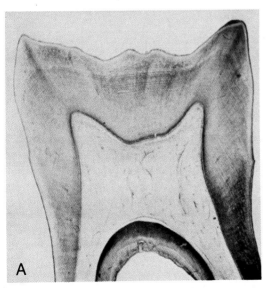 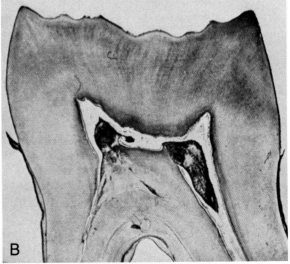

Fig. 10–6. Reductions in the size of the pulp chamber with age. Note that the greatest change is in the height of the pulp chamber, not the mesiodistal width. Note also the decrease in cellular elements of the pulp and the formation of pulp stones with aging of the tooth. *A,* Eight years of age. *B,* Fifty-five years. (From Kronfeld, R.: Histopathology of the Teeth. Philadelphia, Lea & Febiger, 1939.)

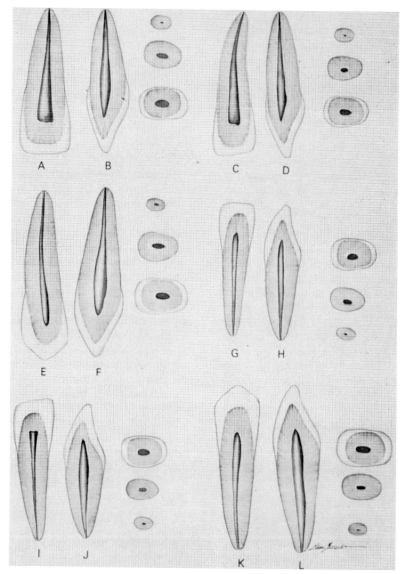

Fig. 10–7. Mesiodistal, labiolingual, cervical, midroot, and apical cross-section views of maxillary central incisors (A and B), maxillary lateral incisors (C and D), maxillary cuspids (E and F), mandibular central incisors (G and H), mandibular lateral incisors (I and J), and mandibular cuspids (K and L).

round in the middle third, and round in the apical third. Lateral canals may be present (24% of specimens), usually in the apical third.[68]

Although the majority of the roots are straight (75%), some may curve distally (8%), mesially (4%), palatally (4%), or labially (9%).[30] The root canal usually follows the direction of the curved root. The palatal and labial curvatures may not be seen in a routine radiograph, unless, radiographs are taken at different horizontal angulations.

The apical foramen is centrally located in the anatomic apex in only 12% of cases, and an apical delta is present in 1% of cases.[68]

Anatomic Relationships in Situ. The labial surface of the root of the maxillary central incisor lies under the labial cortical plate of the maxilla and may fuse with it. Because of the proximity of the labial root surface to the cortical plate, fenestrations and dehiscences may be present, and abscesses may perforate the labial cortical plate. The relationship between the apex of the maxillary central incisor and the osseous plate in the floor of the nasal cavity depends on the height of the face and the length of the root.

Usually, the nasal fossa and the root apex are separated sufficiently that curettage of granulomatous tissue within the surround-

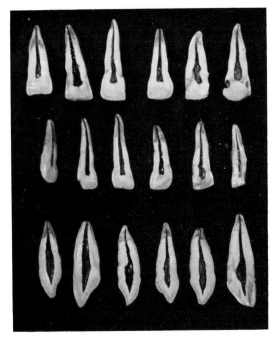

Fig. 10–8. Longitudinal section of maxillary incisors and cuspid teeth showing variations in length, width, and contour of root canals. (Mesiodistal section of incisors and labiolingual section of canine teeth.)

ing cancellous bone does not result in perforation of the floor of the nasal fossa. In some patients, the apex of the root is close to the nasal floor, so an abscess may drain into the nasal fossa or a cyst may bulge into the inferior nasal meatus.[19]

The maxillary central incisor has an average of 2° of mesioaxial inclination and an average of 29° of palatoaxial angulation in its alveolus.[18] The incisive canal parallels the long axis of the maxillary central incisor. The long axis of the tooth serves as a guide for the palatine injection; one should align the barrel of the anesthetic syringe parallel to the tooth and insinuate the needle alongside the papilla.

Access Opening. The shape, size, and coronal extension of the pulp chamber are estimated from the diagnostic radiograph. The internal anatomic structure of the pulp chamber of the maxillary central incisor dictates the shape and size of the access opening.

The enamel is penetrated in the center of the lingual surface at an angle perpendicular to it with a No. 4 round bur in a high-speed contra-angle (Fig. 10–9, A and B). After penetration of the enamel, a No. 4 round carbide bur in a slow-speed contra-angle is directed along the long axis of the tooth until the pulp chamber is reached (Fig. 10–9, C). A "drop" of the bur into the chamber may be felt if the chamber is large enough. The overhanging enamel and dentin of the lingual roof of the pulp chamber are removed, including the pulp horns, with a No. 4 round bur in a slow-speed contra-angle by working from the inside to the outside following the internal anatomy (Fig. 10–9, D). This procedure makes the access cavity walls confluent with the lateral and incisal walls of the pulp chamber and renders the access cavity a lingual extension of the pulp chamber, with a "straight-line" penetration to the apical root canal.

A Gates Glidden drill of appropriate size (usually No. 4) is used to remove the lingual shoulder by working from inside out with light strokes. The lingual shoulder is not an anatomic entity itself, but rather is a prominence of dentin created when the lingual roof is removed (Fig. 10–9, E). By removing the lingual roof and the lingual shoulder of the pulp chamber in an anterior tooth, one gains direct access to the apical area of the root canal (Fig. 10–9, F). Direct access can be verified by placing the straight end of the endodontic explorer into the canal orifice. The explorer should follow the path of the canal without impedance from the walls of the surrounding access preparation.

The shape of the access outline form for all anterior teeth should reflect the shape of the internal anatomic structure of the coronal pulp chamber of each tooth. In maxillary incisors, the access shape is slightly triangular, with the base of the triangle toward the incisal edge (Fig. 10–9, G and H).

The usual anatomic structure of the chamber and root canal in any tooth can be altered by the deposition of reparative or secondary dentin, a response often associated with trauma, caries, restorative procedures, or aging. The pulp chambers of these teeth may be reduced in size or completely calcified. Access preparations can be made as described previously, with the following modifications: Penetrate the enamel in the center of the lingual surface of the tooth at an angle perpendicular to it with a No. 2 round carbide bur in a high-speed contra-angle. After penetration of the enamel, change to a No. 2 round carbide bur in a slow-speed contra-angle, and direct the bur along the long axis of the tooth until the reduced pulp chamber is reached. Enlarge the enamel

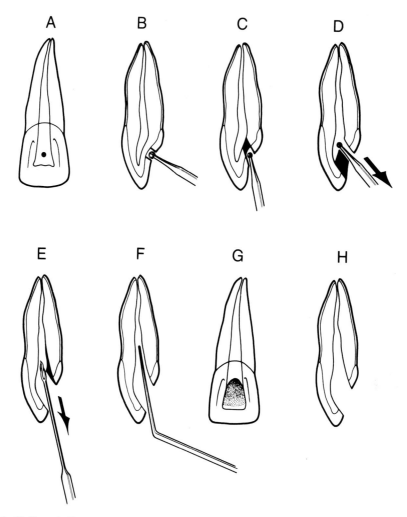

Fig. 10–9. *A,* to *H,* Steps in the access opening of a maxillary central incisor.

portion of the access cavity to an ovoid shape with the greatest diameter incisogingivally. Change to an appropriate-size Gates Glidden drill (No. 3 or 4), and working from the inside to the outside of the chamber, funnel the dentinal walls. The access preparation is completed when it is funnel shaped, smooth, and continuous with the radicular portion of the pulp cavity, and when it provides straight-line access to the apical third of the root canal.[17]

Maxillary Lateral Incisor

Average Tooth Length. The average length of this tooth is 23.1 mm.[54]

Pulp Chamber. The shape of the pulp chamber of the maxillary lateral incisor is similar to that of the maxillary central incisor but smaller (see Fig. 10–7). It only has two pulp horns, corresponding to the developmental mamelons. It is broad mesiodistally, with its broadest part incisally. The division between root canal and pulp chamber is indistinct.

Root and Root Canal. The configuration of the root canal of the maxillary lateral incisor is also conical, but it has a finer diameter than the maxillary central incisor and, occasionally, may have a fine constriction in its course toward the apex. In cross section, the canal is ovoid labiopalatally in the cervical third because of the flatness of the root, ovoid in the middle third, and round in the apical third. Lateral canals occur more frequently in these teeth (26%) than in maxillary central incisors.[68]

The majority of roots have a distal curve (53%), whereas others are straight (30%).

Other roots may curve mesially (3%), palatally (4%), labially (4%), or have an "S-shape" or bayonet curve (6%).[54] The root canal usually follows the direction of the curvature of the root. The apical foramen is centrally located in the anatomic apex in 22% of cases, and an apical delta is present in only 3% of cases.[68]

Anatomic Relationships in Situ. As with the central incisor, the labial surface of the root of the maxillary lateral incisor lies under the labial cortical plate of the maxilla; therefore, fenestrations and dehiscences may be present. As this root curves distally, it may be in the center of the cancellous bone pointing toward the palate, and abscesses arising in this area may drain palatally as well as labially.[19]

The maxillary lateral incisor has an average of 16° of mesioaxial inclination and an average of 29° of palatoaxial angulation in its alveolus.[18]

Access Opening. The access opening for the maxillary lateral incisor is similar to that for the maxillary central incisor, but it is smaller and usually more ovoid. The technique for entry is the same as for the maxillary central incisor, except a No. 2 round bur may be used instead of a No. 4.

Anomalies. The developmental anomaly of dens invaginatus occurs frequently in the maxillary lateral incisor. Also possible is underdevelopment of this tooth, in the form of a "peg lateral," or overdevelopment of the dental tubercle on the lingual surface, the so called "talon cusp." These anatomic anomalies require modifications in the access openings.

Maxillary Cuspid

Average Tooth Length. The average length of this tooth is 26 mm, the longest of human teeth. A specimen 33.5 mm in length has been reported.[54]

Pulp Chamber. The pulp chambers of the maxillary cuspids are the largest of any single-rooted teeth (see Figs. 10–7 and 10–8). Labiopalatally, the chamber is triangular in shape, with the apex toward the single cusp and a broad base in the cervical third of the crown. Mesiodistally, it is narrow, sometimes resembling a flame. In cross section, the chamber is ovoid in shape, with the greater diameter labiopalatally. Only one pulp horn is present, corresponding to one cusp. The division between the pulp chamber and the root canal is indistinct.

Root and Root Canal. The single root canal of the maxillary cuspid is larger than that of the maxillary incisor. It is wider in labiopalatal than in mesiodistal dimension, and on reaching the middle third, it tapers gradually to an apical constriction.

In cross section, the root canal is ovoid in the cervical and middle thirds and generally round in the apical third. Lateral canals are present in 30% of cases.[68]

One report noted straight roots in 39% of cases, whereas in 32% the root curved distally, in 7% it curved palatally, and in 13% it curved labially; 7% had an "S" or bayonet shape, and 2% had dilacerations.[30]

The apical foramen is centrally located in the anatomic apex in 14% of cases, and an apical delta is present in only 3%.[68] In some patients, the apex of the root may be fine and tapered. These roots are difficult to see radiographically, and if the apex undergoes endodontic instrumentation without a consideration of the apical thinness, the apex can be destroyed.

Anatomic Relationships in Situ. The root of the maxillary cuspid is positioned in the cancellous bone of the maxilla between the nasal cavity and the maxillary sinus, called the canine pillar. The labial surface of the root lies under the labial cortical plate and may fuse with it. Because of its great size, it causes the most prominent bulge in the maxilla, called the alveolar or canine eminence. The size and proximity of the root to the cortical plate may produce fenestrations and dehiscences in that plate.

An abscess originating in the maxillary cuspid usually perforates the labial cortical plate below the insertion of the levator muscles of the upper lip and drains into the buccal vestibule. If the perforation occurs above this insertion, the abscess will drain into the canine space and will cause cellulitis.[19]

Apical curettage may be difficult during periradicular procedures because of the length of the tooth. The maxillary cuspid tooth has an average of 6° distoaxial inclination and an average of 21° of palatoaxial angulation in its alveolus.[18]

Access Opening. The access opening for the maxillary cuspid is basically the same as for the maxillary central and lateral incisors. The only variation is that the shape of the access opening is ovoid, as dictated by pulp chamber anatomy. The technique for entry is the same as for the maxillary central and lateral incisors (Fig. 10–10).

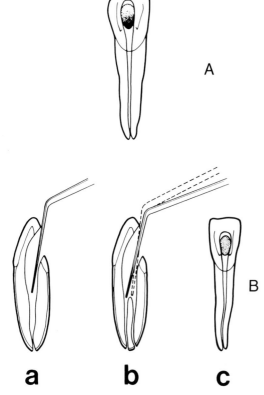

Fig. 10–10. Access opening. *A,* Maxillary cuspid tooth. *B,* Mandibular incisors (a, b, c).

Anomalies. The maxillary cuspid has two roots in rare cases.

Maxillary First Premolar

Average Tooth Length. The average length of this tooth is 21.5 mm.[54]

Pulp Chamber. The pulp chamber of the maxillary first premolar is narrow mesiodistally. It has a pulp horn under each cusp, but both may be missed in routine radiographic projections because of superimposition of one over the other (Figs. 10–11 and 10–12). It is wide buccopalatally, and the buccal pulp horn is more prominent than the palatal in young teeth. The roof of the pulp chamber is coronal to the cervical line. The floor of the pulp chamber is convex, usually with two canal orifices, one buccal and the other palatal, and it lies deep in the coronal third of the root below the cervical line. In cross section, the pulp chamber is wide and ovoid in a buccopalatal dimension.[23]

Roots and Root Canals. The maxillary first premolar has 2 roots in 54.6% of cases (Table 10–2). In 21.9% of the double-rooted cases, the roots are separated, whereas in 32.7%,

the roots are partially fused. Of the total cases in this study, 43% have 1 root and 2.4% have 3 roots. When 2 roots are present, they may diverge as much as 25% from each other.[54]

Regardless of whether maxillary first premolars have 1 or 2 roots, they have 2 root canals at the apex in 69% of cases.[68] When fused roots occur, a groove running in an occlusoapical direction divides the root into buccal and palatal portions, each containing a single root canal. The palatal canal is generally the larger of the 2 canals, it is directly under the palatal cusp, and its orifice can be penetrated by following the palatal wall of the pulp chamber.[23] The buccal canal is directly under the buccal cusp, and its orifice can be penetrated by following the buccal wall of the pulp chamber.[23]

Twenty-six percent of these teeth have only a single root canal at the apex. Of these 26%, only 8% have 1 canal orifice at the pulp chamber and 1 canal exiting at the apex, whereas 18% have 2 orifices in the pulp chamber floor that coalesce to form a single canal at the apex.[68] Transverse channels between the canals are common. In a tooth with a single canal through the length of the root, the canal is ovoid in shape, wider buccopalatally than mesiodistally in the cervical and middle thirds and round in the apical third. When 2 root canals are present, the cervical thirds are ovoid in shape, at midroot they are almost round, and in the apical third they are round and small. Lateral canals may be present in 49.5% of cases, with 11% found in the furcation between the buccal and palatal roots.[68]

In teeth with a single root, the majority of the roots are straight (38.4%), almost an equal number have a distal curve (36.8%), and some curve buccally (14.4%), palatally (2.4%), or have an "S" or bayonet shape (8%).[54] In double-rooted maxillary premolars, the buccal roots are straight in 27.8%, have a buccal curve in 14%, have a palatal curve in 36.2%, have a distal curve in 14%, and have an "S" or bayonet shape in 8% of cases. The palatal roots are straight in 44.4%, have a buccal curve in 27.8%, have a palatal curve in 8.3%, have a distal curve in 14%, and have an "S" or bayonet shape in 5.5% of cases.[54]

The apical foramina are centrally located in 12% of cases, and an apical delta is present only in 3.2% of cases.[68]

Anatomic Relationships in Situ. The maxillary first premolar lies in its alveolar socket below the maxillary sinus and is separated

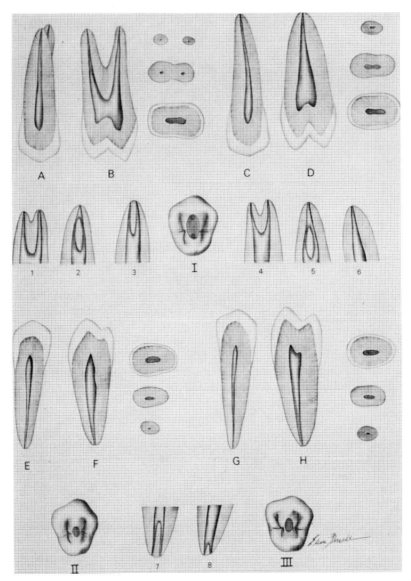

Fig. 10–11. Mesiodistal, buccolingual, cervical, midroot, and apical cross-sectional views of maxillary first premolars (A and B), maxillary second premolars (C and D), mandibular first premolars (E and F), and mandibular second premolars (G and H). Variations in apical root canal anatomy of maxillary and mandibular premolars (1 to 8). Access openings for premolars (I, II, III).

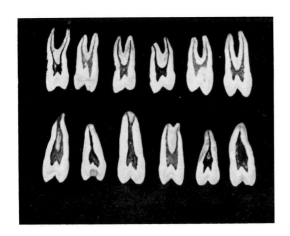

Fig. 10–12. Longitudinal section of maxillary first premolars (top row) and second premolars (bottom row). Note the variations in shape and size of the root canals. (Labiolingual view.)

Table 10–2. Root Canals and Apical Foramina in Maxillary First Premolars

Investigator	Year	Teeth Sample	Method	One Canal and One Foramen (%)	One Canal and Two Foramina (%)	Two Canals and One Foramen (%)	Two Canals and Two Foramina (%)	Three Canals (%)
Pineda and Kuttler[52]	1972	259	In vitro radiographs	26.2	7.7	23.9	41.7	0.5
Green[20]	1973	50	In vitro sections	8.0	—	26.0	66.0	—
Carns and Skidmore[11]	1973	100	In vitro resin casts	9.0	—	13.0	72.0	6.0
Vertucci and Gegauff[71]	1979	400	In vitro clear and dyed sections	8.0	7.0	18.0	62.0	5.0
Bellizzi and Hartwell[2]	1985	514	In vivo radiographs	6.2	—	—	90.5	3.3

(Courtesy of Drs. Gary R. Hartwell and Frank R. Portel of Fort Gordon, Georgia, and Drs. Thomas L. Walker and Carlos E. del Rio of San Antonio, Texas.)

from it by a thin layer of spongy and compact bone. The buccal surface of a single- or double-rooted maxillary first premolar is in close proximity to the buccal cortical plate. The proximity of these roots to the cortical plate may produce a fenestration or a dehiscence in that plate. The palatal root of the double-rooted specimen lies in spongy bone away from the palatal cortical plate.[19] The maxillary first premolar has an average of 10° of distoaxial inclination and an average of 6° of buccoaxial angulation in its alveolus.[18]

Access Opening. By measuring the shape, the size, and the extension of the pulp chamber mesially, distally, and coronally in the diagnostic radiograph, one can determine the approximate size, shape, depth, and location of the coronal access cavity to be prepared. The internal anatomic structure of the pulp chamber of the maxillary first premolar dictates the shape and size of the access opening (Fig. 10–13, A).

Using a No. 2 round carbide bur in a high-speed contra-angle, one penetrates the enamel in the center of the occlusal surface between the buccal and lingual cusps, and the bur is directed into the long axis of the tooth (Fig. 10–13, B). Then a No. 2 round carbide bur in a slow-speed contra-angle, aligned in the long axis of the tooth, is used to penetrate through the dentin into the pulp chamber (Fig. 10–13, C). The operator frequently feels the bur "drop" into the pulp chamber when the chamber is large. Using the radiographic measurement, one penetrates deep enough to remove the roof of the pulp chamber without cutting into the chamber floor; one should avoid an access opening that is too shallow and exposes only the pulp horn tips, which

may appear to be root canal orifices (Fig. 10–13, H and I).

To remove the roof of the pulp chamber, one should place the bur alongside the walls of the chamber and cut occlusally (see Fig. 10–13, D). A tapered cylinder, self-limiting diamond* in a slow-speed contra-angle is used to remove the remaining roof of the pulp chamber (see Fig. 10–13, E). The walls of the access cavity are smoothed and are sloped slightly toward the occlusal surface with this diamond. The divergence of the access cavity walls creates a positive seat for the temporary filling, such as Cavit. The border of this ovoid access cavity should not extend beyond half the lingual incline of the facial cusp and half the facial incline of the palatal cusp (Fig. 10–13, F).

The access cavity preparation for endodontic treatment of a premolar differs from Black's cavity preparation for an occlusal restoration (Class I). In Black's preparation, the ovoid shape runs mesiodistally and encompasses all pits and fissures, whereas the endodontic preparation runs ovoid in a buccolingual direction and permits direct access to the root canal, especially the buccal and lingual canal orifices when more than one canal is present (see Fig. 10–13, G).

Any loose debris is removed by irrigating the access cavity with a 5.2% sodium hypochlorite solution. Excess sodium hypochlorite is removed by suction or is absorbed with 2 × 2 gauze sponges. The pulp chamber should be suctioned dry to permit unimpeded observation of the pulpal floor. The anatomic dark lines in the pulpal floor

*RA, CU3, ½L, Blu-White, Densco, Denver, Colorado.

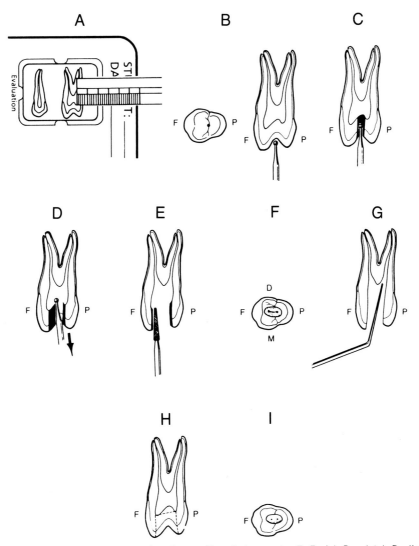

Fig. 10–13. *A* to *I*, Steps in the access opening of a maxillary first premolar. F, Facial; P, palatal; D, distal; M, mesial.

(dentinal map) should be examined and followed with an endodontic explorer to identify the orifices. The orifice of the buccal canal lies beneath the buccal cusp, and the orifice of the palatal canal lies beneath the palatal cusp.[17]

Anomalies. The maxillary first premolar in rare cases has three root canals.[71]

Maxillary Second Premolar

Average Tooth Length. The average length of this tooth is 21.6 mm.[54]

Pulp Chamber. The maxillary second premolar, like the maxillary first premolar, has a narrow chamber mesiodistally showing one pulp horn superimposed over another when it is viewed in this projection (see Figs. 10–11 and 10–12). It is wider buccopalatally than

the maxillary first premolar and shows two pulp horns in this projection, a buccal and a palatal. The roof of the pulp chamber is similar to that of the maxillary first premolar, but the pulp floor is deeper if two canals are present. If one root canal is present, the root canal orifices will be indistinct, but if two canals are present, two distinct orifices will be visible. In cross section, the pulp chamber has a narrow, ovoid shape.[23]

Root and Root Canals. Maxillary second premolars have only a single root in 90.3% of patients (Table 10–3). Only 2% have 2 well-developed roots, whereas 7.7% have 2 roots that are partially fused.[54] The roots are straight in 37.4% of patients; 33.9% have a distal curve, 15.7% have a buccal curve, and 13% have an "S" or bayonet shape.[54]

Table 10–3. Root Canals and Apical Foramina in Maxillary Second Premolars

Investigator	Year	Teeth Sample	Method	One Canal and One Foramen (%)	One Canal and Two Foramina (%)	Two Canals and One Foramen (%)	Two Canals and Two Foramina (%)	Three Canals (%)
Pineda and Kuttler[52]	1972	282	In vitro radiographs	62.8	8.9	19.0	9.3	—
Green[20]	1973	50	In vitro sections	72.0	—	24.0	4.0	—
Vertucci and colleagues[73]	1974	200	In vitro clear and dyed sections	48.0	—	27.0	24.0	1.0
Bellizzi and Hartwell[2]	1985	630	In vivo radiographs	40.3	—	—	58.6	1.1

(Courtesy of Drs. Gary R. Hartwell and Frank B. Portel of Fort Gordon, Georgia, and Drs. Thomas L. Walker and Carlos E. del Rio of San Antonio, Texas.)

One canal is usually present at the apex in about 75% of cases.[73] When 2 canals occur, they may be distinct and separated along the entire length of the root, or they may converge to form a common canal as they approach the apex. Straight canals are found in only 9.5% of these teeth.[73] The majority of canals are curved. They may curve distally, buccally, palatally, mesiodistally, or buccopalatally.[73]

Lateral canals are present in 59.5% of cases; 1.6% occur in the furcation area if 2 roots are present.[68]

In cross section, the canals in the cervical third are ovoid and narrow. In the middle third, when 1 canal is present it is ovoid, and when 2 canals are present they are round; in the apical third, the cross section is round regardless of whether 1 or 2 canals are present. The apical foramen is centrally located in 12% of cases, and an apical delta is present in only 3.2% of cases.[68]

Anatomic Relationships in Situ. The root or roots of the maxillary second premolar are situated below and therefore closer to the maxillary sinus than the maxillary cuspid. The sinus may dip down and surround the tip of the root or roots forming prominences in the sinus floor. The separation between the roots and the sinus may be a thin layer of bone, or bone may be completely absent leaving only the periodontal ligament and the schneiderian membrane of the sinus.[19]

The maxillary second premolar has an average of 19° of distoaxial inclination and an average of 9° of palatoaxial angulation in its alveolus.[18]

Access Opening. The access opening for the maxillary second premolar is basically the same as for the maxillary first premolar.

It is varied only as dictated by the anatomic structure of the pulp chamber.

Anomalies. The maxillary second premolar in rare cases has three root canals.[73]

Maxillary First Molar

Average Tooth Length. The average length of this tooth is 21.3 mm.[54]

Pulp Chamber. The pulp chamber of the maxillary first molar is the largest in the dental arch, with four pulp horns: mesiobuccal, distobuccal, mesiopalatal, and distopalatal (Figs. 10–14 and 10–15). The arrangement of the four pulp horns gives the pulpal roof a rhomboidal shape in cross section. The four walls forming the roof converge toward the floor where the lingual wall almost disappears; the floor of the pulp chamber thus has a triangular form in cross section. The orifices of the root canals are located in the three angles of the floor. Anatomic dark lines in the floor of the pulp chamber connect the orifices.

The palatal orifice is the largest, round or oval in shape and easily accessible for exploration (see Fig. 10–14, C). The mesiobuccal orifice is under the mesiobuccal cusp, is long buccopalatally, and may have a depression at the palatal end in which the orifice of a fourth canal may be present. The mesiobuccal orifice is located by insinuating the tip of a long-shank explorer, Starlite D-11, in a mesiobucco-apical inclination into the point angle created at the juncture of the buccal wall, mesial wall, and subpulpal floor of the pulp chamber. The distobuccal orifice is located slightly distal and palatal to the mesiobuccal orifice and is accessible from the mesial for exploration. The floor of the pulp chamber is in the cervical third of the

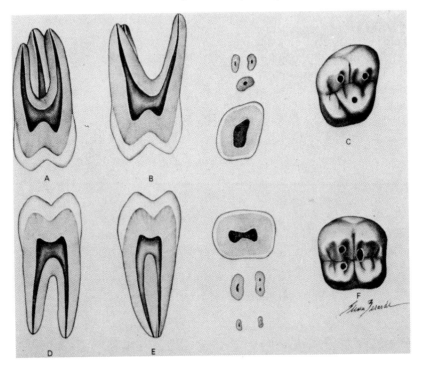

Fig. 10–14. Mesiodistal, buccolingual, and cross-sectional views of a maxillary molar (A and B) and a mandibular molar (D and E), with phantom views of root canal orifices (C and F). The mesial root canals are often located more mesially than shown.

root, and the roof is in the cervical third of the crown.

Roots and Root Canals. The maxillary first molar has 3 roots with, usually, 3 canals situated mesiobuccally, distobuccally and palatally (Table 10–4). The mesiobuccal root is broad in the buccopalatal direction. The majority of the mesiobuccal roots have a distal curve (78%), but some are straight (21%)

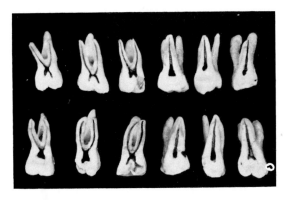

Fig. 10–15. Longitudinal sections of maxillary first and second molar teeth. The first three teeth in a row show the mesiobuccal and distobuccal root canals, and the last three teeth in a row show the palatal canal. (Mesiodistal view.)

and some are "S" or bayonet shaped (1%).[30] The mesiobuccal root has 1 canal and 1 foramen in 64% of cases.[20] It is the narrowest of the 3 canals, flattened in a mesiodistal direction in the orifice but round in the apical third. The mesiobuccal canal is not always patent along its entire length and is divided to form a second root canal in 22% of cases.[20] Clinically, the orifice of the second canal is often difficult to find; when found, it may be difficult to enter even with the finest instrument. Two separate and distinct canals occur in 14% of these teeth[20] (Fig. 10–16). The mesiobuccal root has lateral canals in 1% of cases and apical deltas in 8%.[68] The apical foramen is centrally located in only 14% of cases.[68]

The distobuccal root is small and is more or less round in shape. It is straight in 54% of cases, has a distal curve in 17%, has a mesial curve in 19% and has an "S" or bayonet shape in 10% of cases.[30] The distobuccal root usually has a single root canal, which is a narrow, tapering canal sometimes flattened in a mesiodistal direction, but generally cone shaped, ending in a small, round canal in the apical third. Lateral canals are present in 36% of cases; apical deltas are present in only

Table 10—4.   Root Canals and Apical Foramina in Maxillary First Molars: Mesiobuccal Root

Investigator	Year	Teeth Sample	Method	One Canal and One Foramen (%)	One Canal and Two Foramina (%)	Two Canals and One Foramen (%)	Two Canals and Two Foramina (%)
Weine[76]	1969	208	In vitro sections	48.5	—	37.5	14.0
Pineda and Kuttler[52]	1972	262	In vitro radiographs	39.0	—	12.5	48.5
Pineda[51]	1973	245	In vitro radiographs	41.0	—	17.0	42.0
Seidberg and colleagues[57]	1973	100	In vitro sections	38.0	—	37.0	25.0
Pomeranz and Fishelberg[53]	1974	71	In vivo radiographs	72.0	—	17.0	11.0
Vertucci[68]	1985	100	In vitro clear and dyed sections	45.0	—	37.0	18.0

(Courtesy of Drs. Gary R. Hartwell and Frank B. Portel of Fort Gordon, Georgia, and Drs. Thomas L. Walker and Carlos E. del Rio of San Antonio, Texas.)

2%. The apical foramen is centrally located in only 19% of these teeth.[68]

The palatal root has the largest diameter and is the longest root of the maxillary first molar. It is straight in only 40% of cases. It may curve buccally (55%), mesially (4%), or distally (1%).[23] The operator must be aware that this root may curve in the apical third toward the buccal because such a curvature is not apparent radiographically. Failure to recognize such a curve may lead to perforation of the root if the instruments are not precurved during cleaning and shaping procedures. The palatal canal is ovoid mesio-distally and tapers toward the apex, where it becomes a small, round canal. Lateral canals are present in 40% of these roots, and apical deltas are only seen in 4%.[68] The apical foramen is centrally located in only 18% of cases.[68]

Lateral canals are present not only in the roots (45%), but also in the trifurcation (18%).[68] One may see a divergence of as much as 45° between the palatal and buccal roots.[23]

Anatomic Relationships in Situ. The maxillary first molar lies under the maxillary sinus. The fundus of the alveolar socket containing the root may protrude into the sinus and may produce a small, bony prominence in the floor of the sinus. As in the maxillary second premolar, bony defects in these small prominences may leave only the periodontal ligament and the mucoperiosteal lining of the sinus to separate the roots from the sinus cavity. This close relationship may produce soreness in the maxillary teeth due to maxillary sinusitis; conversely, infection of the sinus may result from pulpal disease.[19]

The divergence of the roots may permit the sinus floor to drop into the trifurcation. The divergence of the roots also brings the buccal surfaces of the mesiobuccal and distobuccal roots and the palatal surface of the palatal root into close proximity to the buccal and palatal cortical plates of bone, respectively. The proximity of the buccal roots to the cortical plate may produce fenestrations or dehiscences. Because of its divergence, the palatal root may extend toward the lateral area of the nasal floor.[19]

Access Opening. The internal anatomy of the pulp chamber of the maxillary first molar dictates the shape and size of the access opening. By determining the shape and size of the chamber, by measuring the extension of the pulp chamber mesially, distally, and coronally on the diagnostic radiograph, and by transposing these measurements to the tooth, one can estimate the approximate size, shape, depth, and location of the coronal access cavity to be prepared (Fig. 10–16, A).

The enamel is penetrated with a No. 4 round carbide bur in a high-speed contra-angle by positioning the instrument in the central fossa and angling it toward the palatal root (Fig. 10–16, B). The bur is directed toward the palatal canal, where the pulp chamber of this tooth is largest (Fig. 10–16, C).

After penetration of the enamel, one uses a No. 4 round carbide bur in a slow-speed contra-angle to penetrate the dentin; the bur is angled toward the palatal root until the pulp chamber is reached (Fig. 10–16, D). A

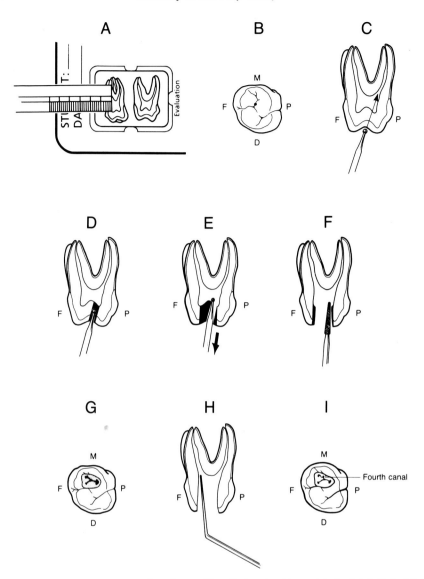

Fig. 10–16. *A* to *I*, Steps in the access opening of a maxillary first molar. M, mesial; D, distal; F, facial; P, palatal.

"drop" of the bur into the pulp chamber may be felt if the chamber is large. In partially calcified chambers, the drop of the bur is not felt, and the operator has to rely on the measurements made from the radiograph to avoid penetration beyond the chamber roof.

Cutting occlusally from within the pulp chamber, one removes the bulk of the roof of the pulp chamber (Fig. 10–16, *E*). The shape and size of the internal anatomy of the pulp chamber guide the cutting. A tapered-cylinder, self-limiting diamond in a slow-speed contra-angle is used to remove the remaining roof of the pulp chamber (Fig. 10–16, *F*). The walls of the access cavity are refined with this diamond to be divergent toward the

occlusal surface, and this divergence creates a positive seat for the temporary filling that prevents its displacement by occlusal forces.

The walls of the access cavity should be confluent with the walls of the pulp chamber and slightly divergent toward the occlusal surface. The access opening is usually triangular, with round corners extending toward, but not including, the mesiobuccal cusp tip, the marginal ridge, and the oblique ridge (Fig. 10–16, *G*). This triangular preparation permits direct access to the root canal orifices (Fig. 10–16, *H*).

Loose debris is removed by irrigation with a 5.2% solution of sodium hypochlorite. Excess sodium-hypochlorite solution is removed by suction or is absorbed with a 2 × 2 gauze. The pulp chamber should be suctioned dry for unimpeded examination of the floor. The anatomic dark lines in the pulpal floor (dentinal map) should be examined and followed with an endodontic explorer, to identify the orifices, as described previously. One should routinely search for a fourth orifice and canal that may be present in the mesiobuccal root[17] (Fig. 10–16, *J*).

Anomalies. Pulp stones may be present in the pulp chamber of the maxillary first molar. Such stones should be identified and removed during access preparation. The pulp stones are reduced in size by grinding and are removed with the help of the endodontic spoon excavator.

Rarely, a second canal is present in the palatal root.

Maxillary Second Molar

Average Tooth Length. The average length of this tooth is 21.7 mm.[54]

Pulp Chamber. The pulp chamber of the maxillary second molar is similar to that of the maxillary first molar, except it is narrower mesiodistally (see Fig. 10–15). Because of this narrower dimension, the roof of the pulp chamber is more rhomboidal in cross section, the floor of the pulp chamber is an obtuse triangle in cross section, and the mesiobuccal and distobuccal canals are closer together and may appear to have a common opening, but they are readily distinguishable from each other. Sometimes, all three canal orifices may be almost in a straight line.[23]

Roots and Root Canals. The maxillary second molar usually has 3 roots, which are closely grouped (Table 10–5). Because of this close grouping, the buccal roots may fuse, and occasionally all 3 roots fuse to form a single conical root. Studies have reported

this characteristic in 46% of cases.[30] The palatal root is usually straight, but in 37% of cases it has a buccal curve.[30] The mesiobuccal root usually curves distally; only 22% of these roots are straight.[30] The distal root is usually straight, but in 17% of cases it has a mesial curve.[30] If 3 roots are present, one usually sees 3 canals, with a fourth canal in the mesiobuccal root less frequently than in the maxillary first molar.[52] If the buccal roots fuse to form 1 buccal root, the tooth may have only 2 canals, 1 buccal and 1 palatal, although it is not unusual to find 3 canals. A tooth with only 1 root usually has only 1 conical root canal.[54]

Fewer lateral canals are present in the roots or in the furcation of the maxillary second molar than in the maxillary first molar. In only 16% of roots are the foramina centrally located, and only apical deltas are seen in 3% of roots.[68]

Anatomic Relationships in Situ. The maxillary second molar usually is more closely related to the maxillary sinus than the maxillary first molar.[19]

Access Opening. The maxillary second molar access opening is basically the same as for the maxillary first molar, with the variations that anatomic structure dictates.

Anomalies. The two most frequent anomalies in the maxillary second molar are the presence of only one root and one canal and the incidence of pulp stones in the pulp chamber.

Maxillary Third Molar

Average Tooth Length. The average length of this tooth is 17.1 mm.[54]

Pulp Chamber. The maxillary third molar anatomically resembles the second molar. The pulp chamber can be similar to that of the maxillary second molar with three canal orifices, but it may also have an odd-shaped

Table 10–5. Root Canals and Apical Foramina in Maxillary Second Molars: Mesiobuccal Root

Investigator	Year	Teeth Sample	Method	One Canal and One Foramen (%)	One Canal and Two Foramina (%)	Two Canals and One Foramen (%)	Two Canals and Two Foramina (%)
Pineda and Kuttler[52]	1972	294	In vitro radiographs	64.6	14.4	8.2	12.8
Pomeranz and Fishelberg[53]	1974	29	In vivo radiographs	62.1	—	13.8	24.1
Vertucci[68]	1985	100	In vitro clear and dyed sections	71.0	—	17.0	12.0

(Courtesy of Drs. Gary R. Hartwell and Frank B. Portel of Fort Gordon, Georgia, and Drs. Thomas L. Walker and Carlos E. del Rio of San Antonio, Texas.)

chamber with four or five root canal orifices or a conical chamber with only one root canal.

Roots and Root Canals. The maxillary third molar may have three well-developed roots that are closely grouped. It may also have fused roots, one conical root, or four or more independent roots. The roots may be straight, curved, or dilacerated, and they may be fully or partially developed.

Root canals vary from one to four or even five in number, depending on the number of roots. One may find a "C-shaped" pulp chamber with a "C-shaped" root canal.

Anatomic Relationships in Situ. The maxillary third molar is closely related to the maxillary sinus and the maxillary tuberosity.

Access Opening. The access opening is similar to that for the maxillary second molar, with modifications for variations in anatomic structure.

Anomalies. The maxillary third molar is a tooth in which anomalies are common, not exceptions.

Mandibular Central Incisor

Average Tooth Length. The average length of this tooth is 20.8 mm.[54]

Pulp Chamber. The mandibular central incisor is the smallest tooth in the arch (see

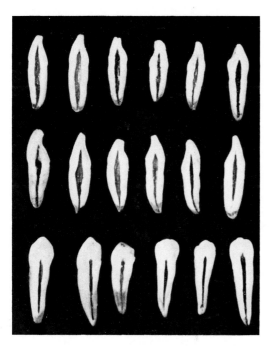

Fig. 10–17. Longitudinal section of mandibular incisor and cuspid teeth. (Labiolingual sections of incisors and mesiodistal sections of cuspid teeth.)

Figs. 10–7 and 10–17). The pulp chamber is small and flat mesiodistally. The three distinct pulp horns present in a recently erupted tooth become calcified and disappear early in life because of constant masticatory stimulus. Labiolingually, the pulp chamber is wide and ovoid in cross section in the cervical third of the crown and tapers incisally.

Root and Root Canals. The mandibular central incisor has 1 root, which is flat and narrow mesiodistally but wide labiolingually (Table 10–6). The root is straight in 60% of cases, or it may have a distal (23%) or labial (13%) curvature.[30] The canal configuration varies from 1 canal exiting in 1 apical foramen, as in 70% of these teeth, 2 canals exiting into 1 apical foramen (5%), or 1 canal bifurcating into 2 canals, coming together, and exiting into 1 apical foramen (22%); conversely, 2 canals may exit into 2 apical foramina (3%)[68] (see Fig. 10–10). From the labiolingual dimension, the canal is broad in the cervical and middle thirds of the root, tapers gradually toward the apex, and forms a constriction in the apical third of the root. In cross section, the canal is ovoid in the labiolingual direction in the cervical third of the root, ribbon-shaped in the labiolingual direction in the middle third, and round in the apical third. The ribbon-shaped configuration in the middle third is due to the flatness of the root in this region. This area is where bifurcations usually occur and where perforation can occur from overinstrumentation.[23]

The mandibular central incisor has lateral canals in 20% of cases and apical deltas in 5%. The apical foramen is situated centrally in the root in 25% of cases.[68]

Anatomic Relationships in Situ. The mandibular alveolar process is thin in the labiolingual direction in the area of the anterior teeth. The roots of the anterior teeth are broad labiolingually, occupy most of the alveolar process, and the labial and lingual surfaces of the roots therefore fuse with labial and lingual cortical plates, respectively. The fundus of the alveolar socket of the anterior teeth is in spongy bone close to the narrow incisive canal, a continuance of the mandibular canal.[19] One sees an average of 2° of mesioaxial inclination and an average of 20° of linguoaxial angulation of the tooth in its alveolus.[18]

Access Opening. The access opening of the mandibular central incisor is made in a similar manner as for the maxillary anterior teeth, with the variations that its smaller size

Table 10–6. Root Canals and Apical Foramina in Mandibular Incisors

Investigator	Year	Teeth Sample	Method	One Canal and One Foramen (%)	One Canal and Two Foramina (%)	Two Canals and One Foramen (%)	Two Canals and Two Foramina (%)
Green[22]	1956	200	In vitro sections	80.0	—	7.0	13.0
Rankine-Wilson and Henry[55]	1965	111	In vitro radiographs	60.0	—	35.0	5.0
Green[20]	1973	500	In vitro sections	79.0	—	17.0	4.0
Madeira and Hetem[41]	1973	1,330	In vitro clear and dyed	88.5	—	11.0	0.5
Benjamin and Dowson[4]	1974	364	In vitro radiographs	59.0	—	40.0	1.0
Vertucci[68]	1985	200	In vitro clear and dyed sections	92.5	—	5.0	2.5

(Courtesy of Drs. Gary R. Hartwell and Frank B. Portel of Fort Gordon, Georgia, and Drs. Thomas L. Walker and Carlos E. del Rio of San Antonio, Texas.)

demands. The shape of the access opening of the mandibular incisor is a long oval, with its greatest dimension oriented incisogingivally. Proper access enables one to explore the cervical third of the root to determine whether a second root canal is present[17] (see Fig. 10–10).

Mandibular Lateral Incisor

Average Tooth Length. This tooth averages 22.6 mm in length.[54]

Pulp Chamber. The configuration of the pulp chamber of the mandibular lateral incisor is similar to that of the mandibular central incisor, but the lateral tooth has larger dimensions (see Fig. 10–7).

Root and Root Canals. Although the root of the mandibular lateral incisor is larger than that of the mandibular central incisor, it has basically the same configuration. The majority of the roots are straight or distally or labially curved, as they are in the central incisor, but the distal curve of the lateral incisors is sharper.[23] The incidence of double root canals at the apex is about the same as in the central incisor, and their anatomy in cross section is also similar. Lateral canals are present in 18% of cases; only 6% have apical deltas. The apical foramen is in the center of the radiographic apex in 20% of cases.[68]

Anatomic Relationships in Situ. The relation of the mandibular lateral incisor to its alveolus is the same as in the mandibular central incisor,[19] except for an average of 17° of mesioaxial inclination and an average of 20° of linguoaxial angulation of the tooth in its alveolus.[18]

Access Opening. The access opening is made in the same manner as for the mandibular central incisor.

Anomalies. Gemination and fusion can occur in mandibular anterior teeth.

Mandibular Cuspid

Average Tooth Length. The average length of this tooth is 25 mm.[54]

Pulp Chamber. The mandibular cuspid resembles the maxillary cuspid, but it is smaller in all dimensions (see Figs. 10–7 and 10–17). The pulp chamber is narrow mesiodistally. When viewed labiolingually, the chamber tapers to a point in the incisal third of the crown, but it is wide in the cervical third. Only one pulp horn is present in the adult tooth. In cross section, the chamber is ovoid in the cervical third. No distinct demarcation exists between the pulp chamber and the root canal.[23]

Root and Root Canals. Although the tooth usually has a single root, it may have 2 (2.3%) (Table 10–7). Most of these teeth have a straight root (68%), but some have curvatures: 20% to the distal, 1% to the mesial, 7% to the labial, and 2% have "S" or bayonet-shaped curves.[54]

The mandibular cuspid usually has 1 canal exiting in 1 apical foramen (78%). In 5% of cases, 2 canals come together and exit in 1 apical foramen; in 18%, 1 canal bifurcates and then coalesces to exit in 1 apical foramen; or 2 canals may exit in 2 apical foramina (2%).[68]

When one root canal is present, a labiolingual view of the root shows a canal that is broad in the middle third and tapers to a

Table 10–7. Root Canals and Apical Foramina in Mandibular Cuspids

Investigator	Year	Teeth Sample	Method	One Canal and One Foramen (%)	One Canal and Two Foramina (%)	Two Canals and One Foramen (%)	Two Canals and Two Foramina (%)
Pineda and Kuttler[52]	1972	187	In vitro radiographs	81.5	—	13.5	5.0
Green[20]	1973	100	In vitro sections	87.0	—	10.0	3.0
Vertucci[68]	1985	100	In vitro clear and dyed sections	80.0	—	14.0	6.0

(Courtesy of Drs. Gary R. Hartwell and Frank B. Portel of Fort Gordon, Georgia, and Drs. Thomas L. Walker and Carlos E. del Rio of San Antonio, Texas.)

constriction in the apical third. It is ovoid in cross section in the cervical and middle thirds of the root and round in the apical third.[23]

Lateral canals are present in 30% of cases; apical deltas occur in 8%. The apical foramen is centrally located in 30% of these teeth.[68]

Anatomic Relationships in Situ. The relation of the mandibular cuspid to the alveolar housing is similar to that of the mandibular central and lateral incisors.[19] One sees an average of 13° of mesioaxial inclination and an average of 15° of linguoaxial angulation of the tooth in its alveolus.[18]

Access Opening. The access opening of the mandibular cuspid is made in a similar manner as for the maxillary cuspid, with variations dictated by a smaller anatomic dimension.

Anomalies. The mandibular cuspid on rare occasions has more than one canal and more than one root.[23]

Mandibular First Premolar

Average Tooth Length. This tooth averages 21.9 mm.[54]

Pulp Chamber. The mandibular first premolar is the transitional tooth between anterior and posterior teeth, and in anatomic structure it resembles both types of teeth (see Fig. 10–11 and 10–18). The mesiodistal width of the pulp chamber is narrow. Buccolingually, the pulp chamber is wide, with a prominent buccal pulp horn that extends under a well-developed buccal cusp. In the young tooth, one sees a small lingual pulp horn that may disappear with age and may give the pulp chamber an appearance similar to that of a mandibular cuspid. The prominent buccal cusp and the smaller lingual cusp give the crown of the mandibular first premolar about a 30° lingual tilt (Fig. 10–19). In cross section, the chamber is ovoid, with

the greater diameter buccolingually. If only one canal is present, no distinct division will be seen between the pulp chamber and the root canal.[23,54]

Roots and Root Canals. The mandibular first premolar usually has a short, conical root (Table 10–8). This root may divide in the apical third into 2 or 3 roots.[54] The root is usually straight (48%), but some roots curve distally (35%), buccally (2%), and lingually (7%), and 7% have an "S" or bayonet shape.[30]

One canal and 1 foramen are present in 70% of cases; 1 canal bifurcates into 2 canals uniting into 1 canal in the apical third and then exiting in 1 foramen in 4% of cases; 1 canal bifurcates into 2 canals and exits in 2 foramina in 24% of cases; 2 canals exit in 2 foramina in 1.5% of cases; and 3 canals exit in 3 foramina 0.5% of cases.[68]

If one canal is present, it will be cone shaped and simple in outline. Mesiodistally, such a root canal is narrow; buccolingually, it is broad and tapers toward the apical third. In cross section, the cervical and middle

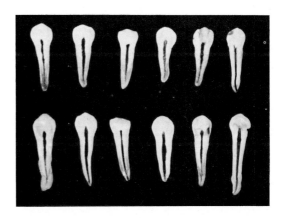

Fig. 10–18. Longitudinal sections of mandibular first and second premolar teeth.

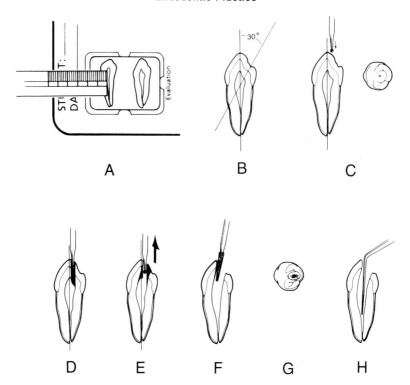

Fig. 10–19. *A* to *H*, Steps in the access opening of a mandibular first premolar.

thirds are ovoid, and the apical third is round.

Lateral canals are present in 44.3% of cases and apical deltas are found in 5.7%. The apical foramen is centrally located in only 15% of these teeth.[68]

Anatomic Relationships in Situ. The mandibular first premolar is closely related to the outer and inner alveolar plates. These plates consist of thick layers of compact bone. The mental canal and foramen are sometimes close to the root apex of the mandibular first premolar; the radiographic appearance may

suggest periapical pathosis.[19] One sees an average of 14° of distoaxial inclination and an average of 10° of linguoaxial angulation of the tooth in its alveolus.[18]

Access Opening. By determining the shape and size and measuring the extension of the pulp chamber mesially, distally, and coronally in the diagnostic radiograph and by transposing these measurements to the tooth, one can estimate the approximate size, shape, depth, and location of the coronal access cavity to be prepared (Fig. 10–19, *A*). The internal anatomy of the pulp chamber

Table 10–8. Root Canals and Apical Foramina in Maxillary First Premolars

Investigator	Year	Teeth Sample	Method	One Canal and One Foramen (%)	One Canal and Two Foramina (%)	Two Canals and One Foramen (%)	Two Canals and Two Foramina (%)	Three Canals (%)
Pineda and Kuttler[52]	1972	202	In vitro radiographs	74.2	23.4	—	1.5	0.9
Green[20]	1973	50	In vitro sections	86.0	—	4.0	10.0	—
Zillich and Dowson[79]	1973	1,287	In vitro radiographs	76.9	—	5.2	17.5	0.4
Vertucci[68]	1985	400	In vitro clear and dyed sections	74.0	24.0	—	1.5	0.5

(Courtesy of Drs. Gary R. Hartwell and Frank B. Portel of Fort Gordon, Georgia, and Drs. Thomas L. Walker and Carlos E. del Rio of San Antonio, Texas.)

dictates the shape and size of the access opening.

The mandibular first premolar has about a 30° lingual tilt of the crown to the long axis of the root (Fig. 10–19, *B*). To compensate for the tilt and to prevent perforations, the enamel is penetrated at the upper third of the lingual incline of the facial cusp with a No. 2 carbide bur in a high-speed contra-angle centered mesiodistally and directed along the long axis of the root (Fig. 10–19, *C*).

The procedure is the same as for the maxillary premolars (Fig. 10–19, *D* to *F*). The resulting access cavity is ovoid, with the walls of the pulp chamber confluent with the access cavity and divergent occlusally. The ovoid preparation should extend buccally and lingually enough to allow the complete removal of the roof of the pulp chamber (Fig. 10–19, *G*). This ovoid access preparation permits exploration for bifurcations or trifurcations in the middle and apical thirds[17] (Fig. 10–19, *H*).

Anomalies. Bifurcations and trifurcations of the roots or root canals are the most common anomalies. They present a challenge during cleaning, shaping and obturation.

Mandibular Second Premolar

Average Tooth Length. The length of this tooth averages 22.3 mm.[54]

Pulp Chamber. The pulp chamber of the mandibular second premolar is similar to that of the mandibular first premolar, except the lingual horn is more prominent under a well-developed lingual cusp (see Figs. 10–11 and 10–18).

Roots and Root Canals. The mandibular second premolar usually has a single root, but on rare occasions 2 to 3 roots are present (Table 10–9). The root has a greater girth and is wider buccolingually than that of the mandibular first premolar. The root of the mandibular second premolar may curve distally (40%), although in 39% of cases it is straight. In 10% of cases it has a buccal curve, in 3% a lingual curve, and in 7% a bayonet curve; 1% has trifurcated root canals.[30] Usually, 1 canal exits in 1 apical foramen (97.5%), but in some roots (2.5%), a single canal may bifurcate exiting in 2 foramina.[68] When 1 canal is present, its configuration is similar to that of the mandibular first premolar.

Lateral canals are present in 48.3% of cases and apical deltas in 3.4%. The apical foramen is centrally located in only 16.1% of these teeth.[68]

Anatomic Relationships in Situ. The relationship of the mandibular second premolar to its mandibular housing is similar to that of the mandibular first premolar, but in closer relationship to the mental foramen.[19] One sees an average of 10° of distoaxial inclination of the root and an average of 34° of buccoaxial angulation of the tooth in its alveolus.[18]

Access Opening. The access opening for the mandibular second premolar is basically the same as for the mandibular first premolar, except the enamel penetration is initiated in the central fossa, and the ovoid access opening is wider mesiodistally, as dictated by the wider pulp chamber.

Anomalies. The mandibular second premolar has two roots in rare cases.

Mandibular First Molar

Average Tooth Length. The average length of this tooth is 21.9 mm.[54]

Pulp Chamber. The roof of the pulp chamber of the mandibular first molar is often rectangular in shape (see Figs. 10–14 and

Table 10–9.   Root Canals and Apical Foramina in Mandibular Second Premolars

Investigator	Year	Teeth Sample	Method	One Canal and One Foramen (%)	One Canal and Two Foramina (%)	Two Canals and One Foramen (%)	Two Canals and Two Foramina (%)	Three Canals (%)
Pineda and Kuttler[52]	1972	250	In vitro radiographs	98.8	1.2	—	—	—
Green[20]	1973	50	In vitro sections	92.0	—	4.0	4.0	—
Zillich and Dowson[79]	1973	906	In vitro radiographs	87.9	—	0.9	10.8	0.4
Vertucci[68]	1985	400	In vitro clear and dyed sections	97.5	2.5	—	—	—

(Courtesy of Drs. Gary R. Hartwell and Frank B. Portel of Fort Gordon, Georgia, and Drs. Thomas L. Walker and Carlos E. del Rio of San Antonio, Texas.)

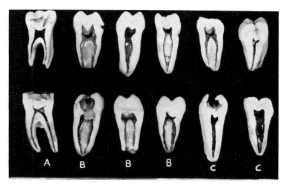

Fig. 10–20. Longitudinal sections of mandibular first and second molar teeth. In the mesiodistal sections (A), note the difference in the size of the pulp chambers. The buccolingual sections show the mesial (B) and the distal (C) root canals.

10–20). The mesial wall is straight, the distal wall round, and the buccal and lingual walls converge to meet the mesial and distal walls and to form a rhomboidal floor. The roof of the pulp chamber has four pulp horns; mesiobuccal, mesiolingual, distobuccal, and distolingual. These four pulp horns recede with age, with a resulting decrease in the size of the pulp chamber. The roof of the pulp chamber is located in the cervical third of the crown just above the cervix of the tooth, and the floor is located in the cervical third of the root.

Three distinct orifices are present in the pulpal floor: mesiobuccal, mesiolingual, and distal (see Fig. 10–14). The mesiobuccal orifice is under the mesiobuccal cusp and is usually difficult to find and to enter if not enough tooth structure is removed. To penetrate this orifice, insert a long-shank explorer, Starlite D-11, in a mesiobucco-apical inclination into the point angle created at the juncture of the mesial wall, buccal wall, and subpulpal floor of the pulp chamber. The mesiolingual orifice is located in a depression formed by the mesial and lingual walls. This orifice can be explored from a distobuccal direction. A groove usually connects the orifices of the mesiobuccal and mesiolingual canals. The mesiobuccal and mesiolingual orifices may be close together under the mesiobuccal cusp. The distal orifice, which is oval in shape, with the widest diameter buccolingually, can be explored by starting from a mesial direction. If the distal orifice is penetrated in a marked distobuccal or distolingual direction, one should seek an additional orifice and canal in the distal root. The multiple orifices in the distal root are usually found in the buccal and lingual portion of the ovoid coronal root canal.

Roots and Root Canals. Usually, 2 well-differentiated roots are present in the mandibular first molar, 1 mesial and 1 distal (Table 10–10). Both roots are wide and flat buccolingually, with a depression in the middle of the root buccolingually. This anatomic characteristic may be accentuated in the mesial root. A third root is found in some cases, either distally or mesially (5.3%).[54] The mesial root curves distally in 84% of cases and is straight in 16%. The distal root is straight in 74% of cases, curves to the distal in 21%, and curves to the mesial in 5%.[30]

Although the mandibular first molar has 2 roots, 3 canals are usually present. The mesial root has 2 canals that exit in 2 foramina in 41% of cases, 2 canals that coalesce to exit in 1 foramen in 28%, 2 canals that coalesce to form 1 canal and bifurcate and exit in 2 foramina in 10%, 1 canal that exits in 1 foramen in 12%, and 1 canal that bifurcates and exits in 2 foramina in 8%. In rare cases, 3 canals exit in 3 foramina.[68]

The distal root has 1 canal exiting in 1 foramen in 70% of cases, 1 canal bifurcating and exiting in 2 foramina in 8%, 2 canals coalescing and exiting in 1 foramen in 15%, 2 canals exiting in 2 foramina in 5%, and 2 canals coalescing to form 1 canal and later bifurcating to exit in 2 foramina in 2% of cases.[68] When 2 canals are present in either root, they may converge toward and exit in 1 foramen, or they may have interconnecting lateral canals between them that form a single ribbon canal ending in 1 foramen.

In cross section, all three canals are ovoid in the cervical and middle thirds and round in the apical third. Two canals present in the distal root are usually round in cross section from the cervical third to the apical third.[23]

Lateral canals are present in the furcation in 23% of cases, in the mesial root in 45%, and in the distal root in 30%. Apical deltas are present in the mesial root in 10% of cases and in the distal root in 14%. When only 1 apical foramen is present, it is centrally located in 22% of cases in the mesial root and in 20% of cases in the distal root.[68]

Anatomic Relationships in Situ. The mesial root of the mandibular first molar is in close proximity to the buccal cortical plate, whereas the distal root is centrally located. The apex of the roots of mandibular first molars may be close to the mandibular

Table 10–10. Root Canals and Apical Foramina in Mandibular First Molars

Investigator	Year	Teeth Sample	Method	Roots	One Canal and One Foramen (%)	One Canal and Two Foramina (%)	Two Canals and One Foramen (%)	Two Canals and Two Foramina (%)	Three Canals (%)
Skidmore and Bjorndahl[62]	1971	45	In vitro resin casts	Mesial	6.7	—	37.8	55.5	—
				Distal	71.1	—	17.7	11.2	—
Pineda and Kuttler[52]	1972	300	In vitro radiographs	Mesial	12.8	—	30.2	57.0	—
				Distal	73.0	—	12.7	14.3	—
Vertucci[68]	1985	100	In vitro clear and dyed sections	Mesial	12.0	8.0	28.0	51.0	1.0
				Distal	70.0	8.0	15.0	7.0	—

(Courtesy of Drs. Gary R. Hartwell and Frank B. Portel of Fort Gordon, Georgia, and Drs. Thomas L. Walker and Carlos E. del Rio of San Antonio, Texas.)

canal, or they may be at some distance from it, depending on the length of the roots and the height of the body of the mandible.[19]

Reported is an average of −58° of buccoaxial inclination of the roots of the first mandibular molar in its alveolus.[18]

Access Opening. The access opening for the mandibular first molar follows the anatomic features of the pulp chamber. The enamel and dentin are penetrated in the central fossa with the bur angled toward the distal root, where the pulp chamber is largest (Fig. 10–21). The preparation follows the procedures outlined for the maxillary molar. The access opening is usually trapezoidal with round corners or rectangular if a second distal canal is present (Fig. 10–21, H). The access opening extends toward the mesiobuccal cusp, to uncover the mesiobuccal canal, lingually slightly beyond the central groove, and distally slightly beyond the buccal groove.[17]

Anomalies. The mandibular first molar may have three roots. Pulp stones may be present in the pulp chamber.

Mandibular Second Molar

Average Tooth Length. This tooth averages 22.4 mm in length.[54]

Pulp Chamber. The pulp chamber of the mandibular second molar is smaller than that of the mandibular first molar, and the root canal orifices are smaller and closer together (see Fig. 10–20).

Roots and Root Canals. The majority of the mandibular second molars have 2 roots (71%), but teeth with 1 root (27%) and teeth with 3 roots (2%) are seen (Table 10–11). In single-rooted teeth, 53% of the roots are straight, but they may curve distally (26%), lingually (2%), or have an "S" or bayonet shape (19%). If 2 roots are present, the mesial root usually curves distally (61%), but it can

be straight (27%), curved buccally (4%), or have an "S" or bayonet shape (7%). The distal root is usually straight (58%), but it may curve distally (18%), mesially (10%), buccally (4%), or have an "S" or bayonet shape (6%).[30]

Three root canals are usually present in the mandibular second molar. The most frequent variation is the presence of only 2 canals. The mesial root has 1 canal and 1 foramen in 27% of cases, 1 canal bifurcating and exiting in 2 foramina in 9% of cases, 2 canals exiting in 2 foramina in 26% of cases, and 2 canals coalescing and exiting in 1 foramen in 30%. The distal root has 1 canal exiting in 1 foramen in 92% of cases, 1 canal bifurcating and exiting in 2 foramina in 1% of cases, 2 canals exiting in 2 foramina in 4% of cases, and 2 canals coalescing and exiting in 1 foramen in 3% percent of cases.[68] When the mesial root of the mandibular second molar has two canals, they often join near the apex to exit as a single foramen. In cross section, all 3 root canals are small and ovoid in the cervical and middle thirds and round in the apical third.

Lateral canals are present in the mesial root in 49% of cases and in the distal root in 34% of cases. Apical deltas are present in the mesial root in 6% of cases and in the distal root in 7%. Lateral canals are present in the furcation in 11% of these teeth. When a single apical foramen is present, it is centrally located in 19% of cases in the mesial root and in 21% of cases in the distal root.[68]

Anatomic Relationships in Situ. The position of the mandibular second molar in its alveolar housing is basically the same as that of the mandibular first molar, except the mesial root is more centrally located and the distal root is closer to the lingual cortical plate. The relationship between the apex of the root and the mandibular canal may be closer.[19] One sees an average of −52° of buc-

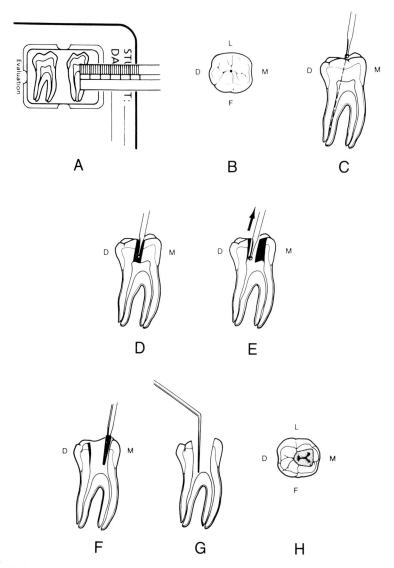

Fig. 10–21. *A* to *H*, Steps in the access opening of a mandibular first molar. L, lingual; F, facial; D, distal; M, mesial.

Table 10–11.   Root Canals and Apical Foramina in Mandibular Second Molars

Investigator	Year	Teeth Sample	Method	Roots	One Canal and One Foramen (%)	One Canal and Two Foramina (%)	Two Canals and One Foramen (%)	Two Canals and Two Foramina (%)
Pineda and Kuttler[52]	1972	300	In vitro radiographs	Mesial	58.0	—	20.6	21.4
				Distal	73.0	—	12.7	14.3
Vertucci[68]	1985	100	In vitro clear and dyed sections	Mesial	27.0	9.0	38.0	26.0
				Distal	92.0	1.0	3.0	4.0

(Courtesy of Drs. Gary R. Hartwell and Frank B. Portel of Fort Gordon, Georgia, and Drs. Thomas L. Walker and Carlos E. del Rio of San Antonio, Texas.)

coaxial inclination of the roots of the second molar in its alveolar housing.[18]

Access Opening. The access opening for the mandibular second molar is created as for the mandibular first molar, with the variations that a smaller tooth demands. Because of the buccoaxial inclination, it is sometimes necessary to reduce a large portion of the mesiobuccal cusp to clean and shape the mesiobuccal canal.

Anomalies. The mandibular second molar may have a third root, or it may have one conical root with one conical canal. Pulp stones may be present in the pulp chamber.

Mandibular Third Molar

Average Tooth Length. The average length of this tooth is 18.5 mm.[54]

Pulp Chamber. The pulp chamber of the mandibular third molar anatomically resembles the pulp chamber of the mandibular first and second molars. It is large and possesses many anomalous configurations such as "C-shaped" root canal orifices.[23]

Roots and Root Canals. The mandibular third molar usually has two roots and two canals, but occasionally one root and one canal or three roots and three canals. The root canals are generally large and short.[23]

Anatomic Relationships in Situ. The alveolar socket of the mandibular third molar may project onto the lingual plate of the mandible. The apex of the root may be in close proximity to the mandibular canal.[19]

Access Opening. The access opening for the mandibular third molar is created as for the mandibular first and second molars, with the variations that anatomic structure dictates.

Anomalies. The mandibular third molar frequently has a complex anatomic structure.

ANOMALIES OF PULP CAVITIES

Certain developmental anomalies of the pulp cavities may render the execution of endodontic procedures difficult or impossible. In hereditary opalescent dentin (dentinogenesis imperfecta), the pulp cavities may be small or even obliterated. Hyperparathyroidism may cause pulp calcification and loss of lamina dura. Hypofunction of the pituitary gland may lead to retarded eruption of teeth and to open root apices. Dentinal dysplasia is a hereditary condition characterized by obliteration of the pulp chamber and defective root formation. In contradistinction to dentinal dysplasia, taurodontism is characterized by a short tooth and a much larger than normal pulp chamber (Fig. 10–22). It may be a throwback to ancient man because a large pulp chamber is characteristic of Neanderthal man. Taurodontism is probably due to a lack of invagination of the epithelial root sheath during development. It may be considered an ethnic or familial trait because it occurs in family groups, such as in Eskimos. In some cases of dentinal dysplasia, the root development is disturbed, with obliteration of the root canals.[29,39,56]

Dens in Dente

Dens in dente is an invagination within the crown or root of the lingual surface of the tooth (Fig. 10–23). This invagination creates a space within the tooth that is lined with enamel and communicates with the oral cavity. This malformation or anomaly may occur in any anterior tooth, but it is most often observed in maxillary lateral incisors. At times, more than one tooth is affected. Invagination of the lingual enamel of maxillary incisor teeth often causes widening of the pulp chamber. Such teeth are predisposed to decay because of the anatomic malformation, and pulp disease may result before the root apex is fully developed. Intentional filling of the defect may prevent pulp involvement in such cases.

Dens Evaginatus

Dens evaginatus is a developmental anomaly that produces an extra cusp-like struc-

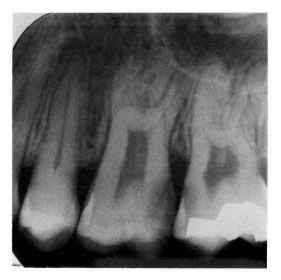

Fig. 10–22. Taurodontism, characterized by short roots and a large pulp chamber. (Courtesy of T.L. Walker, San Antonio, Texas.)

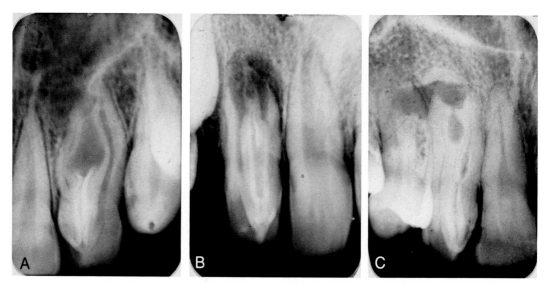

Fig. 10–23. *A* to *C*, Varieties of dens in dente.

ture, usually in the area of the transverse
ridge of premolars (Fig. 10–24). It is formed
during early tooth development by the proliferation and evagination of the enamal epithelium into the stellate reticulum, with
resulting protuberance of enamel and dentin
with a pulp horn. The cusp-like structure is
subject to wear or fracture that exposes the
pulp, with the sequelae of pulp and periapical disorders. Although this anomaly is predominantly found in persons of Mongolian
ancestry, it has been reported in Caucasians.
The majority of cases reported have been in
premolars, but incisors, cuspids, and molars
have also been involved. Dens evaginatus can
occur unilaterally or bilaterally.[7,59,60]

A palatal developmental groove may be
present in maxillary central and lateral incisors (Fig. 10–25). This groove, which appears
as an invagination of the enamel, originates
in the cingulum of the incisors and ends apically at various levels of the root. It is
believed that it is an attempt by the tooth bud
to form a second root. Once the integrity of
the periodontal attachment is broken in the
area of the anomaly, a probable linear periodontal defect will develop to the level of
the groove apically. The result is a self-per-
petuating periodontal defect for which the
eventual treatment is tooth extraction. Radiographically, the lesion created by the anomaly produces a radiolucency along the length
of the groove. This radiolucency can be differentiated from a vertical root fracture by the
clinical presence of the developmental
groove.[61]

TEMPORARY FILLING

The multivisit approach to endodontic
therapy requires the placement of a temporary filling to seal the access cavity between
visits to the endodontist. The purpose of the
temporary filling is to seal the access cavity
and thereby to prevent the contamination of
the root canal system by saliva, with its bacterial flora, food, and foreign materials, and
to prevent any intracanal medication from
leaking.

An ideal temporary filling material should
meet the following requirements: (1) it
should hermetically seal the cavity peripherally; that is, be impervious to bacteria and
to the oral fluids; (2) it should harden within
a few minutes after insertion in the cavity;
(3) once set, it should withstand the forces
of mastication; (4) it should be easy to manipulate; (5) it should be easy to remove; and (6)
it should harmonize with the color of tooth
structure. At present, no material meets all
the requirements satisfactorily.

From the standpoint of producing a her-
metic seal, the zinc-oxide-eugenol cements
are probably the best. Although they are not
always strong enough to withstand the forces
of mastication, this disadvantage can be overcome by increasing the bulk of the restoration
and by designing the access cavity with
sound, divergent walls. An objection to a
zinc-oxide-eugenol cement is its slow setting
time. Deformation of the filling, while setting, may cause contamination of the root
canal by saliva. The addition of 0.5 to 1.0%

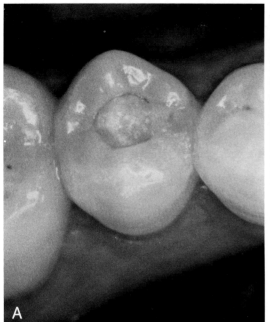

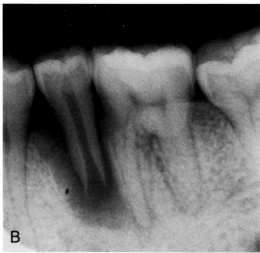

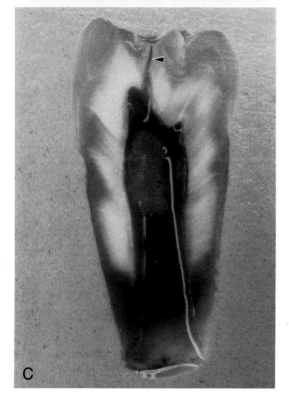

Fig. 10–24. *A*, Dens evaginatus showing a cusp-like structure in the area of the transverse ridge. *B*, Radiograph from another patient showing an immature apex and a periapical area of radiolucency. *C*, Buccolingual ground section showing an area of pulp extension in the cusp-like structure (arrow). (From Senia, E.S., and Regesi, J.A.: Oral Surg., *38*:465, 1974.)

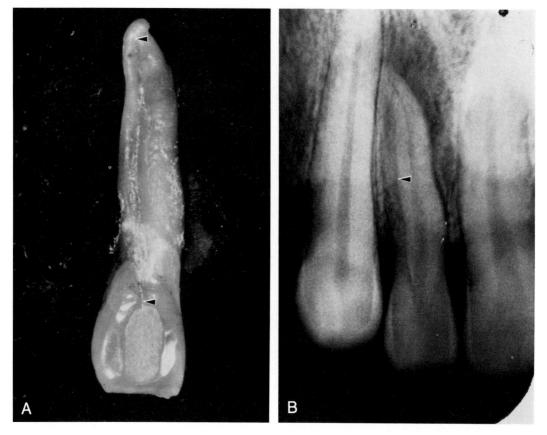

Fig. 10–25. Gross (*A*) and radiographic (*B*) views of a palatal developmental groove in a maxillary lateral incisor. Note that the groove (arrows) originates in the cingulum and ends in the apex of the root. (Courtesy of E.S. Senia, San Antonio, Texas.)

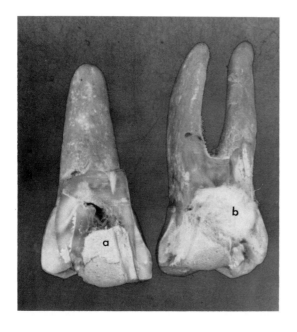

Fig. 10–26. Section of a maxillary first molar showing a temporary filling of Cavit (a) and two cotton pellets (b). (From Weber, R.T., et al.: Oral Surg., *46*:123, 1978.)

zinc acetate accelerates the setting time of zinc oxide-eugenol and prevents its deformation.

IRM,* a polymer-reinforced zinc-oxide-eugenol material can be used in temporary fillings. Although this material has greater surface hardness than zinc-oxide-eugenol cement, it softens on contact with intracanal medications, such as metacresylacetate, camphorated chlorophenol or formocresol.[48] In an in vitro study in which Cavit† and IRM were placed in contact with camphorated chlorophenol, IRM proved to be a more effective seal against microorganisms.[6]

Another satisfactory preparation for temporary fillings is Cavit, a zinc oxide-polyvinyl preparation. It is simply squeezed from a tube as needed and forms a reasonably hard temporary filling if the patient is instructed not to chew on it for at least an hour. Nine temporary filling materials were tested for leakage using a dye, and only zinc oxide-eugenol and Cavit prevented leakage.[50] In a later series of tests of 12 temporary filling materials, only Cavit, zinc oxide-eugenol, and Kwikseal maintained a leak-proof cavity when tested with either a dye or a test organism.[49] The sealing qualities of Cavit seem to be based on the material's ability to expand while setting.[78]

Cavit is a hydrophilic compound that sets in the presence of moisture. For this reason, it should not be used in vital teeth because it may desiccate dentin and thereby produce sensitivity in the teeth.[78] To prevent leakage, a thickness of Cavit of at least 3.5 mm should be used,[75] and long periods of time between appointments predispose the tooth to leakage.[36]

Two kinds of temporary seals are frequently used. The double seal consists of a medicated cotton pellet sealed in the pulp chamber by an inner seal of temporary stopping and an outer seal of Cavit, IRM, or zinc-oxide-eugenol cement. The single seal consists of a medicated cotton pellet in the pulp chamber covered by another dry cotton pellet and sealed with Cavit, IRM, or zinc-oxide-eugenol cement (Fig. 10–26).

BIBLIOGRAPHY

1. Barrett, M.T.: Dent. Cosmos, 67:581, 1925.
2. Bellizzi, R., and Hartwell, G.: J. Endod., 11:37, 1985.
3. Bellizzi, R., and Hartwell, G.: J. Endod., 9:246, 1983.
4. Benjamin, K.A., and Dowson, J.: Oral Surg., 38:122, 1974.
5. Bernick, S., and Nedelman, C.: J. Endod., 1:88, 1975.
6. Blaney, T.D.: J. Endod., 7:453, 1981.
7. Bhaskar, S.N.: Synopsis of Oral Pathology, 6th Ed. St. Louis, C.V. Mosby, 1981.
8. Burch, J.G., and Hulen, S.: Oral Surg., 34:262, 1972.
9. Burke, J.H.: U.S. Navy Med. News Lett., 52:16, 1968.
10. Carlsen, O.: Tandlaegebl., 72:787, 1968.
11. Carns, E.J., and Skidmore, A.E.: Oral Surg., 36:880, 1973.
12. Chapman, C.E.: J. Br. Endod. Soc., 3:52, 1969.
13. Coolidge, E.D., and Kesel, R.G.: Endodontology, 2nd Ed. Philadelphia, Lea & Febiger, 1956, p. 132.
14. Cutright, D.E., and Bhaskar, S.N.: Oral Surg., 27:678, 1969.
15. Davis, S.R., et al.: Oral Surg., 34:642, 1972.
16. DeDeus, Q.D.: J. Endod., 1:361, 1975.
17. Del Rio, C.E., and Canales, M.L.: A Sophomore Pre-Clinical Laboratory Course. San Antonio, University of Texas Dental School, 1985.
18. Dempster, W.T., et al.: J. Am. Dent. Assoc., 67:779, 1963.
19. DuBrul, E.L.: Sicher's Oral Anatomy, 7th Ed. St. Louis, C.V. Mosby, 1980.
20. Green, D.: Oral Surg., 35:689, 1973.
21. Green, D.: Morphology of the Endodontic System, 1969.
22. Green, D.: Oral Surg., 9:1224, 1956.
23. Green, D.: Oral Surg., 8:743, 1955.
24. Grove, C.J.: Dent. Cosmos, 74:451, 1932.
25. Gutierrez, J.H.: Oral Surg., 25:108, 1968.
26. Hampson, E.L., and Atkinson, A.M.: Br. Dent. J., 116:546, 1964.
27. Walkoff, O., and Hess, W.: In Lehrbuch des konservierenden Zahnheilkünde. Edited by W. Hess. Leipzig, J.A. Barth, 1954, p. 273.
28. Hess, W., and Zürcher, E.: The Anatomy of the Root Canals of the Teeth of the Permanent and Deciduous Dentitions. New York, Wm. Wood, 1925.
29. Hoggins, G.S., and Marsland, E.A.: Br. Dent. J., 92:305, 1952.
30. Ingle, J.I., and Taintor, J.E.: Endodontics, 3rd Ed. Philadelphia, Lea & Febiger, 1985.
31. Kelsten, L.B.: J. Am. Dent. Assoc., 40:120, 1950.
32. Kereskes, K., and Tronstad, L.: J. Endod., 3:74, 1977.
33. Kirkham, D.B.: J. Am. Dent. Assoc., 91:353, 1975.
34. Kronfeld, R.: Histopathology of the Teeth. Philadelphia, Lea & Febiger, 1939, p. 233.
35. Kuttler, Y.: J. Am. Dent. Assoc., 50:544, 1955.
36. Lamers, A.C., et al.: Oral Surg., 49:541, 1980.
37. Lane, A.: J. Br. Endod. Soc., 7:9, 1974.
38. Laws, A.J.: N. Z. Dent. J., 67:186, 1971.
39. Logan, J., et al.: Oral Surg., 75:317, 1962.
40. Lowman, J.V., et al.: Oral Surg., 36:580, 1973.
41. Madeira, M.C., and Hetem, S.: Oral Surg., 36:589, 1973.
42. Madeira, M.C., et al.: Rev. Fac. Araçatuba, 2:27, 1973.
43. Marshall, F.J., et al.: Oral Surg., 13:208, 1960.
44. Molven, O.: Oral Surg., 35:232, 1973.
45. Nalbandian, J., et al.: J. Dent. Res., 39:598, 1960.
46. Nicholls, E.: Oral Surg., 16:839, 1963.
47. Nosonowitz, D.M., and Brenner, M.R.: N.Y. J. Dent., 43:12, 1973.
48. Olmsted, J.S.: J. Endod., 3:342, 1977.
49. Parris, L., and Kapsimalis, P.: Oral Surg., 17:771, 1964.

---

*L.D. Caulk, Milford, Delaware.
†Premier Dental Products, Norristown, Pennsylvania.

50. Parris, L., and Kapsimalis, P.: Oral Surg., *13*:982, 1960.
51. Pineda, F.: Oral Surg., *36*:253, 1973.
52. Pineda, F., and Kuttler, Y.: Oral Surg., *33*:101, 1972.
53. Pomeranz, H.H., and Fishelberg, G.: J. Am. Dent. Assoc., *88*:119, 1974.
54. Pucci, F.M., and Reig, R.: Conductos Radiculares. Buenos Aires, Editorial Medico-Quirurgica, 1944.
55. Rankine-Wilson, R.W., and Henry, P.: J. Am. Dent. Assoc., *70*:1162, 1965.
56. Rushton, M.: Guy's Hosp. Rep., *89*:369, 1939.
57. Seidberg, B.H., et al.: J. Am. Dent. Assoc., *87*:852, 1973.
58. Seltzer, S., et al.: Oral Surg., *22*:375, 1966.
59. Senia, E.S., and Regesi, J.A.: Oral Surg., *38*:465, 1974.
60. Shafer, W.G., et al.: Oral Pathology, 4th Ed. Philadelphia, W.B. Saunders, 1983.
61. Simon, J.H.S., et al.: Oral Surg., *31*:833, 1971.
62. Skidmore, A.G., and Bjorndahl, A.M.: Oral Surg., *32*:778, 1971.
63. Skillen, W.G.: J. Am. Dent. Assoc., *19*:719, 1932.
64. Stewart, G.G.: Current Therapy in Dentistry. St. Louis, C.V. Mosby, 1970, p. 95.
65. Sycaras, S.: Odontostomatol. Prog., *24*:99, 1970.
66. Thomas, N.G.: J. Nat. Dent. A., *8*:11, 1921.
67. Van de Voorde, H., et al.: Ill. Dent. J., *44*:179, 1975.
68. Vertucci, F.J.: Oral Surg., *58*:589, 1985.
69. Vertucci, F.J.: J. Am. Dent. Assoc., *89*:369, 1974.
70. Vertucci, F.J.: U.S. Navy Med., *63*:29, 1974.
71. Vertucci, F.J., and Gegauff, A.: J. Am. Dent. Assoc., *99*:194, 1979.
72. Vertucci, F.J., and Williams, R.G.: Oral Surg., *38*:308, 1974.
73. Vertucci, F.J., et al.: Oral Surg., *38*:456, 1974.
74. Von der Lehr, W.N., and Marsh, R.A.: Oral Surg., *35*:105, 1973.
75. Weber, R.T., et al.: Oral Surg., *46*:123, 1978.
76. Weine, F., et al.: Oral Surg., *28*:419, 1969.
77. Wheeler, R.C.: Pulp Cavities of the Permanent Teeth. Philadelphia, W.B. Saunders, 1976.
78. Widerman, F.H., et al.: J. Am. Dent. Assoc., *82*:378, 1971.
79. Zillich, R., and Dowson, J.: Oral Surg., *36*:738, 1973.

11 Preparation of the Root Canal: Equipment and Technique for Cleaning, Shaping, and Irrigation

Endodontic treatment can be divided into three main phases: biomechanical preparation of the root canal (cleaning and shaping), disinfection, and obturation. The initial step for cleaning and shaping the root canal is proper access to the chamber that leads to straight-line penetration of the root canal orifices. The next step is exploration of the root canal, extirpation of the remaining pulp tissue or gross debridement of necrotic tissue, and verification of the instrument depth. This step is followed by proper instrumentation, irrigation and debridement, and disinfection (sanitization) of the root canal. Obturation usually completes the procedure.

The importance of adequate canal cleaning and shaping, rather than reliance on antiseptics, cannot be overemphasized. Histologic examination of pulpless teeth in which root canal therapy has failed often shows that the canals were only superficially cleaned. At times, not even the pulp tissue had been removed (Fig. 11–1). Cleaning and shaping the root canal comprise the most important phase of endodontic treatment. Other aspects of treatment cannot be neglected, however, because they are all interrelated and contribute to the success of endodontic therapy.

The objectives of cleaning and shaping are twofold: (1) to debride and disinfect (sanitize) the root canal system; and (2) to contour the root canal walls and apical tip, for the purpose of sealing the root canal completely with a condensed, inert filling material. To help achieve these objectives, each individual root canal should be examined radiographically and explored with endodontic instruments. The examination should include an assessment of canal length, shape, size, curvature, entrance orifice, location of

foramina, bifurcations, and presence of calcifications or obstructions.

A root canal that has been cleaned and shaped should be a continuous tapering cone, with the narrowest cross-sectional diameter apically and the widest diameter coronally. The walls should taper evenly toward the apex and should be confluent with the access cavity, to give the prepared root canal the "quality of flow," that is, a shape that permits plasticized gutta-percha to flow against the walls without impedance.[124]

The preparation of an apical matrix, that is, an artificially produced ledge in the apical root canal, is designed to prevent the extrusion of the obturating materials into the periapex and to produce an effective apical seal following condensation. When preparing the apical matrix, one should avoid enlarging the apical foramen, transporting it to a different position on the root tip, perforating the root tip, or blocking the root canal with pulpal and dentinal debris. The apical matrix becomes the apical terminus of the shaped canal against which the endodontic filling is condensed.

Theoretically, the canal preparation should extend apically to the cementodentinal junction. This junction is located at or near the greatest constriction (minor diameter) of the apical foramen (see Fig. 11–27). The continuous deposition of the cementum causes the position of the apical foramen to deviate from the center of the root apex an average of 0.2 to 0.5 mm.[54] The distance of the minor diameter of the foramen from the cemental surface is an average of 0.5 mm in young teeth and 0.75 mm in mature teeth (Fig. 11–2).[144] Consequently, the determi-

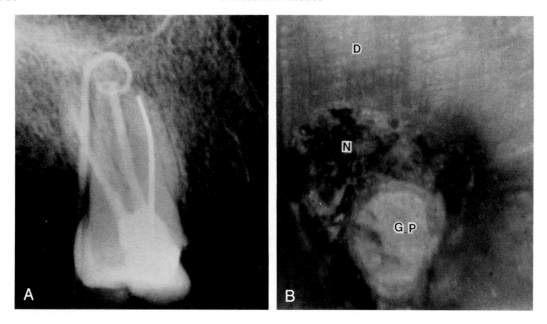

Fig. 11–1. *A*, Radiograph of a maxillary right second molar shows the palatal root as the origin of a sinus tract. *B*, Histologic examination of the palatal root shows necrotic tissue and debris as the cause of failure. D, dentin; N, necrotic tissue; GP, gutta-percha filling.

nation of the dentinoenamel junction in vivo is arbitrary and is based on radiographic interpretation, tactile sensation, and a knowledge of pulpoperiapical anatomy. Most clinicians prefer to terminate instrumentation and obturation within 0.5 mm (±0.5 mm) of the radiographic apex.

LOCAL ANESTHESIA

At the start of root canal therapy, local anesthesia is used. Other agents used in the past for extirpating pulp painlessly include arsenic, paraformaldehyde, and diathermy.

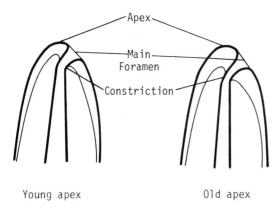

Fig. 11–2. In the young apex, the apical constriction is located 0.5 mm from the cementum surface; in the old, 0.75 mm (Kutler[81]). The main foramen is located an average of 0.2 to 0.5 mm from the radiographic apex (Green[54]).

All these methods are inadequate and time consuming and, with the advent of local anesthesia, archaic. Anesthesia, like any medication, should not be administered without a thorough knowledge of the patient's medical and dental history. Any prior allergic reactions or untoward episodes during dental treatment must be investigated and evaluated, to avoid any future reaction to medication.

Infiltration Anesthesia

Infiltration anesthesia is the injection of a local anesthetic into the soft tissues in the region of the root apex. Infiltration is probably the simplest, safest, and fastest method of producing anesthesia for removal of a dental pulp. The injection of an anesthetic stops any pain and makes pulp removal possible. The injection is made as for removal of a tooth; one inserts the needle into the mucobuccal fold slightly mesial of the tooth to be anesthetized and carries it toward the root apex until bone is encountered. An effective, long-lasting anesthetic solution such as 2% lidocaine (Xylocaine) with 1:100,000 epinephrine is preferred, although other local anesthetics are also effective. The Committee on Medical Education of the American Heart Association and the Council on Dental Therapeutics of the American Dental Association have approved a report of a conference at which it was stated that: "The concentrations of vasoconstrictors normally used in dental local anesthetic solutions are not contraindicated in patients with cardiovascular disease when administered carefully and with preliminary aspiration."[4a] Generally, one carpule of the anesthetic solution (1.8 ml) is sufficient, but administration of more anesthetic solution is often required for pulp extirpation than for extraction of a tooth.

A palatal injection for maxillary teeth is unnecessary in most cases, but at times, adequate anesthesia cannot be obtained without it because of innervation of the pulp by fibers from the periodontal ligament. Despite care in injection, complete anesthesia may not follow. A subperiosteal injection should then be made, by inserting the needle near the apex of the tooth, just under the periosteum, and slowly depositing about 0.5 ml of anesthetic solution.

Anesthetic techniques described in this text are limited to those necessary for painless endodontic treatment. For a more comprehensive understanding of local and general anesthesia, one should consult other texts specifically on that subject.

Block (Conduction) Anesthesia

Because of the dense buccal alveolar plate, infiltration anesthesia alone is ineffective in the mandibular posterior region of the mouth, particularly for the removal of pulps in molar and premolar teeth. In such cases, block, or conduction, anesthesia of the inferior alveolar and long buccal nerves should be used. At times, however, the inferior alveolar nerve may be difficult to anesthetize because of its anomalous distribution; for example, it may give off a branch that runs anterior to the mandibular foramen and enters the mandible through an opening anterior and inferior to the foramen.[28] The long buccal nerve (buccinator) injection that follows the original block injection is delayed until lip symptoms occur, signifying that the initial injection was effective. When the injection is properly executed, it is probably the most effective method for producing the anesthesia necessary for removal of a pulp, particularly in posterior teeth. A modified technique for injecting the inferior alveolar nerve by inserting the needle about half an inch higher than the place of the conventional injection has also been used. It has been reported that complete anesthesia was obtained in all cases with this technique.[23]

Because the buccal nerve is above the level of the inferior alveolar nerve, it is possible to anesthetize both nerves by diffusion of solution from one injection.

The Gow-Gate mandibular block is another type of mandibular block anesthesia. It differs from the inferior alveolar block in that the anesthesia is deposited in the lateral aspect of the neck of the condyle below the insertion of the lateral pterygoid muscle instead of in the mandibular sulcus. Advocates of the Gow-Gate technique claim a higher success rate than with the conventional technique, although the onset of anesthesia is longer.[89] This technique can be used either routinely or when the conventional technique fails to produce anesthesia. The endodontist may also use other forms of regional anesthesia: posterior superior alveolar, infraorbital, greater palatine, nasopalatine, maxillary or second-division blocks. These nerve blocks are indicated when infiltration anesthesia is inadequate.

Techniques to Augment Infiltration and Conduction Anesthesia

At times, it is difficult to obtain adequate anesthesia with an injection of a local anesthetic solution because of the inflamed state of the pulp. The reason for the inefficiency of the anesthetic solution in areas of inflammation may be the increase in peripheral nerve activity,[17,19] or a decrease in pH of the inflamed tissues that allows few anesthetic molecules to reach the nerves and thereby prevents full anesthesia.[88] When infiltration or block anesthesia fails, other techniques can be used to induce complete anesthesia.

Intrapulpal Anesthesia

If sensitivity of the tooth persists following infiltration or block anesthesia, intrapulpal anesthesia may be administered. This direct injection into the body of the exposed pulp can be done only if the exposure of the pulp is large enough to admit a hypodermic needle. Too large an exposure, however, may cause a backflow of solution, with little or no solution entering the pulp to anesthetize it. This problem can be prevented by introducing the needle into the root canal until it binds and by forcing the anesthetic solution into the radicular pulp. In many cases, it is necessary to bend the needle, to penetrate the root canals. A drop or two of anesthetic solution is quickly discharged into the pulp, and the resulting anesthesia is effective and immediate.

In a double-blind study, Birchfield and Rosenberg found that it was immaterial whether a local anesthetic or sterile saline solution was used for intrapulpal anesthesia, provided the syringe needle fitted tightly into the cavity and penetrated the pulp.[12]

Periodontal Ligament Injection

The periodontal ligament or intraligamentary injection is used to augment incomplete dental anesthesia. It is considered an intraosseous injection because of the distribution of the anesthetic in the medullary spaces adjacent to the periodontal ligament.[131] In some patients, it causes a transient decrease in blood pressure and an increase in heart rate. These cardiovascular changes are manifested clinically as palpitations and anxiety. This injection is not recommended for patients with cardiovascular diseases.[132]

The objective of this injection is to anesthetize the periodontal ligament of the tooth undergoing endodontic therapy and thereby to block the pulpal nerves. Damage to the periodontal ligament from this injection is minimal and is usually confined to the crestal area where the needle penetrates. The injured periodontal ligament has shown rapid recovery in experiments in monkeys.[152]

Special pressure syringes have been developed for the intraligamentary injection (Fig. 11–3). These syringes are manufactured to deliver a preset volume of anesthetic (0.14 to 0.22 ml) with minimal effort and without breaking the anesthetic carpule. A short 27- or 30-gauge needle is inserted interproximally with positive pressure as deeply as possible along the root of the tooth, with the bevel of the needle toward the crestal bone. In posterior teeth, the needle is bent to a convenient angle, and the trigger is squeezed, to deliver around 0.2 ml intraligamentally alongside the mesial and distal roots of multirooted teeth. The onset of anesthesia is immediate, and the effect lasts an average of 27 min when using 2% lidocaine containing epinephrine 1:50,000. Lidocaine containing no epinephrine lasts an average of 1 min.[77]

This technique is most frequently used in mandibular molars and is approximately 92% effective.[151] The ability to anesthetize a single tooth makes this technique invaluable in the diagnosis of diffuse pain of unknown origin (anesthetic test).

PULPECTOMY

Once adequate coronal access has been gained, the next step is pulp extirpation from the chamber and root canals. The pulp chamber and root canal may contain a vital, partially vital, or necrotic pulp. Pulpectomy, or pulp extirpation, is the complete removal of a normal or diseased pulp from the pulp cavity of the tooth. The operation is sometimes inappropriately referred to as devitalization. When the tooth has been left open for drainage, and when food or other debris has accumulated in the pulp cavity, in addition to the residual necrotic pulpal debris, the removal of this material from the pulp cavity is referred to as debridement (Fig. 11–4).

In pulpectomy, the pulp is literally torn from the root canal when it is extirpated. This procedure leaves a lacerated wound. The reaction comprises hemorrhage, inflammation, and repair. Although pain can occur, it is frequently minimal and can be controlled with mild analgesics.

The tooth from which a pulp is removed or missing has been referred to as devital, avital, or even "dead." The term pulpless is preferred because it correctly describes the condition; tooth vitality is not related to the presence or absence of pulp tissue.

Another common misconception is that the endodontally treated tooth will turn "black." Although discoloration cannot always be prevented, it can be prevented in most cases. During pulpectomy, every effort should be made to prevent infiltration of blood into the dentinal tubules because this is one of the principal causes of discoloration. Frequent irrigation and debridement of the root canal and pulp chamber with sodium-hypochlorite solution (5.2%) will help to prevent this major cause of tooth discoloration.

Because the removal of a vital pulp is dreaded by many patients, the dentist should alleviate the patient's fears and should ensure that the operation is painless. Only a pulp that has been completely anesthetized should be extirpated.

Technique for Pulpectomy and Gross Debridement

The tooth to undergo root canal therapy is identified by penetrating the enamel at the site of the access cavity. The rubber dam is applied, and the field of operation is disinfected; that is, the tooth, clamp, and rubber dam are scrubbed with a sterile cotton-tip

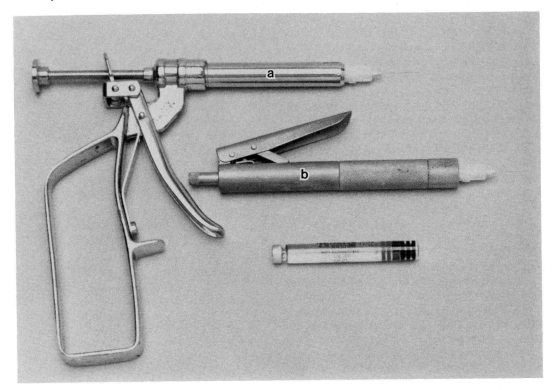

Fig. 11–3. Special pressure syringes developed for intraligamentary injection: Peri-press (Universal Dental Implements, Fanwood, New Jersey) (a) and PDL-Intraligamentary (Special Products, Inc., Santa Cruz, California) (b).

applicator saturated with a 5.2% solution of sodium hypochlorite. The access cavity is completed as described in Chapter 10. In posterior teeth, after complete removal of the roof of the pulp chamber, the coronal pulp is removed with sharp endodontic spoon excavators. The chamber is irrigated with a 5.2% solution of sodium hypochlorite and is dried with suction. Next, the canal orifices are located by probing with endodontic explorers along the anatomic grooves located in the chamber floor or at the point angle formed by the walls and floor of the pulp chamber and leading to the root canals.

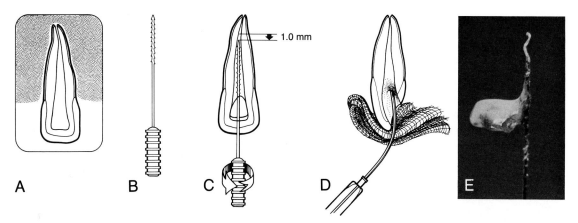

Fig. 11–4. Gross debridement. *A,* Radiograph (schematic view) is studied for anatomic variations and size of the image of the root canal. *B,* A broach is selected to fit the apical third of the root canal loosely. *C,* The broach is introduced into the root canal to the point of unforced contact with the walls of the canal; it is then withdrawn 1 mm, is rotated 360° to engage the pulp tissue, and is withdrawn to remove the pulp. *D,* The root canal is copiously irrigated with a 5% solution of sodium hypochlorite, to remove loose debris and blood. *E,* Extirpated pulp of a maxillary first molar. (*E,* Courtesy of G. Walters, San Antonio, Texas.)

These anatomic grooves, sometimes called the dentinal map, unite the canal orifices, which are at the end of the grooves. The grooves are darker than the floor of the pulp chamber (Fig. 11–5).

In teeth with one root canal in which the pulp chamber is confluent with the root canal, the orifice is easily located in the center of the tooth; the maxillary central incisors, lateral incisors, and cuspids are such teeth. The mandibular central and lateral incisors may have a buccal and a lingual canal. The orifice of the lingual canal in these teeth may be difficult to find because it is located lingually under the cingulum.

The maxillary first premolar usually has two canals, one buccal and one lingual. The orifices of the buccal and lingual canals are continuous, respectively, with the buccal and lingual walls of the pulp chamber. The floor of the pulp chamber of this tooth is convex, it lies deep in the coronal third of the root, and the orifices are connected by a dark groove.

The maxillary second premolar and the mandibular first and second premolars usually have one root canal, and their orifices are in the center of the tooth. Because these teeth may have two canals, the operator should search for this anatomic variation routinely.

The maxillary first molar usually has three canals, with a pulpal floor that is generally triangular in shape. At the corners of the triangle are three orifices connected by dark grooves. The palatal orifice is round or oval,

usually found in the center of the mesial half of the tooth, and is located and penetrated by inserting an exploratory instrument from the buccal wall of the access cavity, aimed apically and palatally. The mesiobuccal orifice, found under the mesiobuccal cusp, is located and penetrated by inserting an exploratory instrument from the distopalatal area of the access cavity in a mesiobuccal-apical direction. If a fourth canal is present, its orifice is generally located palatal to the mesiobuccal orifice. The distobuccal orifice, found under the distobuccal cusp and distal to the mesiobuccal orifice, is located and penetrated by inserting an exploratory instrument from the mesiopalatal area of the access cavity in a distobuccal-apical direction.

The maxillary second molar is similar to the maxillary first molar, but with a smaller pulp chamber. More anatomic variations occur in this tooth than in the maxillary first molar.

The mandibular first molar usually has a triangular floor with three orifices in the angles of the triangle connected by dark grooves (Fig. 11–5). The distal orifice has an elliptic shape in the buccolingual dimension and is in the center of the tooth buccolingually. If this orifice is either buccal or lingual in position, a second canal will probably be present. One may see a single orifice with two canals emerging from it. The mesiobuccal orifice is located under the mesiobuccal cusp, and the mesiolingual orifice is located in line mesially with the mesiobuccal orifice and mesially to the distal orifice. An anatomic variation seen in the mesial portion of the first mandibular molar is the presence of only one mesial orifice under the buccal cusp containing one or two canals. The distal orifice is located by inserting an exploratory instrument from the mesial part of the access cavity in a distoapical direction. The mesiobuccal orifice is penetrated with an exploratory instrument by probing from the distolingual part of the access cavity in a mesiobuccal-apical direction. The mesiolingual orifice is found by probing from the distobuccal in a mesiolingual-apical direction. The second mandibular molar is similar to the first mandibular molar, but it has more anatomic variations.

The operator must be familiar with the anatomic variation encountered in the different teeth and must search for them in every tooth

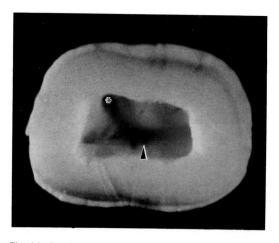

Fig. 11–5. Anatomic groove (arrow) on the pulpal floor of a mandibular first molar uniting the root canal orifices (*). The roof of the pulp chamber and one-third of the crown have been removed.

using radiographs and visual and tactile exploration.

In some instances, reactions of the pulp to inflammatory changes have caused calcification and blockage of an orifice or of most of the root canal. Radiographs taken at different angulations provide useful information on the extent of the calcification and the feasibility of opening the root canal. A blocked orifice can be opened by picking out the calcified tissue with a sharp endodontic explorer or by removing the blockage using slow-speed, small, round burs. If the foregoing procedures are not successful, a chelating agent, ethylenediaminotetraacetic acid (EDTA), is sealed in the chamber for 24 hours. The chelating agent may soften the dentin that is covering the orifice, so it can be removed and the orifice opened by picking with an endodontic explorer. Root canals that are partially calcified can be opened by cautious penetration of the calcified canal

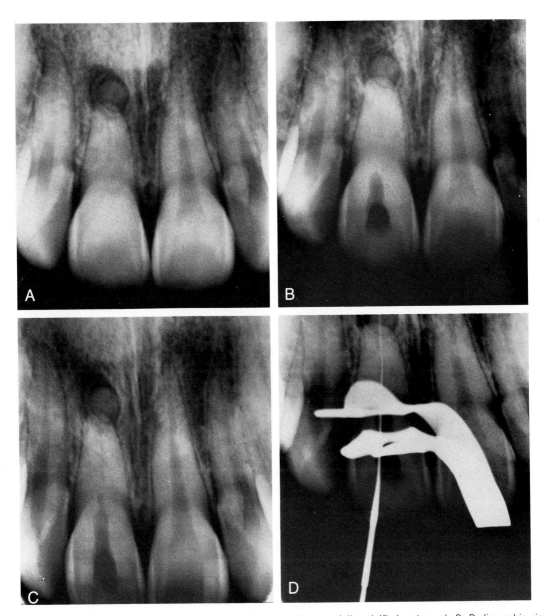

Fig. 11–6. *A*, Radiograph of a maxillary right central incisor with a partially calcified root canal. *B*, Radiographic view of an access cavity created for treatment of this tooth. *C*, Radiographic view after cautious penetration with small, round burs, to reach a patent root canal. (The progress of penetration with sequentially smaller burs was monitored radiographically.) *D*, The patency of the root canal is established. (Courtesy of J. Alexander, San Antonio, Texas.)

with small round burs, the penetration monitored by successive radiographs in order to avoid root perforation, until the canal is patent (Fig. 11–6).

Once the canal is penetrated, it should be explored with a smooth broach or small endodontic instrument. The true working length of the tooth should also be determined. Insert an instrument to the estimated working length of the root canal, that is, a length calculated from the diagnostic radiograph from a selected occlusal spot to a point arbitrarily designated as the dentinocemental junction (constricture) in the apical root tip of the tooth. Verify the position of the instrument radiographically, and adjust the estimated length to an exact working length that becomes the terminus of the root canal for instrumentation and obturation. This terminus is usually short of the radiographic apex, within 0.5 mm.

Pulpectomy and gross debridement of the root canal are the next steps in cleaning and shaping of the root canal. One should use a barbed broach, which is a short-handled endodontic instrument used for the extirpation of the entire pulp and for the removal of necrotic debris, absorbent points, cotton pledgets, and other foreign material from the root canal (Fig. 11–7). It is manufactured from a tapered, round, soft iron wire in which angle cuts are made into the surface to produce barbs. Barbed broaches are available in a variety of sizes, from triple extra fine (XXXF) to extra coarse (XC). Barbed broaches break easily, especially if they bind in the root canal. To avoid binding and breakage, many clinicians initiate root canal exploration and instrumentation with small reamers and files. Macerated pulp tissue is removed, and the root canal is debrided using irrigation and aspiration. Barbed broaches are not

inserted into the root canal until the canal has been enlarged throughout up to a size No. 20 or 25 reamer or file. This precaution prevents accidental binding of small and easily broken broaches.

The selection of a suitably sized broach for the removal of the pulp and gross debridement is important. A barbed broach that is too wide does not permit removal of all the pulp tissue, or it may force the pulp apically as the broach is inserted in the canal. It may also bind in the canal as it is rotated and may thereby break, or the barbs may become embedded in the dentin as the broach is withdrawn. On the other hand, if the broach is too narrow, it will not engage the pulp tissue sufficiently to allow its removal.

By comparing the size of the broach with the size of the last instrument used in the root canal or an estimated size of the image in a radiograph, one should select a barbed broach that fits loosely into the apical third of the root canal (see Fig. 11–4). The root canal is irrigated with a 5.2% solution of sodium hypochlorite, and the barbed broach is introduced until one notes unforced contact with root canal walls. The broach is withdrawn about 1 mm and is rotated 360° to engage the pulp tissue; it is withdrawn again to remove this tissue.

When the root canal is unusually wide, as in young teeth, even a coarse barbed broach may not be able to engage and remove the massive pulp tissue. In such cases, two fine barbed broaches are inserted into the canal and are rotated at the same time until the pulp tissue is engaged and removed.

Hemorrhage following pulp removal is controlled by means of copious irrigation with a 5.2% sodium-hypochlorite solution, followed by drying of the canal with suction and sterile absorbent points. Each point

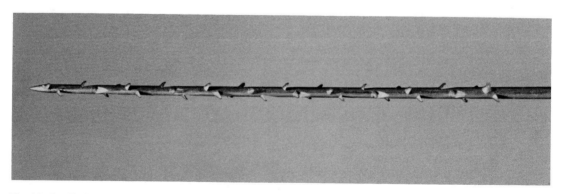

Fig. 11–7.   Barbed broach used for extirpation of the pulp and gross debridement of the root canal.

should remain in the root canal for about a minute and should not touch the pulp stump. When hemorrhage is persistent, the presence of a tag or remnant of pulp tissue left behind in the root canal should be suspected. One must also look for an additional untreated canal or root perforation. Every effort should be made to remove all the pulp tissue at one time. If pulp fragments remain, they should be removed by repeating the procedure with the appropriate barbed broach or during the cleaning and shaping of the root canal with files and irrigation.

A barbed broach can be cleaned by scrubbing with a bur brush. Another effective method of cleaning a broach that has tissue tags or necrotic debris in its barbs is to place it in a 5.2% sodium-hypochlorite solution for half an hour. The tissue or necrotic debris will completely dissolve. The broach is then rinsed in running water, is air dried, and is sterilized in dry heat. Because broaches are inexpensive, except when one is broken and blocking a root canal, and difficult to clean, it seems judicious to discard them rather than to clean them.

Repair Following Pulpectomy

Whenever pulp is extirpated, the residual tissue in or around the tooth is wounded. The resulting inflammatory process causes some degree of tenderness in the tooth. Repair can be separated into four phases: (1) initial necrosis or sloughing; (2) formation of granulation tissue; (3) connective tissue framework; and (4) repair with homologous tissue. When the pulp is severed at its most constricted portion, hemorrhage follows. A clot of fibrin covers the residual tissue stump, as well as the shreds of tissue still adhering to the canal wall.

An inflammatory reaction follows pulp removal, with rapid mobilization of polymorphonuclear leukocytes that form a protective barrier. Shortly afterward, the macrophages appear on the scene and engulf and digest foreign material introduced during the operation as well as dead tissue cells and microorganisms. On the fibrin framework, fibroblasts proliferate to initiate repair. On the surface of the root canal near the apical foramen, an ingrowth of connective tissue from the periodontal ligament may occur, followed by resorption of dentin and deposition of secondary cementum. If the pulp stump should be injured by mechanical instrumentation or chemical irritation, the inflammatory reaction may be acute and may extend into the periapical tissue for some distance. This phenomenon accounts for the periodontitis occasionally produced following pulpectomy. In that case, resorption of periapical tissue and even of the dentinal surface near the apical foramen may occur. Repair follows after subsidence of the inflammatory reaction, except cementoblasts may enter the root canal and may lay down secondary cementum where resorption had taken place. At the same time, a fibrous callus forms in the periodontal tissue and approximates the end of the root canal filling.

IRRIGATION

One of the most neglected phases of endodontic treatment is the removal of minute fragments of organic debris and dentinal shavings from the root canal. A principle of surgery is that before a wound is ready for disinfection, all necrotic material and debris must be removed. Many dentists fail to appreciate the importance of this basic rule of surgery and rely principally on drug therapy, rather than on thorough cleaning and irrigation of the root canal. The need for cleaning and shaping and the importance of removing resultant debris, as well as pulp remnants, are often ignored. Thorough debridement and cleaning are as necessary in endodontic treatment as in surgery.

The importance of cleaning and shaping of the root canal cannot be overemphasized.

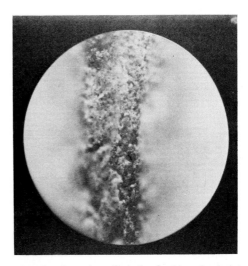

Fig. 11–8. Ground section of a freshly extracted tooth from which the pulp was "completely" removed, showing the irregular surface of the root canal with fragments of pulp tissue attached to the canal surface. Magnification ×60.

The irregularities in dentin provide areas in which bacteria live, and the tags of tissue provide pabulum on which they thrive (Fig. 11–8). During and following cleaning and shaping, the canal should be irrigated to wash out fragments of pulp tissue and dentinal shavings that have accumulated. Much debris and organic tissue, which are present more often than one realizes, are removed by the flushing action of the irrigating solutions. Irrigation may also be used to wash out food debris when the canal has been left open for drainage during the acute stage of an alveolar abscess.

Several investigators have shown that unless adequate irrigation is part of the canal cleaning process, debris will be left behind regardless of the irrigant used;[5,142] moreover, the clearance of debris from the canal was proportional to the amount of irrigant used. Other studies have shown that frequent irrigation of the canal is mandatory, and irrigation is more complete in properly enlarged canals.[115] Penetration of the irrigant is more effective in canals with larger diameters than in smaller apical constrictions.[126] In pulpectomy, the irrigant solution flows only as far as the insertion of the instrument, but in pulpless teeth, it not only fills the entire canal, but can also leak into the periapex.[121] These investigators point out that the irrigating solution should be constantly exchanged to maintain its efficiency. High-volume ultrasonic irrigation systems have been developed. These systems enhance the penetrating and debriding action of the irrigant by ultrasonic activation.

Through the years, different irrigating solutions have been recommended. A stream of hot water (140 to 176° F) discharged from an insulated syringe,[113] physiologic saline solution,[5] a 30% solution of urea,[15] ureaperoxide solution in glycerin,[135] a solution of chloramine,[27] sodium hypochlorite, and sodium hypochlorite in conjunction with ethylenediaminotetraacetic (EDTA) acid are just a few.

Unless irrigation is part of the canal cleaning process, debris will be left behind.[5,147] Of a number of solutions studied, none was more effective than a 5.2% solution of sodium hypochlorite.[61] It completely dissolved an entire pulp in 20 min to 2 hours, whereas the next most effective solution required at least 24 hours to accomplish the same result. Although this solvent action of sodium hypochlorite on tissue has been con-

firmed,[96] other investigators have found sodium hypochlorite less effective in narrow than in wide root canals[126] (Fig. 11–9).

Sodium hypochlorite, a reducing agent, is a clear, straw-colored solution containing about 5% of available chlorine. The solution should be kept in a cool place, away from sunlight. Popular household bleaching agents, such as Clorox or Purex, are usually 5.2% solutions of sodium hypochlorite and are satisfactory.

If the canal is filled with the solution during the entire cleaning and shaping procedure, the irrigant will act as a lubricant, solvent of pulp tissue, antiseptic, and bleach.

No unanimity of opinion exists as to which concentration of sodium hypochlorite should be used in root canal therapy. On the basis of published data,[51,65,69,119,120,141,142,153] we believe that a 2.6 to 5.2% solution is an effective concentration for use as a solvent of organic tissue in the root canal. A 50% dilution of a commercial preparation (Clorox) with distilled water gives a solution of 2.6% sodium hypochlorite.

Sodium hypochlorite is not only a pulp solvent and root canal irrigant, but also it has significant antimicrobial properties. Disinfection by means of sodium hypochlorite is initially slow, but increases progressively.[63] Destruction of bacteria takes place in two phases: (1) penetration into the bacterial cell; and (2) chemical combination with the protoplasm of the bacterial cell that destroys it. Sodium hypochlorite was the most effective among five halogen antiseptics tested,[134] but its effectiveness was reduced when diluted.[128]

Alternate irrigations with sodium hypochlorite and hydrogen peroxide have been advocated. Their interaction in the canal produces a transient but energetic effervescence that mechanically forces debris and microorganisms out of the canal. At the same time, the oxygen liberated in an active state assists in destroying anaerobic microorganisms. Sodium hypochlorite is the most effective irrigant for removing loose debris.[72] The combination with hydrogen peroxide seems to reduce the tissue-solvent property of sodium hypochlorite.[72] No significant difference is found between cleanliness of a canal irrigated with sodium hypochlorite and that of a canal irrigated with hydrogen peroxide.[39] The advantages of alternating solutions of hydrogen peroxide, 3%, and sodium hypochlorite, 5.2% are: (1) the effervescent

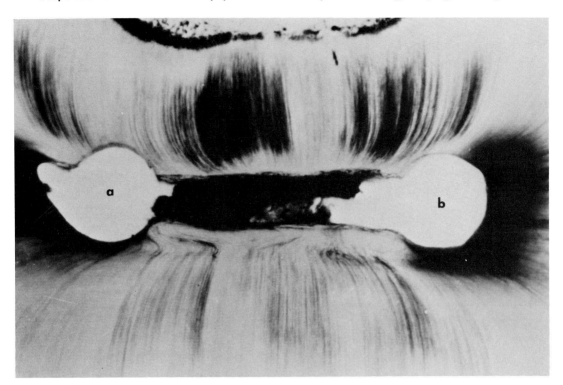

Fig. 11–9.   Cross section of the mesial root of a mandibular first molar showing root canals 5 mm from the apex. A smaller amount of pulp tissue was removed in side a of the isthmus, as compared to side b, which was treated with a 5.2% solution of sodium hypochlorite. (Courtesy of S. Senia, San Antonio, Texas.)

reaction, in which it mechanically "bubbles" and pushes debris out of the root canal through the least-resistant orifice into the chamber; (2) the solvent action of the sodium hypochlorite on the organic debris of the pulp tissue; and (3) the disinfecting and bleaching action by both solutions. One should always use sodium hypochlorite last because hydrogen peroxide can react with pulp debris and blood to form gas. Any gas trapped within the tooth will cause continuous pain.

EDTA, a chelating agent, has been used as an irrigating solution. This solution has removed the smear layer of dentin and left virtually no debris on the surface of the dentin.[47,86] The smear layer is a combination of dentin, pulpal, and bacterial debris. Some clinicians advocate the removal of the smear layer by irrigating the canal with EDTA followed by sodium hypochlorite.[69,75] The properties and uses of EDTA in endodontics are discussed later in this chapter.

Technique

The technique of irrigation is simple. The only instrument required is a disposable plastic pipette or glass syringe with an endodontic notched needle (Fig. 11–10). The needle should be bent to an obtuse angle, to reach the canals of posterior as well as anterior teeth. The solution used for irrigation is 5.2% sodium hypochlorite. The needle is inserted partway into the root canal. It should not be inserted so it binds. Sufficient room between needle and canal wall allows for the return flow of the solution and avoids forcing of solution into the periapical tissue. In many cases, in upper anterior teeth, the needle can be inserted for a distance of half the length of the canal without binding, although one does not need to advance the needle that far into the canal (Fig. 11–11).

When one is certain that the needle does not bind, the solution should be ejected from the syringe with little or no pressure on the plunger. The object is to wash out the canal and not to force the solution under pressure into the periradicular tissues. During the cleaning and shaping of the root canal, care should be taken that the canals are always full of fresh solution.

In narrow root canals, the tip of the needle is placed near the root canal orifice, and the

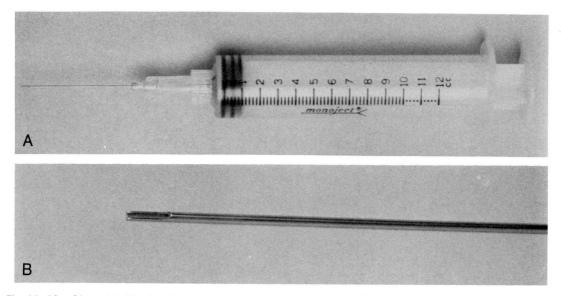

Fig. 11—10. Disposable 12-ml syringe (A) with notched needle (B). The notched needle lessens the pressure from the forceful ejection of the irrigating solution. (Courtesy of Monoject-Winthrop Laboratories, New York.)

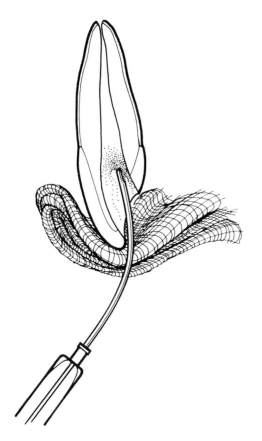

Fig. 11—11. Curved irrigating needle is partially inserted into the root canal without binding. The irrigating solution drains out of the canal and is absorbed on a sterile gauze sponge, to monitor the removal of debris from the root canal.

irrigant is discharged until it fills the pulp chamber. The solution is then pumped into each root canal with a root canal file.

A perforated irrigating needle has been developed to deliver irrigant 360° in the root canal. It is claimed that large volumes of the irrigant solution have "physically removed more material when delivered by the perforated irrigation needle."[48] A disadvantage of the perforated needle is that it is delicate and bends out of shape easily.

The return flow of solution is caught on a gauze sponge or is aspirated. Irrigation should be followed by thorough drying of the root canals after the completion of cleaning and shaping. Most of the residual irrigating solution may be removed from the root canal by holding the needle of the syringe in the canal and withdrawing the plunger slowly. Final drying should be effected with absorbent points.

Compressed air must not be used for drying the root canal because tissue emphysema may result if an air bubble penetrates the periapical tissues. Several cases of emphysema have been reported as a result of drying the root canal with compressed air.[87,110,127,129] The emphysema may last as long as a week. The death of a child has been associated with the use of compressed air in the root canal.[116]

INSTRUMENTS

Root canal instruments may be divided into four types according to their function.

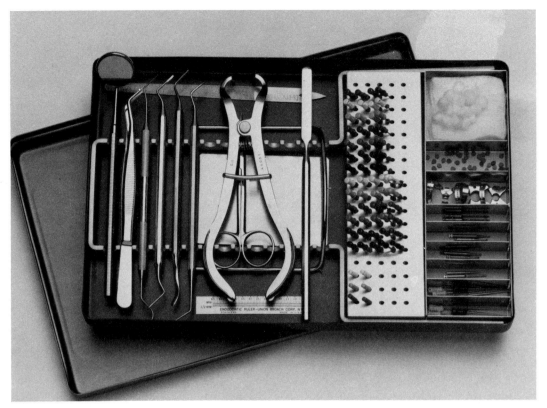

Fig. 11–12. Endodontic instrument kit, designed by C.E. del Rio, Columbus Dental, Columbus, Ohio. A root canal instrument tray that can be dry-heat sterilized, containing root canal instruments, burs, stops, cotton sponges and pellets, rubber dam clamps, forceps, frame scissors, ruler, file, spatula, and other operative instruments.

Figure 11–12 shows an endodontic instrument kit. The first use is *exploring*, to locate the canal orifice and to determine or assist in obtaining patency of the root canal. Examples are smooth broaches and endodontic explorers (Fig. 11–13). Second, instruments are used for *debridement*, to extirpate the pulp and to remove debris and other foreign material. An example is the barbed broach (see Fig. 11–7). The third use is for *shaping*, to shape the root canal laterally and apically. Examples are reamers and files (Fig. 11–14). Fourth, instruments are used for *obturating*, to cement and pack gutta percha into the root canal. Examples are pluggers, spreaders, and lentulo spirals (Fig. 11–15).

Standardization

At one time, root canal instruments were made according to the whim of manufactur-

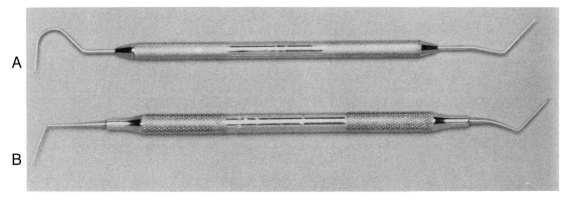

Fig. 11–13. Endodontic explorers. *A*, No. 23–16. *B*, No. 16.

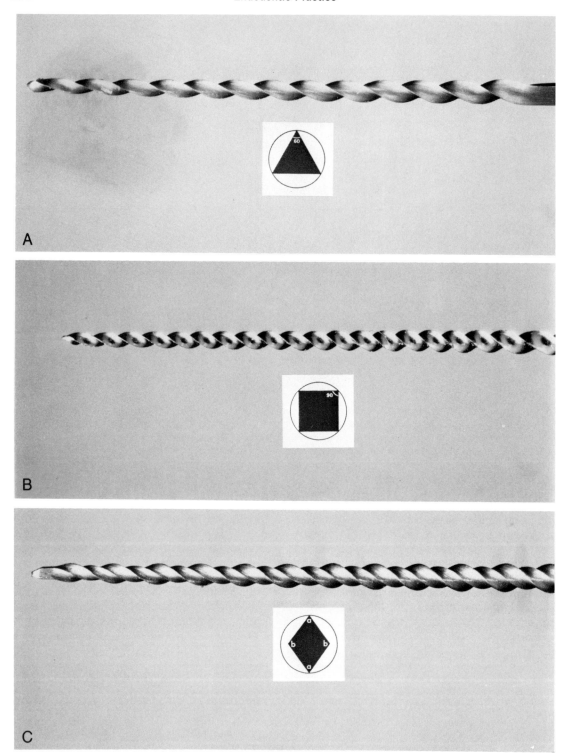

Fig. 11–14. Endodontic instruments used for cleaning and shaping the root canal. *A*, K-reamer, traditionally made from a triangular blank. *B*, K-file, traditionally made from a square blank. *C*, K-flex file, traditionally made from a diamond-shaped blank.

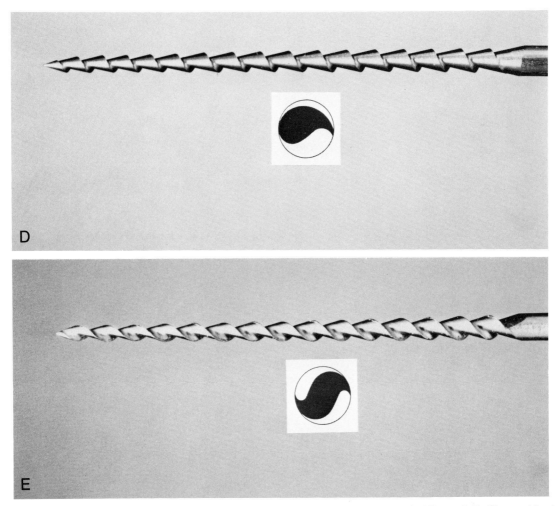

Fig. 11–14 Continued. *D*, Hedstroem file, machined from a round blank to produce spiral flutes. *E*, Unifile, machined from a round blank to produce a double helix.

ers, with no definite specifications regarding diameter, taper, or length of the cutting blades. Significant differences in widths of instruments supposedly of the same size were found when they were measured with a micrometer-measuring microscope.[55] Ingle and LeVine, using an electronic microcomparator, found variations in diameter and taper for the same sizes of instruments.[74] They suggested a definite increment in diameter as the size progressed while maintaining a constant taper of all blades regardless of size (Fig. 11–16). Essentially, their recommendations were as follows: (1) instruments shall be numbered from 10 to 100, the numbers to advance by 5 units to size 60, then by 10 units to size 100; (2) each number shall be representative of the diameter of the instrument in hundredths of a millimeter at the tip; for example, No. 10 is $^{10}/_{100}$ or 0.1 mm at the tip,

No. 25 is $^{25}/_{100}$ or 0.25 mm at the tip, and No. 90 is $^{90}/_{100}$ or 0.9 mm at the tip; and (3) the working blade (flutes) shall begin at the tip, designated site D_1, and shall extend exactly 16 mm up the shaft, terminating at designated site D_2. The diameter of D_2 shall be $^{32}/_{100}$ or .32 mm greater than that of D_1, for example, a No. 20 reamer shall have a diameter of .20 mm at D_1 and a diameter of 0.20 plus 0.32 or 0.52 mm at D_2. This sizing ensures a constant increase in taper of 0.02 mm per mm for every instrument regardless of size. (Note: the increased diameter of D_2 over D_1 was originally designated as $^{30}/_{100}$ or 0.3 mm.)

Other specifications were added later: the tip angle of an instrument should be 75 ± 15°, instrument sizes should increase by 0.05 mm at D_1 between Nos. 10 and 60, for example, Nos. 10, 15, and 20, and they should

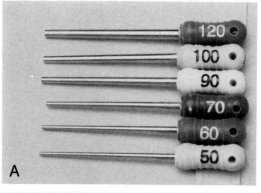

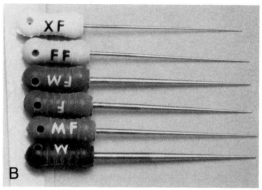

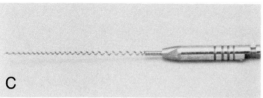

Fig. 11–15. *A*, Finger pluggers used for vertical compaction of gutta percha. *B*, Finger spreaders used for lateral compaction of gutta percha. *C*, Lentulo spiral used to deliver sealer or paste to the root canal.

increase by 0.1 mm from No. 60 to 150, for example, Nos. 60, 70, and 80; Nos. 06 and 08 have been added for increased instrument selection. In addition, instrument handles have been color coded for easier recognition (Table 11–1).

Stainless steel root canal instruments are used more often today than carbon steel instruments because they are more flexible and are therefore less likely to fracture when strained (deformed), and they are less susceptible to corrosion, usually caused by contact with sodium-hypochlorite solution. The finer sizes of reamers and files have low resistance to torque (pressure used to rotate instrument for cutting and shaping) and break using less force than larger instruments when they bind in a root canal. As a result, most small instruments are manufactured from square blanks, which are more resistant to torque fractures, and large instruments are manufactured from triangular blanks, to improve their cutting efficiency.[35,106]

An adequate supply of instruments should be available for any eventuality in the course of an endodontic operation. This recommendation refers not only to various kinds of instruments, but also to an adequate number of instruments.

Instruments are available in lengths of 21, 25, 28, and 30 mm. Ordinarily, instruments 25 mm long are used, but occasionally, 21-mm instruments are needed for molars, especially when the patient cannot open the

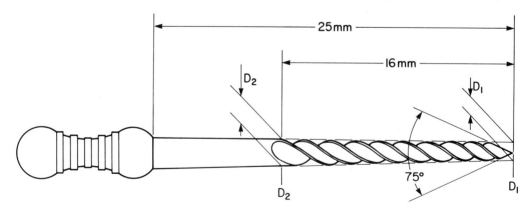

Fig. 11–16. Specifications for an endodontic instrument. D_1, Diameter at the tip, in hundredths of millimeters; D_2, Diameter in hundredths of millimeters at the end of the cutting blade, that is, 16 mm from D_1. The taper of the instrument from D_1 to D_2 is in increments of 0.02 mm in width per millimeter of length. The tip angle of the instrument should be $75 \pm 15°$.

Table 11–1.   Specifications of Files and Reamers

Nearest Old Number	Color Code	New Number	Diameter*	
			D_1 (mm)	D_2 (mm)
000	Pink	6	.06	.38
00	Gray	8	.08	.40
0	Purple	10	.10	.42
1	White	15	.15	.47
2	Yellow	20	.20	.52
3	Red	25	.25	.57
4	Blue	30	.30	.62
5	Green	35	.35	.67
6	Black	40	.40	.72
—	White	45	.45	.77
7	Yellow	50	.50	.82
—	Red	55	.55	.87
8	Blue	60	.60	.92
9	Green	70	.70	1.02
10	Black	80	.80	1.12
11	White	90	.90	1.22
—	Yellow	100	1.00	1.32
12	Red	110	1.10	1.42
13	Blue	120	1.20	1.52
14	Green	130	1.30	1.62
15	Black	140	1.40	1.72
—	White	150	1.50	1.82

*Distance on the shaft between D_1 and D_2 is 16 mm.

mouth wide, and 28- and 30-mm instruments are necessary for cuspids and other teeth in which a 25-mm instrument cannot reach the apical foramen. Reamers are also available in 40-mm lengths for use in preparing root canals for endodontic implants.

Instruments for Cleaning and Shaping

The following sections describe the physical and functional properties of reamers and files.

Physical Characteristics of Reamers and Files

In the early 1900s, the Kerr Manufacturing Company designed and manufactured new K-type endodontic instruments to improve the efficiency of root canal preparation. The reamers were used with a pushing-rotating motion (torque), and files were used with a rasping or pulling motion. Originally manufactured from round, tapered piano wire (carbon steel), most instruments are now manufactured from a variety of stainless steel blanks. The stainless steel wire is ground along its long axis into a 4-sided (square cross-section) or 3-sided (triangular cross-section) tapered shaft that is twisted into flutes extending 16 mm from the top to the tip of the cutting blade. The number of flutes twisted into each blade of a similar-sized instrument determines whether that instrument is a reamer (less flutes) or a file (more flutes). For example, a No. 30 reamer may have 15 flutes per 16-mm blade, and a No. 30 file may have 22 flutes per 16-mm blade. The traditional reamer, manufactured from a triangular blank (see Fig. 11–14, *A*), and file, manufactured from a square blank (see Fig. 11–14, *B*), are still made by a few companies; however, most manufacturers make reamers and files from similar blanks, and such reamers and files differ only in the number of flutes along their blade. Heuer reported that files are manufactured from blanks twisted to produce tighter flutes (1.93 to 0.88 mm), and reamers are manufactured with looser flutes (0.80 to 0.28 mm).[72] Because the use of square blanks results in instruments that resist fracture more effectively than those made from triangular blanks, square blanks are generally used for smaller, fragile instruments. When instrument fracture is no longer a critical factor, such as in larger instruments, triangular blanks are used because the triangular-blanked instruments cut approximately 2.5 times more efficiently.[106]

Reamers and K-type files do not break unless they have an undetected defect in the steel shaft or until the instrument is strained or deformed, that is, rotated on its axis when bound in a root canal for several 360° twists. The more flexible the instrument steel, the more full turns a blade can withstand before breaking. If an instrument is used with a maximum turn of 90°,[83] and if it is withdrawn periodically for inspection, the chance of instrument fracture is obviously reduced. Once an instrument is deformed, however, it does not continue to cut under pressure; instead, it continues to deform until it fractures.[106] Once deformed, the instrument must be discarded. The instrument temper is not affected by salt or glass-bead sterilization, and, contrary to a common misconception, few instruments become dull before they deform.

Recently, rhomboidal or diamond-shaped blanks have been twisted to produce a file called K-flex* (see Fig. 11–14, C) The manufacturer claims that this design increases the flexibility and cutting efficiency of the instrument. The rhomboidal blank produces alternating high and low flutes that are supposed to make the instrument more efficient in removal of debris.

Hedstroem files, also known as H-files, are manufactured from a round stainless steel wire machined to produce spiral flutes resembling cones or a screw. This instrument has a higher cutting efficiency than K-instruments, but it is fragile and fractures easily (Fig. 11–14, D).

Unifiles are machined from round stainless steel wire by cutting two superficial grooves to produce flutes in a double-helix design. They resemble the Hedstroem file in appearance, are less subject to fracture, but they are less efficient (see Fig. 11–14, E).

Functional Characteristics of Reamers and Files

Traditionally, reamers were used with a rotating-pushing motion, limited to a quarter- to a half-turn, and disengaged with a pulling motion when bound. Following the cleaning and shaping of the root canal with a small reamer and reaming to the root apex (working length), the same-size file was inserted into the root canal to the apex, laterally pressed against one side of the canal wall, and withdrawn with a pulling motion, to file the dentinal wall. The file was rein-

serted, and the procedure, known as circumferential filing, was repeated circumferentially around the walls of the canal until the next-size reamer could be used (Fig. 11–17). In narrow root canals, reamers were used alternately with files in sequence of sizes to produce a uniformly instrumented and enlarged canal.[86,120] Frequent irrigation facilitated instrumentation, debrided the canal, and helped to disinfect the canal. From time to time, dentinal debris, clogging the flutes of the instrument, was removed by squeezing the blade between layers of gauze and turning the instrument counterclockwise (Fig. 11–18). Before reinserting the instrument, it was inspected for deformation and resterilized in the salt sterilizer.

Many clinicians now use both reamers and files with a push turn (reaming) and a pull stroke (filing) in one continual motion. The same precautions for use prevail, however; that is, use a quarter- to a half-turn only, do not force an instrument that binds, debride and inspect the blade periodically, instrument in a wet field, use a sequence of sizes and return to a smaller instrument periodically to prevent packing of debris in front of the instrument tip and to avoid ledging, confine instruments within the root canal by using instrument stops and avoid forcing debris into the periapical tissue, clean and dry root canal instruments, and sterilize instruments after every use before placing them in their case.

LENGTH DETERMINATION

The radiograph plays an important role in cleaning and shaping because it permits the operator to form a visual conception of the internal tooth structure and periradicular tissue. The original diagnostic radiograph can now be studied and measured to estimate the working length of the tooth, from occlusal surface to root apex. This length is later verified by inserting instruments to the estimated working length in each root canal and taking an instrumentation radiograph (Fig. 11–19). The exact working length for each canal is determined by adjusting the length of insertion so the tip of the instrument ends 0.5 mm from the root apex. Table 11–2 gives the average length of teeth.

The radiograph is an exact "road map" of the anticipated journey between the access opening into the pulp chamber and the apical root foramen. The clinician must learn to

---

*Kerr Manufacturing Co., Romulus, Michigan.

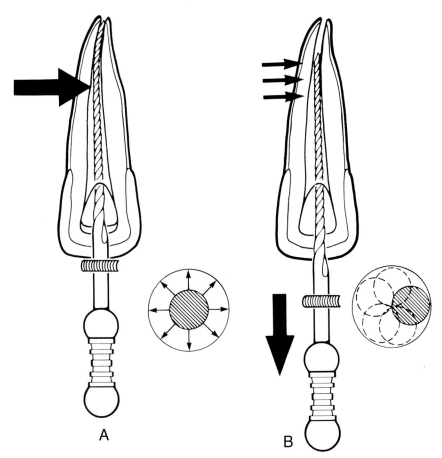

Fig. 11–17.   *A* and *B*, Circumferential filing is the technique of inserting the file into the root canal to the desired length, engaging it into the dentin wall by applying lateral pressure, and withdrawing it. This procedure is performed around all the walls of the root canal.

interpret the radiograph, to assist in instrument selection for exploration of the complicated root canal system. One can measure the distance between the roof and the floor of the pulp chamber and the occlusal surface, to determine the depth of the access cavity and thus to avoid inadvertent perforations. One notes the presence of atypical anatomy, the number of canals and roots, curvatures, bifurcations, lateral canals, pulp stones, obstructions such as root canal fillings, posts, or broken instruments, resorptions, decay, and periodontal disease, for example, and uses endodontic skills effectively and successfully to complete the cleaning, shaping, and disinfecting of all root canals in preparation for obturation.

Diagnostic or exploratory instruments are usually Nos. 10 to 20 K-files. These instruments are flexible enough to follow root canal curvatures and to fit into fine tortuous canals and are stiff enough to be inserted through debris and tissue until they reach the root apex. When an instrument is removed from the canal, the operator should examine it for curvatures that were not apparent by tactile sensation or radiographic examination; examples are a buccal curvature in the palatal canal of a maxillary first molar or a palatal curvature in a maxillary lateral incisor. One should record any observed anatomic variations and use this information for cleaning, shaping, and filling the root canal.

The setting of an instrument stop to the exact working length for each canal is valuable in confining instruments to a root canal, to prevent trauma or forcing of debris and bacteria into the periradicular tissue. Stops can be made by inserting an instrument blade through a small piece of rubber dam or rubber band. Commercial stops made of metal, silicone rubber, and plastic are also available. Teardrop silicone-rubber stops have an added advantage because they do not have

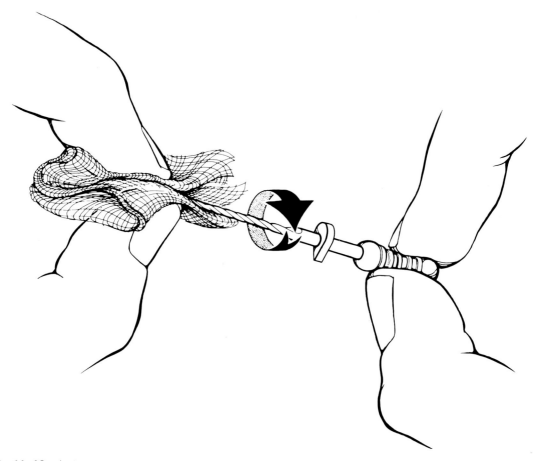

Fig. 11–18. Instruments are cleaned of debris by holding the blade between layers of gauze under digital pressure and turning it counterclockwise.

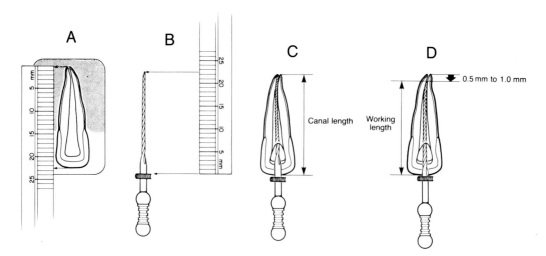

Fig. 11–19. *A*, The length of the tooth is measured on the diagnostic radiograph (schematic view). *B*, This measurement is transferred to a diagnostic instrument prepared with a silicone stop, the instrument is placed in the root canal, and a radiograph is made. *C* and *D*, The root canal and working lengths are determined from the radiograph.

Table 11–2.   Average Length of Teeth

	Maxillary (mm)	Mean*	Mandibular (mm)	Mean*
Central incisor	23	23.7	20.5	21.8
Lateral incisor	22	23.1	21	23.3
Cuspid	26.5	27.3	25.5	26.0
First premolar	20.5	22.3	20.5	22.9
Second premolar	21.5	21.3	22	22.3
First molar	20.5	22.3	21	22.0
Second molar	20	22.2	20	21.7

*Bjorndahl and colleagues have computed the mean anatomic measurements to be approximately 1 mm greater than the above measurements,[13] but it is safer to be slightly short in estimating tooth length, to avoid damaging periapical tissue.

to be removed from the instrument during sterilization at 450° F. In addition to designating the working length, the teardrop tip can be positioned to indicate instrument curvature, a prepared gentle curvature made on the instrument blade that facilitates insertion of the instrument into a canal orifice and penetration to the root apex in fine, tortuous canals (Fig. 11–20). The desired curvature is attained by grasping the blade with a gauze sponge and bending the instrument in a gentle slope (Fig. 11–21, *A* and *B*).

Initially, the K-file is inserted into the root canal through the access cavity with a slight wiggling motion, to bypass any obstruction or debris, and is gently teased along the entire canal length until it has been inserted to the estimated working length of the canal. A radiograph is taken to compare the exact position of the instrument in the root canal with the measured depth of insertion. If necessary, the measured length is adjusted so that the instrument tip is inserted up to 0.5 mm from the radiographic apex. This procedure completes the tactile exploration of the root canal and establishes the exact working length to be used during sequential instrumentation of the root canal (Fig. 11–21, *C* and *D*).

If a change of tactile sensation during exploration of the root canal suggests that the instrument is at the apical constricture, even though it seems short of the estimated working length, one should take a radiograph to verify the location of the instrument tip. Once the exact length between the reference point on the tooth surface and the apical constricture (or 0.5 mm short of the root apex) is known, the instrument stops should be adjusted accordingly, so subsequent sequential instrumentation will end within the root canal at the established terminus.

Reference points in anterior teeth are usually the incisal edges, and in posteriors, they are the cusp tips. The reference point must be a definite and reliable point or surface, to ensure exactness in all subsequent measurements. Incisal edges or cusps that are undermined or fractured should be ground until a sound surface is attained.

A radiograph is made with the snug-fitting K-file in position, to determine the length of

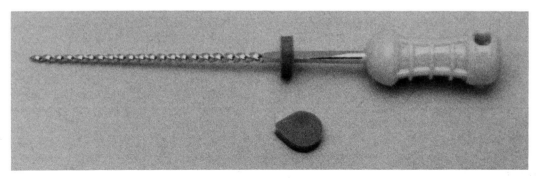

Fig. 11–20.   Teardrop silicone stops are placed at right angles to the shaft of the instrument, to obtain accurate measurements.

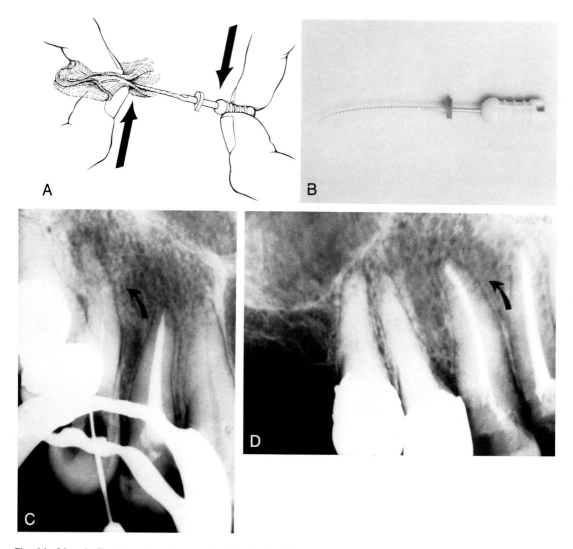

Fig. 11–21. *A,* Files are curved by grasping the blade with a gauze sponge and bending the blade until the desired curvature is attained. The directional silicone stop is set to indicate the direction of the curve. *B,* Instrument with a gentle curve, for exploring straight root canals. *C,* A file inserted in the root canal of a cuspid tooth meets with an obstruction against the wall because of the "S-shaped" configuration of the root canal (arrow). When the file was gently bent, it became possible to clean and shape the root canal up to the apex. *D,* Radiograph showing a completed root canal filling of the tooth shown in *C,* following the curvature of the root canal to the apex (arrow).

the root canal. The canal length is the distance from the apical exit of the root canal to the reference point on the crown of the tooth (see Fig. 11–19). If the K-file is 1 mm longer or shorter than the radiographic foramen of the canal, one should add or subtract the necessary length to obtain the root canal length, but if the difference is greater than 1 mm, one should make the necessary adjustment on the K-file and take another radiograph (Fig. 11–22).

Two length-determination radiographs may be necessary at times, one at the normal angulation, the other at a 20° mesial or distal horizontal angulation. The tridimensionality gained from these 2 views allows better visualization of the configuration of the root canal and its terminus. When 2 root canals are present in a single root, for example, the mesial root of a mandibular molar or 2 roots aligned in the same plane, such as in the maxillary first premolar, 2 radiographs from different angulations will separate the images of the root canals.

The working length should be arbitrarily established 0.5 mm to 1.0 mm shorter than

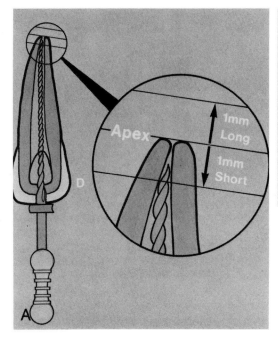

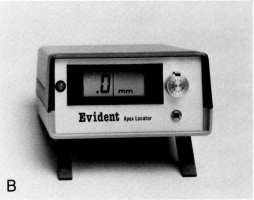

Fig. 11–22. *A*, If a length-determination radiograph shows an instrument 1 mm too short or too long in relation to the foramen, the problem can be corrected without further radiography. *B*, Evident Apex Locator. (Courtesy of Evident Dental Co., London.)

the measured canal length because the actual length of the tooth is 1.2 mm less than the radiographic image and the apical foramen is approximately 0.3 mm short of the actual root tip (see Fig. 11–19).[148] Certain anatomic studies have reported the dentinocemental junction about 0.4 to 0.7 mm away from the root apex.[14,81] Although the dentinocemental junction is a variable, it is always short of the root apex, and for this reason, instruments should stop at least 0.5 to 1.0 mm short of the canal length. The size of the last instrument used in the root apex is variable and depends on the following: (1) the apical size of the root, because if the root tip is fine, overzealous instrumentation can fracture the apical root tip; (2) apical root curvature, because if the curvature is pronounced, overinstrumentation can distort the apical foramen, spatially displace it, perforate the apical root tip, remove the established apical stop within the canal, and result in instrument fracture; and (3) the ability of the operator to gain direct access to the root apex; that is, if more curvatures are present in a root canal, smaller, flexible instruments must be used. In addition, all instruments must be confined within the root canals, to avoid irritating the periapical tissues with the instrument tip, initiating an immunocomplex reaction, or causing a transient bacteremia by microbes pushed out of the root canal into the periradicular tissues, especially danger-

ous if the patient has a history of valvular or cardiac disease.[7,10]

When apical resorption is evident in a radiograph, the working length should be reduced 1.5 to 2.0 mm in case the apical constricture has been destroyed by the resorption. In such an event, an apical stop is created short of the radiographic apex to prevent overinstrumentation and subsequent overfilling of the root canal.

Electronic Method

In recent years, electrical devices have been developed for determining the length of a tooth without resorting to radiography. This working length is determined by comparing the electrical resistance of the periodontal membrane with that of the gingiva surrounding the tooth, both of which should be similar.[138,139] A probe, such as a file, is attached to an electronic instrument with an electric cord and is inserted through the root canal until it contacts the surrounding periodontal ligament (soft tissue). When the probe touches the soft tissues of the periodontal membrane, the electrical-resistance gauges for both gingiva and periodontal ligament should have similar readings. By measuring the depth of insertion of the probe, one may determine the exact working length of the root canal (Fig. 11–22).

The audiometric method, a variation on the principle of electrical resistance of comparative tissue, uses low-frequency oscillation sound to indicate when similarity to electric resistance has occurred by a similar sound response. By placing an instrument in the gingival sulcus and inducing an electric current until sound is produced, and then repeating this by placing an instrument through the root canal until the same sound is heard, one can determine the length of the tooth.

Electronic measurement of tooth length is only effective in 80 to 90% of cases, as compared with the radiographic method.[14,18,22,76,82,107,112,125,153] A discrepancy can occur when tags of necrotic tissue are left inside a root canal, when the instrument in the canal comes in contact with a metallic restoration, when a pulp stone is present, and when a foreign substance is present in the root canal. Radiographs are still the most accurate means of determining root canal length.[20]

Xeroradiography, with its property of edge enhancement (edge contrast), makes the anatomic structures of the tooth and periradicular tissues appear sharper (Fig. 11–23). This sharpness leads to faster and easier visualization of the structures and position of the diagnostic instrument in the root canal and allows a more accurate interpretation of canal length and apical exit of the root canal.[22]

Cleaning and Shaping

Cleaning and shaping the root canal consist of removing the pulp tissue and debris from the canal and shaping the canal to receive an obturating material. Using sequentially larger sizes of files and irrigating and disinfecting the canal to clear it of debris, one shapes the canal to receive a well-condensed filling that seals the root canal apically and laterally, to prevent any leakage.

In cleaning and shaping a root canal, the following rules should be observed: (1) direct access should be obtained along straight lines; (2) the length of the tooth should be accurately determined; (3) instruments should be used in a sequence of sizes with periodic recapitulation, returning to smaller sizes to avoid blockage and ledging; (4) instruments should be used with a quarter- to a half-turn and withdrawn with a pull stroke; (5) barbed broaches should be used cautiously, and only when the root canal is wide enough to permit their insertion and rotation without binding; (6) instruments should be fitted with instrument stops; (7) the apical portion of a root canal, 3 to 4 mm, should be enlarged at least 3 sizes greater

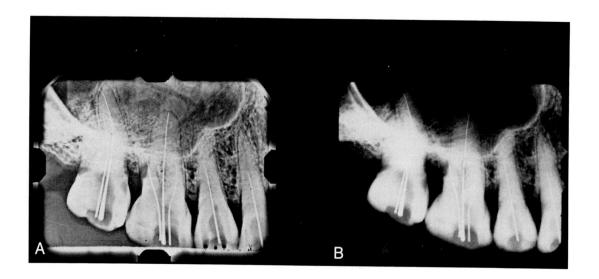

Fig. 11–23. Xeroradiograph (A) and radiograph (B) of a human skull. Note the sharpness of the anatomic structures in the xeroradiograph. (Courtesy of P. San Marco and S. Montgomery, San Antonio, Texas.)

than the first instrument that binds and until the walls are tapered without irregularities; (8) the remainder of the root canal should be enlarged using a step-back technique; (9) one must not force an instrument if it binds; (10) instruments should be checked for deformation and discarded if strain is present; (11) all instrumentation should be done using sterile instruments in a wet canal; (12) debris should not be forced through the apical foramen; and (13) instruments should be confined to the root canal, to prevent trauma to periapical tissue.

Use of Instruments in Size Sequence

Instruments should be used in sequence of sizes. Small instruments should precede large ones. To prevent breakage of instruments and to avoid ledge formation in cleaning and shaping of the root canal, instruments must be used in sequence of sizes. Root canals enlarged by successive sizes of hand instruments are more effectively prepared than by other means.[79] It is desirable to begin with a fine instrument and follow it with the next large size until the largest size for that particular canal is used. Returning to a smaller instrument from time to time before advancing to a larger size (recapitulation) helps to prevent the packing of dentin filings and ensures patency of the root canal through to the apical foramen.

Adequate Enlargement of Root Canals

What constitutes complete and adequate root canal preparation: how large, how wide? The answer is often dictated by the anatomic structure and accessibility of the canal, as well as by the skill of the operator. Inadequate preparation limits the ability of the operator to clean, debride, disinfect, and fill the canal. Overzealous preparation leads to iatrogenic problems, unnecessary weakening of the tooth and susceptibility to fracture, perforations, spatial movement of the apical foramen, and even root-tip fracture.

In the past, two guidelines were considered sufficient for instrumentation: (1) enlarge a root canal at least three sizes beyond the size of the first instrument that binds; (2) enlarge the canal until clean, white dentinal shavings appear in the flutes of the instrument blade. To prepare a root canal adequately, more is required. Root canals should be enlarged, regardless of initial width, to remove irregularities of dentin and to make the walls of the canal smooth and

tapered. Ideally, the minimum size to which a root canal should be enlarged is that corresponding to a No. 25 or 30 instrument in the apical portion and a No. 40 or larger in the midline and coronal portion of the root canal.

The surface of a root canal is irregular and is interspersed with recesses, crevices, and fissures, the result of deposition of secondary and reparative dentin. Root canals should be widened for four reasons: (1) to remove microorganisms on the canal surface mechanically;[58] (2) to remove pulp tissue, because even when a vital pulp is extirpated, tags of pulp tissue and odontoblasts cling to the canal wall and are not removed with the body of the pulp; they later undergo necrosis and provide an environment for bacterial growth; (3) to increase the capacity of the root canal, to permit irrigating solutions to reach the apical third of the root canal for effective debridement;[125] (4) to shape the root canal to receive gutta-percha, because the wider the canal, the easier it is to fill it, particularly if it is a narrow canal initially.

Root canals are often inadequately enlarged.[62] Preparation of a root canal to three sizes larger than the original instrument that bound at the working length is inadequate.[64] A study has shown that for root canals to be effectively irrigated, they should be enlarged to at least the size of a No. 40 file, although this may not be possible always in the apical 3 or 4 mm. The prepared root canal should be smooth and large enough to allow adequate debridement and obturation. The color of dentinal shavings is no indication of the presence of infected dentin or organic debris. Enlarging the root canal with three subsequent sizes of files may be sufficient in some cases, whereas in others, twice that size may not be enough. The degree of enlargement depends to some extent on the width and configuration of the root canal. The canal of a narrow tooth, such as a lower incisor, cannot be enlarged as much as the canal of a lower cuspid.

Precautions in Instrumentation

A root canal instrument should not be forced if it binds. To force an instrument is to invite breakage. Only controlled finger pressure should be used in manipulating an instrument in the root canal. The instrument should be coaxed, rather than forced. Both reamers and files should be withdrawn and examined from time to time, to make certain that the instrument is intact and that the flutes of the blade on the instrument are still uniformly spaced and are not deformed (Fig. 11–24).

All instrumentation of the root canal should be done in a wet canal, with an antiseptic irrigating solution applied for this purpose. Root canal instruments cut dentin more effectively in a wet environment,[147] just as a bur cuts faster in a wet cavity. Moreover, as the root canal instrument is withdrawn from the canal, the wet debris and dentin chips cling to the instrument and are removed from the canal. Furthermore, the presence of the irrigant disinfects the canal while it facilitates its enlargement. Although any aqueous antiseptic solution may be used for this purpose, we prefer a 5.2% sodium-hypochlorite

solution because it is an effective solvent of necrotic pulp tissue and organic debris. Root canal instruments should be used with care in the apical third of the canal, so as not to force debris or infected material beyond the root apex or traumatize the periapical tissue. All root canal instruments should be fitted with stops, to prevent their being forced through the apical foramen. Studies show that when instrumentation is confined to the root canal, it rarely produces bacteremia.[7,10]

Step-Back Method

In the step-back (flare, telescopic) preparation of the root canal, each consecutively larger root canal instrument used for shaping the canal wall is placed short of the apex, once the canal has been enlarged in the apical

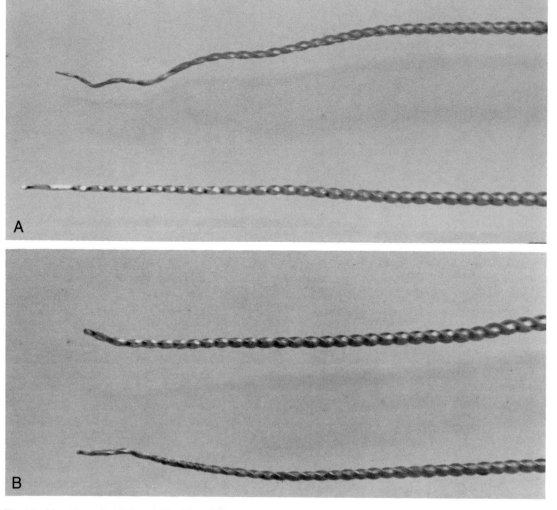

Fig. 11–24. Unraveled flutes of files (*A*) and files with fractured tips (*B*) This damage occurred during instrumentation of root canals. (From Montgomery, S., et al.: J. Endod., *10*:45, 1984.)

third to at least a No. 25 or 30 instrument (Fig. 11–25).

This method of canal preparation has some advantages over the conventional method, namely: (1) it is less likely to cause periapical trauma; (2) it facilitates the removal of more debris;[24,123,150] (3) the greater flare that results from instrumentation facilitates packing of additional gutta-percha cones by either the lateral or the vertical condensation method; (4) the development of an apical matrix or stop prevents overfilling of the root canal; (5) greater condensation pressure can be exerted, which often fills lateral canals with the sealer.

Straight Root Canals

Cleaning and shaping of the root canal begin on completion of gross debridement and determination of the exact working length. The canal and chamber is flooded with a 5.2% solution of sodium hypochlorite; the excess solution is removed by aspiration or is collected on a cotton roll or gauze sponge. All sterilized instruments have stops positioned on the blade set to the working length (Fig. 11–25, *A*). The file is inserted directly through the canal orifice to the desired length; precurving of the file is not necessary in a straight canal. The file is engaged against the dentinal wall with lateral pressure and is withdrawn. This procedure, circumferential filing, is repeated around the entire perimeter until all the walls are instrumented (Fig. 11–25, *B*). The entire canal is then irrigated with sodium hypochlorite, and all the solution and debris are aspirated out of the canal. The file is inspected for deformation, resterilized after cleaning its flutes by squeezing a cotton sponge around the blade while rotating the file counterclockwise, and the filing procedure is repeated (see Fig. 11–18). Once the area of the apical foramen is clean, the apical third of the preparation is started.

The stops of the larger files should be set

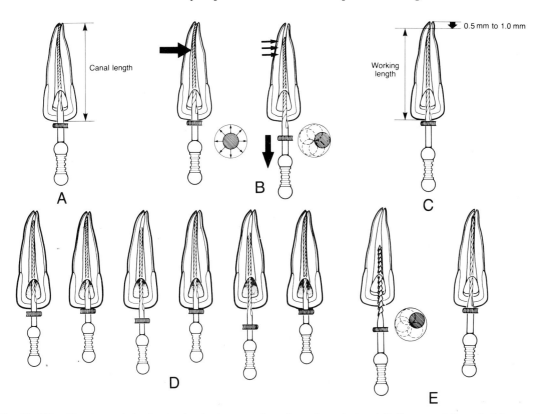

Fig. 11–25. Cleaning and shaping in step-back preparation of a root canal. *A* and *B*, The area of the apical foramen is cleaned and shaped circumferentially the length of the root canal. *C*, The apical third of the preparation is cleaned and shaped circumferentially to a working length. Cleaning and shaping the body of the root canal are begun when the apical preparation is to a minimum size-25 file and the larger files do not reach the working length. *D*, Recapitulation, a term used during instrumentation of the body of the root canal, refers to a return to the last file used in the apical preparation, to maintain the patency of the apical segment while one cleans and shapes the body of the root canal. *E*, The body of the root canal is finished with Hedstroem files.

0.5 to 1.0 mm short of the canal length, to establish the working length (Fig. 11–25, C). The procedure of circumferential filing should be repeated using the larger files in sequentially increasing sizes. Each new file should fit all the way to the working length before one begins circumferential filing. Using an instrument short of the working length can result in ledging and packing of dentin in front of the instrument. Circumferential filing is continued in a wet canal, and all instruments are kept short of the apical terminus. One should return to smaller instruments periodically (recapitulation) to smooth the canal walls, to prevent packing of dentinal debris, and to permit insertion of larger instruments to their working length without their binding in the dentinal walls of the canal.

The original size, anatomic shape, and accessibility of the canal determine the size of the largest file to be used in the apical preparation. When the apical preparation is enlarged to the size of a No. 30 file or larger, and the next subsequent size will not reach the working length, the preparation of the apical third is finished (Fig. 11–25, C). The size of the last file used to form the apical dentinal matrix must be recorded.

To prepare the body of the canal, the largest file that did not attain the working length is inserted until it makes unforced contact with the walls of the canal, and the walls are filed circumferentially once at this new length (Fig. 11–25, D). Forcing of files apically beyond the first point of contact creates ledges. The canal is irrigated with a 5.2% solution of sodium hypochlorite. The last file used in the apical preparation is reinserted to the working length, and the walls of the canal are circumferentially filed again, to maintain the patency of the apical segment (Fig. 11–25, D).

All instrumentation is performed in combination with copious irrigation to prevent blockage of the canal with dentinal or pulp debris, but cautiously, to prevent forcing of irrigating solution beyond the apical foramen. The body of the canal is instrumented with at least three to four larger files, with recapitulation between each size.

A Hedstroem file, also called an H-file, one or two sizes larger than the previous file, is used to finish the instrumentation of the coronal third of the root canal (Fig. 11–25, E). Recapitulation is continued after each use of the Hedstroem file, to prevent blockage of the canal. Instrumentation is finished when the walls are smooth and clean and when the preparation shows continuous taper in an apical direction.

If necessary, a radiograph can be taken of the last file used to prepare the apical third, to verify the proper termination of the working length in the prepared canal. With continuous recapitulation, a larger file than the last one used to prepare the apical third can be placed to working length without binding. The size of the file that fits the apical third of the preparation without binding is recorded and is used as a reference for selecting the size of the primary cone to be used for obturation of the root canal.

Curved Root Canals

In shaping a curved root canal, one should always precurve the file blade before instrumentation. This procedure facilitates the insertion of the instrument to its working length and prevents ledging of the canal walls. The curvature of the blade can be estimated by reviewing the diagnostic radiograph and by observing the anatomic features of the root canal. The curve is prepared by grasping the blade with a gauze sponge and carefully bending the blade until the desired curvature is attained. Bending the blade with pliers may damage the flutes, and using bare fingers to bend the blade leaves epithelial cells containing bacteria in the flutes (Fig. 11–26). The directional silicone stop should be set to indicate the direction in which the file has been curved.

The area of the apical foramen is circumferentially cleaned with a precurved No. 10 file to the canal length as previously described. Small files, Nos. 8, 10, and 15, can be used in curved root canals without any modifications other than precurving. Because of their flexibility, these files maintain their given curvature, whereas less-flexible files, No. 20 and larger, need to be modified to avoid altering the shape of the curved canal in its apical third. Less-flexible curved instruments may overcut the outer surface of the curved canal and may produce an elliptic preparation in the apical third that is difficult to obturate. This elliptic preparation is cone-shaped, with the apex or elbow toward the middle third of the canal and the base or "zip" toward the cementum surface.[154] If the instrument remains within the confines of the root canal, the elliptic preparation will produce internal transportation of the fora-

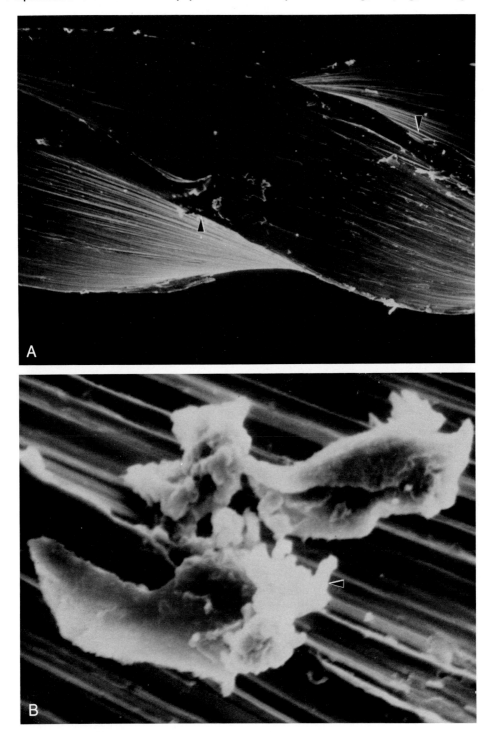

Fig. 11—26.   *A*, Destruction of cutting edge (arrows) after using cotton pliers to bend a file. *B*, Epithelial cells with bacteria (arrow) after bending a file with the fingers. (From Segall, R., et al.: Oral Surg., *44*:786, 1972.)

men, and if the instrument is outside the confines of the root canal, it will produce external transportation of the foramen (Fig. 11–27).

After cleaning the area of the apical foramen, an apical matrix is developed, using instruments that are further modified by dulling the flutes of the outer portion of the curve in the apical segment of the file (Fig. 11–28). This procedure makes the instrument more fragile; however, it prevents the transportation of the apical foramen during instrumentation because the instrument is less efficient in its cutting ability. The flutes are dulled with a sterile diamond file or a sandpaper disc.

Circumferential instrumentation is performed in the apical third using precurved, customized instruments. All circumferential filing follows guidelines similar to those used for all instrumentation: always use instruments sequentially; do not force the preceding file, to reach the apical terminus; do not use instruments in a dry canal; repeatedly irrigate the canal with sodium hypochlorite; clean, recurve, and resterilize all instruments in a hot-salt or glass bead sterilizer before reinserting them into the root canal; and monitor the progress of instrumentation by taking periodic radiographs when needed. The apical third of the canal and the matrix are adequately prepared when a file larger than that used to instrument the apical third cannot be inserted into the terminus of the preparation and provided the canal is enlarged at least to the size of a No. 25 or 30 file, to facilitate the obturation.

The body of the canal, that is, the middle and cervical thirds, is cleaned and shaped by introducing the next-larger file until one notes unforced contact with the dentinal walls. If contact occurs in the curved portion of the root canal, the file should be curved, and the flutes adjacent to the outer portion of the curve in the area of contact should be dulled. One should continue the circumferential instrumentation of the body of the canal with the sequential use of at least three or four larger files, followed by recapitulation with the last apical file, as previously described. The cervical third of the root canal is circumferentially instrumented with Hedstroem files one or two sizes larger than the last K-file used.

The technique previously described applies only to root canals with a gentle curvature (Fig. 11–29). Curved canals that are narrow, have a double curve, or are dilacerated need special modifications for cleaning and shaping.

Narrow Curved Root Canals

The apical segment of the root canal is cleaned and shaped with a prepared No. 10 file to canal length. If the next prepared file (No. 15) binds firmly 1 mm or 2 mm short of the working length, it should not be forced apically beyond this point of contact (Fig. 11–30, *A*). The No. 15 file is removed, and the canal is irrigated with a 5.2% solution of sodium hypochlorite. Because the next-size file needed is not available commercially, the operator can create one by cutting off part of the instrument tip of the No. 10 file. All standardized instruments taper 0.02 mm in diameter per 1 mm of blade length; cutting off 1 mm of the tip of No. 10 file converts it into a No. 12 file.[154]

The stainless steel tip of a file can be cut with sharp iris scissors (Fig. 11–30, *B*). A diamond file is used to re-establish and to smooth the instrument tip (Fig. 11–30, *C*). The instrument is curved as needed, is sterilized, and is ready for use in the apical third of the preparation. It may be necessary to modify subsequent instruments in this same manner, to effect an apical preparation that is at least as large as a size No. 25 or 30 file. Cleaning and shaping of the root canal proceed as previously described.

Double-Curved Root Canals

Double-curved or bayonet-shaped canals are cleaned and shaped with one main variation. When the area of the apical foramen has been cleaned and shaped with a prepared No. 10 file, the middle third curve is eliminated by filing it with a Hedstroem file that straightens out the enlarged canal (Fig. 11–31). A small Hedstroem file is introduced into the root canal until the junction of the middle and apical thirds is reached. The inner portion of this curve is then filed away.

After filing the inner portion of the curve of the middle third once with the Hedstroem file, one should recapitulate with a prepared No. 10 file to the working length to maintain the patency of the root canal. The root canal is irrigated, and the file is cleaned, recurved, and resterilized. This procedure is repeated until the curve is eliminated. Care should be taken not to overinstrument the inner portion of the middle third, to avoid perforation.

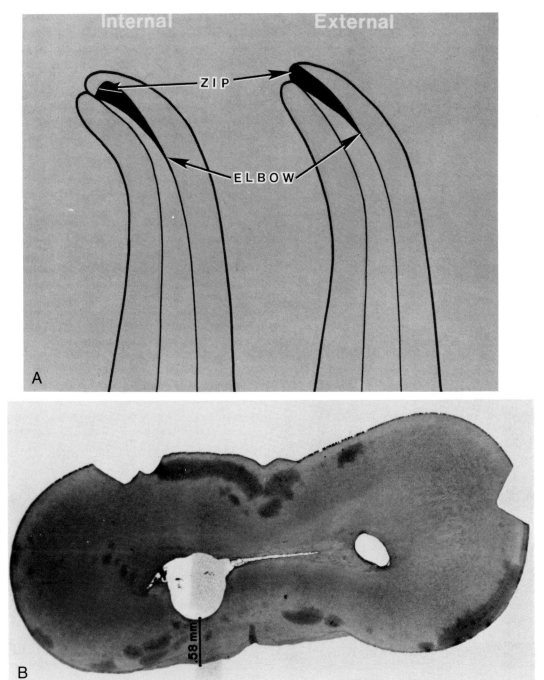

Fig. 11–27. *A,* Internal and external transportation of the foramen. *B,* Histologic cross section of the mesial root of a mandibular molar showing transportation of the canal toward the furca. Note that the distal wall is only 0.58 mm from the exterior of the root. (From Hill, R.L., and del Rio, C.E.: J. Endod., 9:517, 1983.)

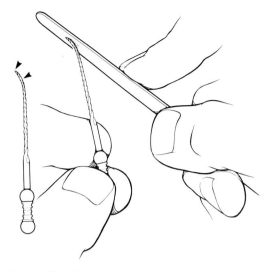

Fig. 11–28. Modification of an instrument to prevent transportation of the foramen in curved root canals, The K-file flutes on the outer portion of the curve (arrows) are dulled with a diamond file.

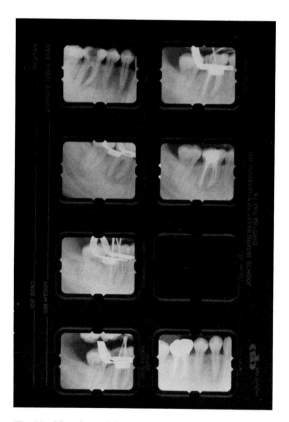

Fig. 11–29. Curved root canals of a mandibular first molar are cleaned and shaped by the step-back technique and are obturated with gutta-percha. (Courtesy of J.V. Bucher, San Antonio, Texas.)

Instrumentation of the apical third of the root canal follows.

Dilacerated Root Canals

Dilacerated or extremely curved canals can be instrumented by enlarging the middle and cervical third of the root canal first. Then the apical segment can be cleaned with a prepared file to canal length. A small Hedstroem file is inserted to the beginning of the dilaceration. Without forcing the file apically, circumferential filing is performed once, and the canal is irrigated and refiled to working length with a prepared No. 10 file. One should repeat this procedure until the middle and cervical thirds are open wide enough that the apical third can be instrumented without forcing the instruments. When the cervical and middle thirds of the canal are open, one should prepare a No. 15 file by dulling the flutes on the outer portion of the apical third and the inner portion of the middle third of the curved instrument (Fig. 11–32). This procedure prevents transportation of the apical foramen and overinstrumentation in the dilacerated area. The apical third is cleaned and shaped as previously described.

MECHANICAL INSTRUMENTATION

Engine-Driven Instruments

Engine-driven instruments can be used for opening root canals; however, they should not be used for canal preparation except as a last resort. The rapid revolution of an engine-driven reamer, file, or broach can create a ledge, a perforation, or an obstruction, especially when the instrument breaks after it binds, particularly in the apical region, where the root canal is narrow. An engine-driven instrument is less likely to enable one to follow a curvature in the root canal than a hand-operated instrument (Fig. 11–33). If an engine-driven instrument is used to gain access to the periapical region, it should be run in a reducing handpiece whose speed is about one-tenth the usual number of revolutions per minute. With reduced speed, the chance of breakage is lessened. If an instrument is used in a contra-angle handpiece, such as when a reducing handpiece is not available, the engine should be run at the slowest possible speed.

Two engine-driven contra-angle handpieces are available, namely, the Giromatic

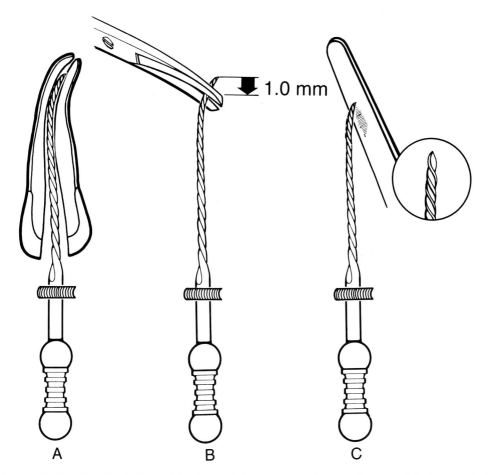

Fig. 11–30. Modification of an instrument to clean and shape narrow root canals. *A*, Sequentially larger file is found to be short of the working length. *B*, One millimeter is cut off a smaller file. *C*, The tip is re-established with a diamond file; the smaller file thereby becomes an intermediate-sized file.

and the Racer. The Giromatic handpiece activates a stainless steel barbed broach or reamer in the root canal through a 90° reciprocating arc at a speed up to 1000 cycles/min. This instrument may pack the dentinal shavings in the canal. Other shortcomings of this instrument and its integration in endodontic practice have been discussed in the literature.[41] When compared with hand instrumentation, the Giromatic was found to be less effective for preparing root canals.[146] Root canals prepared by hand instruments were superior in shape and smoothness. Less time was required to eliminate the morphologic irregularities and to develop an apical matrix in the canal with hand instruments than with automated instruments.[103] Other studies concluded that hand instrumentation was more effective in removing dentinal debris,[97] and the Giromatic preparation took longer and had a tendency to create ledges and to produce flaring at the apex.[155]

The Racer contra-angle handpiece uses a standard file and oscillates the file in the root canal. The instrument's length can be adjusted to the working length using this contra-angle. A major disadvantage of this instrument is that debris may be forced ahead of the instrument, with resulting clogging of the canal or pushing of debris into periapical tissue. When engine-driven instruments are used, access to the apical foramen must be made first with hand instruments. In fact, whether the Giromatic or the Racer is used, access to the apical foramen must always be made with hand reamers or files. Ring found that root canals could not be enlarged with the Racer instrument in 13% of cases.[117] Another report on the Giromatic handpiece stated that narrow root canals of molars could not be enlarged in about 70% of cases.

Power-Driven Instruments

Two types of power-driven reamers are used in endodontics: Gates Glidden drills

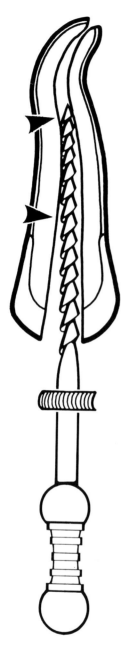

Fig. 11–31. Variation in cleaning and shaping for double-curved or "S-shaped" root canals. A small Hedstroem file is used to reduce the middle-third curve of the root canal (arrows) and leaves only the apical curve to be instrumented.

and the Peeso reamers. The Gates Glidden drill has a long, thin shaft ending in a flame-shaped head, with a safe tip to guard against perforations (Fig. 11–34). The flame head cuts laterally and is used with gentle, apically directed pressure. The long shaft is designed to break at the neck, the narrowest diameter that lies adjacent to the handpiece. If the drill binds during use, it will fracture at the neck of the shaft and will extrude from the tooth. The fractured segment is easily removed by grasping the broken shaft with pliers and pulling it out of the tooth. The Gates Glidden drill is used to remove the lingual shoulder during access preparation of anterior teeth, to enlarge root canal orifices, and to clean and shape the cervical third of root canals in the step-back preparation.

The Peeso reamer has long, sharp flutes connected to a thick shaft (Fig. 11–35). It cuts laterally and is primarily used for the preparation of post space when gutta-percha has been removed from the obturated root canal. Although many clinicians use Peeso reamers to remove the gutta-percha filling during post preparation, it is not advisable to do so and thereby to risk disturbing the apical seal, accidentally removing all the gutta-percha, or perforating the root.

Both Gates Glidden drills and Peeso reamers are made of hardened carbon steel that corrodes easily. These aggressive cutting instruments are inflexible and should be used at slow speed and with extreme caution, to prevent overinstrumentation and perforations.

Ultrasonic and Sonic Instruments

Ultrasonic and sonic instruments have been developed for cleaning and shaping root canals. The ultrasonic instrument consists of a piezoelectric ceramic unit that generates ultrasonic waves, which activate a magnetostrictive stack handpiece. The handpiece holds a K-file or a specially designed diamond file that, when activated, produces movements of the shaft of the file between 0.001 and 0.004 in. at a frequency of 20,000 to 25,000/sec[75] (Fig. 11–36).

This oscillating movement produces the cutting action of the file and creates an ultrasonic wave of sodium-hypochlorite irrigant solution, which is delivered along the side of the file into the root canal. The ultrasonic vibration produces heat that increases the chemical effectiveness of the irrigating solution.[30] It also produces cavitation, that is, the growth and collapse of bubbles, with a resulting increase in the mechanical cleansing activity of the solution.[33] Because of this increase in thermal and mechanical activity of the irrigating solution delivered into the root canal, removal of debris and tissue from the isthmus and removal of the smear layer are more efficient. The bactericidal action of the irrigating solution also increases.[32]

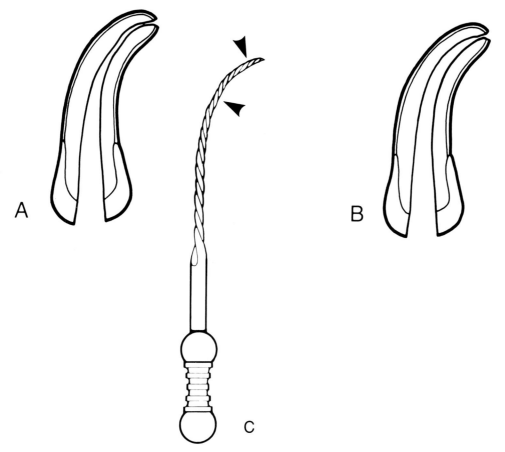

Fig. 11—32. Modification of an instrument to clean and shape a dilacerated root canal. *A* and *B*, Root canal before and after cleaning and shaping. *C*, The flutes of a small, curved file are dulled on the outer portion of the apical third and on the inner portion of the middle third (arrows) of the root canal.

Before ultrasonic instrumentation, the apical third of the root canal should be hand instrumented to at least the size of a No. 15 file. In curved root canals, a precurved No. 15 endosonic file is introduced into the canal to working length (1 mm short of the apical foramen) and is activated. If the instrument is activated short of the working length, it will create a ledge. After activation, the file is moved in a circumferential manner with a smooth push-pull stroke along the walls of the canal (combined with copious sodium-hypochlorite irrigation) for a period of one min. This procedure is repeated with Nos. 20 and 25 files. The straight portion of the canal, usually found in the middle and coronal parts of the root, is circumferentially instrumented with the diamond file using copious irrigation for at least 1 min. On completion of the ultrasonic instrumentation, the terminus of the preparation is checked with a No. 25 hand file.[39]

The ultrasonic file should be inserted into the root canal to the working length before one activates the file's cutting motion, to prevent ledge formation, and the apical third of the canal should be filed cautiously, to prevent transportation of the apical root canal and foramen. Because the automatic irrigation of the canal with sodium-hypochlorite solution produces a fine mist that can irritate the eyes and respiratory systems of both patient and operator, appropriate precautions should be taken.[21,144] Sonic handpieces operate at 1500 to 6500 cycles/min when filing inside root canals (Fig. 11—37). They are similar in shape and weight to dental handpieces and are attached to existing air and water lines. These instruments are used in a manner similar to the ultrasonic system in instrumentation of the root canals. The only difference is that the sonic system uses water as an irrigant and does not usually require diamond files for the flare of the preparation.[6,144]

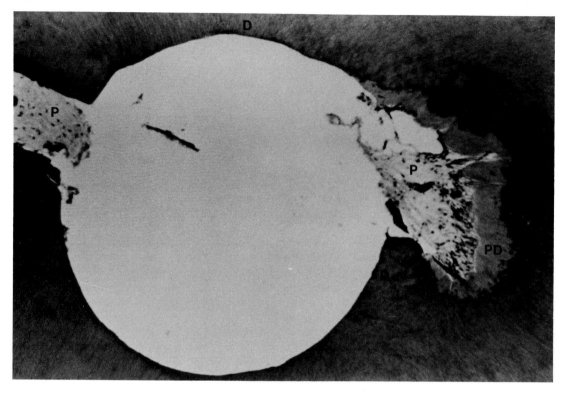

Fig. 11—33. Histologic cross section of the mesiolingual root canal of a mandibular first molar. The root canal was cleaned and shaped with an engine-driven instrument. Note the overprepared dentinal walls (D) of the root canal and the pulp tissue (P) and predentin (PD) left in the root canal. (From Hill, R.L., and del Rio, C.E.: J. Endod., 9:517, 1983.)

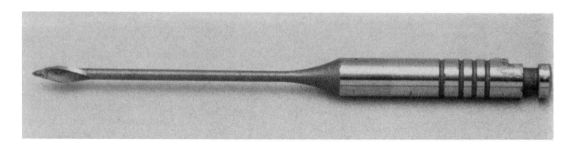

Fig. 11—34. Gates-Glidden drill. Note the flame-shaped head with a safe tip.

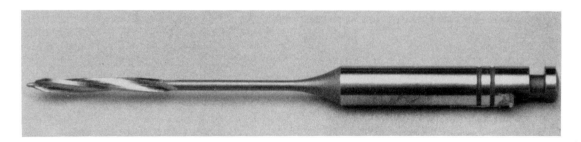

Fig. 11—35. Peeso reamer. Note the long, sharp flutes and the safe tip.

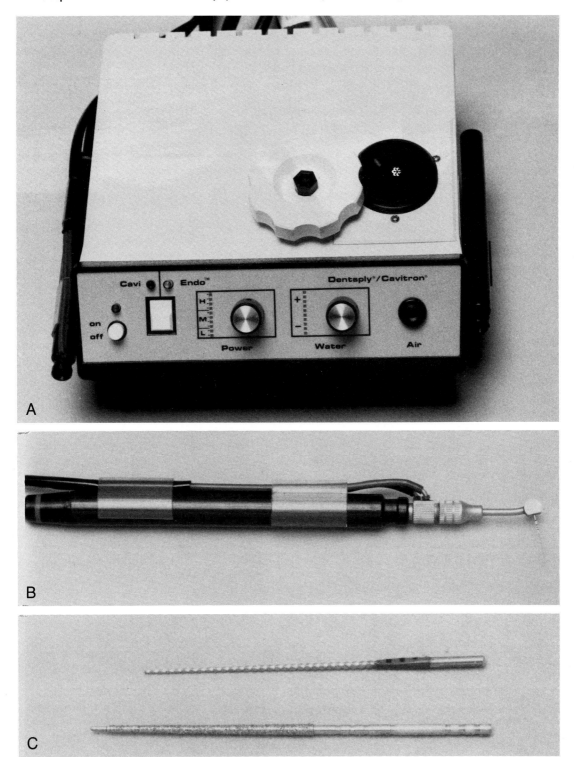

Fig. 11–36. Endosonic System. *A*, Ultrasonic unit with an irrigant reservoir (*). *B*, Magnetostrictive stack handpiece. *C*, Specially designed K-file and diamond file. (Courtesy of L.D. Caulk Division, Milford, Delaware.)

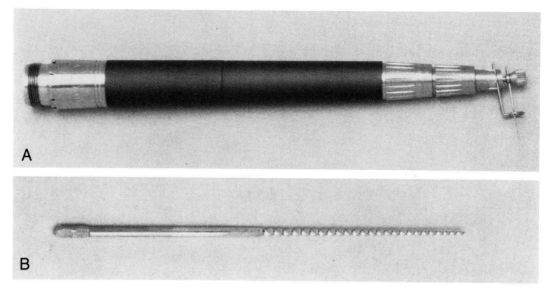

Fig. 11–37. *A,* Endostar 5 is a sonic vibratory endodontic handpiece for cleaning and shaping root canals. *B,* Specially designed K-file. (Courtesy of Syntex Dental Products, Valley Forge, Pennsylvania.)

The new ultrasonic and sonic instrumentation systems are still being evaluated. Although they are in the early stages of development, they appear to have a bright future in endodontic practice for cleaning and shaping of root canals.

PROCEDURAL PROBLEMS OF CLEANING AND SHAPING

Accidental Perforation

Perforations can be avoided by studying the anatomic structure and inclination of the tooth both in the patient's mouth and on the radiograph. One should note any deviation from the normal, such as mesial or distal inclination of the tooth, overlapping of teeth, malalignment of the tooth in the arch in relation to adjacent teeth, abnormal width and shape of root canals, unusual height of crowns in posterior teeth especially if under a splint, and so on. In anterior teeth, the direction of the bur in gaining access to the pulp chamber should be parallel to the long axis of the tooth in all planes, whereas in molar teeth, the bur should be directed toward the largest canal orifice, yet limited to the level of the chamber roof, as measured in the diagnostic radiograph; one thereby avoids the furcation area where most perforations occur. The floor of the pulp chamber of molar teeth may also be perforated in an effort to locate the root canal orifices (Fig. 11–38).

Iatrogenic perforation of the pulp chamber floor or wall, or of the root, may inadvertently occur as a result of misdirection of a bur during access preparation, overinstrumentation of a curved root (apical perforation), overinstrumentation of the coronal root canal (lateral root perforation), and post preparation. Perforation is always followed by hemorrhage because of damage to the periodontal ligament, and the bleeding is sometimes difficult to control. Multirooted teeth are probably perforated because of the anatomic configuration of their roots and canals, the inclination of the tooth, and their difficult accessibility, whereas anterior teeth are accidentally perforated more often during post preparation.

When a perforation occurs, the first step is to control the hemorrhage. This is done by irrigating the cavity and pulp chamber with sterile water or anesthetic solution and then packing a moist, sterile cotton pellet into the pulp chamber and holding it under pressure for 2 or 3 min. On removal of the packing, the location of the perforation becomes apparent, and visibility for locating the root canal orifices is improved. If the packing does not control the bleeding, a cotton pellet saturated with a vasoconstrictor (Racellet) should be applied with pressure to the perforated area until the bleeding stops.

Next, one should locate all the canal orifices and insert files into all the canals. This procedure prevents blockage of the canal ori-

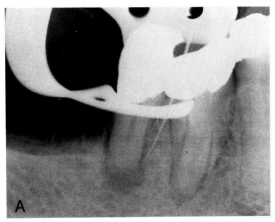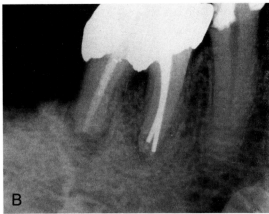

Fig. 11–38.   A, Perforation of the bifurcation of a lower molar. B, The perforation has been walled off with amalgam. Note the apparent loss of bone in the bifurcation adjacent to the sealed perforation.

fices when the filling used to seal the perforation is packed into the chamber. Once this filling sets, the instruments are removed, to leave the root canal orifices patent and accessible.

The repair of a perforation depends on the excellence of the seal between the tooth root and periradicular tissues. Iatrogenic perforations are treated in a manner similar to pathologic perforations, such as caused by internal or external resorption, by induction of a calcific barrier over the perforated foramen, to condense a gutta-percha seal that will not leak and will not hinder periradicular tissue repair. Calcium-hydroxide paste is used most often for this purpose.

When insertion of calcium-hydroxide paste over a series of visits for several months is not feasible or practical, a perforation can be sealed simply and rapidly in a single visit. The calcium-hydroxide paste (Dycal or Life) is packed into the perforation and is allowed to set for a few minutes, followed by amalgam, which is gently packed over the calcium hydroxide by means of a plugger with a diameter slightly larger than that of the perforation. The seal is wiped with a cotton pellet, to ensure adequate marginal adaptation and thereby to prevent leakage. After the initial set of the amalgam, the root canal instruments placed in the canals to protect their patency are removed. Any free amalgam particles are washed loose with a stream of sterile anesthetic solution and aspirated with a suction tip positioned alongside the perforated areas.

When the root of an anterior tooth is perforated, a similar technique may be used, except when the perforation is in the middle third of the canal and the calcium-hydroxide technique has failed to induce a calcific barrier (Fig. 11–39). In such cases, access must first be gained to the root canal. The instrument is left in the canal, or a gutta-percha cone is placed in the canal. A flap is raised, clear access is obtained through the bone to expose the perforation in the root, the perforation is packed with amalgam against the instrument in the canal to prevent clogging of the canal, the flap is coapted and sutured, and the instrument is removed (Fig. 11–40). The root canal is then treated in a routine manner. If the perforation is palatal, surgical access should be gained from the palate.

When the apical third of a curved root is perforated, especially when a periapical area of rarefaction is also present, a periradicular surgical procedure should be considered as an alternative. If the perforation is close to the root apex, the tooth can be treated in the usual manner and monitored for repair and healing; surgical treatment can be deferred until such time as it becomes necessary. If a periapical surgical procedure is not feasible, another alternative to extraction might be intentional replantation.

Cavit has been recommended for filling perforated areas, based on a successful result reported in 88% of 183 cases that were followed from 6 months to 10 years.[67] We prefer using calcium-hydroxide paste to stimulate the formation of a calcific barrier in the defect whenever possible.

Obstruction by Calcification within the Root Canal

The course, length, and diameter of the root canal can be estimated from the radio-

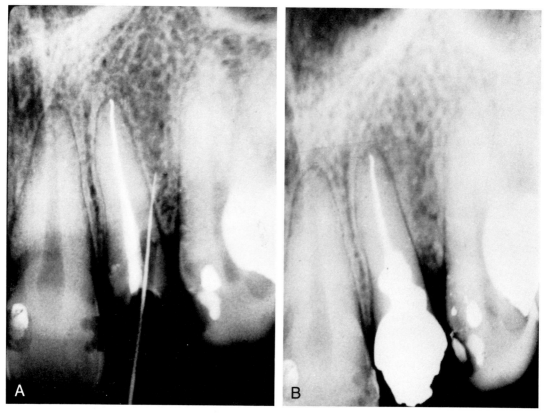

Fig. 11–39. *A,* Perforation resulting from preparation of a root canal for a post. *B,* The perforation was walled off internally with amalgam, and a casting was made later.

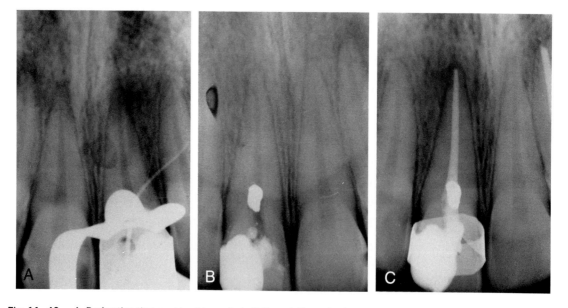

Fig. 11–40. *A,* Perforation that could not be walled off through the pulp chamber because of its location. *B,* After raising of a mucoperiosteal flap and the placement of a gutta-percha cone in the root canal, amalgam was condensed into the cavity against the gutta-percha. The gutta-percha cone was then removed, and the root canal was treated routinely. *C,* The completed root canal filling after routine endodontic treatment.

graph. Radiographs should be carefully studied before endodontic treatment is begun, to judge accessibility of the apical foramen, to determine the presence of any obstructions, and to find solutions for these problems. Occasionally, a pulp stone occludes a root canal. If the stone is in the pulp chamber, as most of them are, its removal will usually be simple.

When a pulp stone seems to occlude the entire root canal, one should patiently explore the canal with a fine instrument, and with an apically directed rotary motion one should attempt to bypass the obstruction. If the procedure is successful, one should widen the canal by cutting the stone with both rotary and translational forces, preferably a withdrawal-filing pull stroke against the stone itself. When a pulp stone that was lying free in the canal becomes wedged and cannot be bypassed, one should use an engine-driven instrument, to grind away at the stone with small, round, long-shank burs.

When the apical end of the root canal is apparently closed and presents an effective barrier against the passage of a fine root canal instrument, the presence of cementum closing off the apical foramen should be suspected. A close scrutiny of the radiograph should be made for any sign of a root canal. If none is apparent, and if no area of rarefaction is present, and the tooth is asymptomatic, no attempt should be made to create an opening through the apical foramen. In such cases, it must be assumed that the foramen has become sealed with secondary cementum. If the tooth is symptomatic, however, or if an area of rarefaction is present, even though it may appear to be partially calcified, apical access must be obtained, to negotiate the canal throughout its entire length to reach the periapical tissues (see Fig. 11–6). This objective may be accomplished by persistent, patient instrumentation with the aid of EDTA.[60] In some cases, however, it may be necessary to perform a root resection and to place a retrograde filling in the root apex.

Broken Instruments in the Root Canal

Another obstruction, which sometimes makes the apical foramen inaccessible, is the presence of broken instruments in the root canal. Nothing is more annoying or disheartening to a dentist than the discovery of a broken instrument in the root canal, and yet, this anxiety can be prevented in most cases by careful examination of instruments for deformation before use and the replacement of used instruments with new ones. If in doubt, throw the instrument out. The extra cost is negligible when compared to the distress, time, and difficulty of attempting to remove a fragment of an instrument, followed by an embarrassed explanation to a patient that a broken instrument is lodged inside a root canal.

Instrument breakage can be practically eliminated by taking the following precautions: Examine new instruments under magnification to look for any defects in manufacturing. If defects are found, such as unraveled or distorted flutes or defective tips, discard the instruments. Instrument sizes No. 8, 10, 15, and 20 are easily deformed and should be examined after each use and discarded if distorted. Instruments larger than No. 25 may be used a number of times if they do not show, under magnification, effects of stress. Every operator should expect to deform several instruments during cleaning and shaping of most root canals and should be prepared to discard these instruments immediately (see Fig. 11–24). At times, it may be necessary to discard more than half a dozen new instruments in preparing difficult canals of molar teeth.

If an instrument breaks in a root canal, try to remove the fractured segment by bypassing it with a smaller instrument and pulling it out (Fig. 11–41, A). If the instrument remains wedged or lodged in the canal, attempt to bypass the broken fragment, again with a smaller instrument (Fig. 11–41, B). If the procedure is successful, the canal should be cleaned, shaped, and obturated with gutta-percha incorporating the instrument fragment in the filling material.

At times, a broken instrument in a root canal cannot be bypassed. In such cases, the canal should be cleaned and shaped to the instrument level and obturated. If the instrument seals the canal close to the root apex and if the apical area was normal prior to the breakage, it may remain normal despite the presence of a fractured instrument and a short-filled canal. If an area of rarefaction was originally present, however, the area will usually persist, and a periradicular surgical procedure should be considered[57] (Fig. 11–41, C).

Teeth with broken instruments and without areas of rarefaction should be observed radiographically every 6 months. In the event

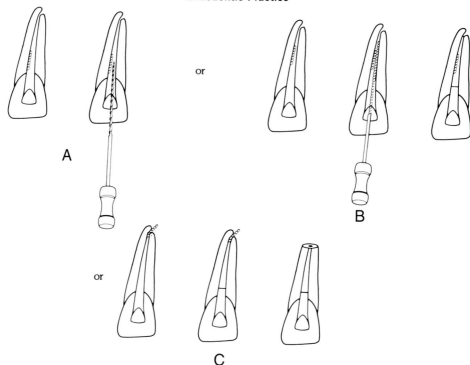

Fig. 11–41. *A*, Fractured segment of an instrument can sometimes be removed by bypassing the segment with a Hedstroem file, engaging the segment, and pulling it out. *B*, If the segment cannot be removed, one should attempt to bypass it, clean and shape the root canal, and incorporate the segment into the obturation. *C*, If the instrument segment is in the apical area, the root canal should be cleaned and shaped to the instrument segment, it should be obturated, and an apicoectomy should be considered.

of bone changes, periradicular surgery and placement of apical amalgam should be considered. When an instrument fragment extends beyond the root apex, it should be removed surgically, and the root end should be sealed with a retrograde amalgam if the orthograde canal filling does not seal the root apex satisfactorily.

Every tooth containing a fractured instrument should not be considered a failure. In a study of 53 cases, the tooth containing the fractured instrument healed in most cases.[36]

Obstruction by Obturating Materials

When retreatment of a tooth previously treated endodontally becomes necessary, the filling material must be removed or bypassed; otherwise, salvaging the tooth from extraction may require an endodontic surgical procedure. Because most teeth to be retreated are sealed with gutta-percha, silver cones, or paste, the following sections discuss the removal of these materials from root canals.

Gutta-percha

Gutta-percha and cement can be removed by the application of mechanical force, in the form of instrumentation, by heat, to sear and soften the gutta-percha, and by solvents such as xylol or chloroform (Fig. 11–42). Gutta-percha is removed from the pulp chamber by heating an excavator blade or plastic instrument blade and searing the exposed gutta-percha. The canal orifices are reopened mechanically by forcing a No. 20 or 25 file through the orifice, or a Gates Glidden drill can be used, cautiously, to remove the gutta-percha obstructing the orifice. The safest method for removing gutta-percha from the orifice and middle root canal is to use a solvent, such as chloroform, which softens the gutta-percha and permits its removal through sequential instrumentation, using files with periodic recapitulation to prevent blockage or perforation of the canal. Xylol or chloroform, administered a few drops at a time, is carried into the pulp chamber by means of a glass syringe; the operator must use caution because these solutions frequently escape from the syringe needle without any apparent pressure on the plunger. The final segments of gutta-percha are removed by embedding a hot file into the apical gutta-percha and withdrawing it once the instrument

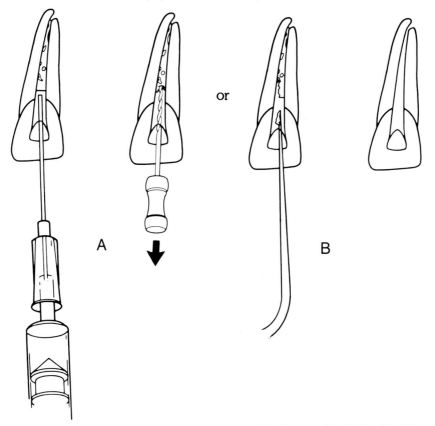

Fig. 11–42. Gutta-percha can be removed by the solvent action of chloroform or xylol with the aid of files (*A*) or by means of a heated instrument with the aid of files (*B*).

cools. The file blade is heated in a hot salt or glass-bead sterilizer, not through flaming. The heat condensor* is an excellent device that delivers controlled heat inside the root canal, softens the gutta-percha, and facilitates its removal. One must avoid forcing fragments of gutta-percha and debris into the periapical tissues.

Silver Cone

A silver cone is not removed as easily as a gutta-percha cone unless the butt end of the silver cone extends into the pulp chamber. In such cases, chloroform or xylol is first used to soften the cement; then, the butt end of the silver cone is vibrated with an ultrasonic scaler (Cavitron) to break the cementing media. The cone is then grasped with a pair of narrow-beaked (Stieglitz) pliers and is removed (Fig. 11–43). If the silver cone extends only slightly into the pulp chamber, it can often be removed by vibration with an

ultrasonic scaler until it becomes loose. One should insert an excavator blade or Caufield silver-cone retriever between the cone and the canal orifice and pry it out (Figs. 11–44 and 11–45). When a silver cone is completely embedded in the root canal, a small, round bur rotated alongside the cone may loosen it.

Paste

Medicated-paste root canal fillings usually require some mechanical pressure with an instrument to penetrate the filling material for removal. Penetration into the paste can be assisted with the liberal application of xylol or chloroform. Depending on the consistency of the paste, the filling may be easy or difficult to remove by sequential instrumentation and recapitulation alone.

Ledge Formation

Ledge formation is frequently the result of careless instrumentation. It is usually caused by use of a large instrument out of sequence and insertion of the instrument short of the working length, or by use of a straight or

---

*L.D. Caulk Co., Milford, Delaware.

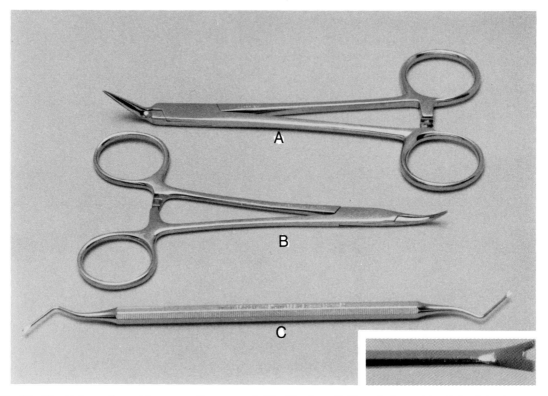

Fig. 11–43. Instruments used to remove silver cones. *A*, Stieglitz pliers. *B*, Mosquito hemostats. *C*, Caufield silver point retriever (the inset shows a higher magnification of the tip).

inflexible instrument in a curved root canal. Attempted instrumentation of a tooth through a poorly designed access cavity may prevent direct access to the apical third of the root canal; that is, the access curvature in the coronal part of the canal may prevent the negotiation of an instrument through the apical canal curvature in a fine, tortuous canal and may result in ledge formation. Ledges and blocked canals are recognized when the instrument cannot be reinserted to its established working length.

To remove a ledge inside a root canal, locate its position by inserting an instrument until it is blocked, and verify the depth of insertion by taking a radiograph. Once the ledge has been located, irrigate the canal copiously in sequence with an organic tissue solvent (sodium-hypochlorite solution) and an inorganic solvent or chelating agent (EDTA). Explore the ledged area with a small file, No. 10 or 15, in which a severe curvature has been made from the tip extending about 1 to 3 mm up the blade. When the ledge is reached, the instrument is retracted slightly and rotated to allow the curved tip to bypass the ledge, and the instrument is teased api-

cally past the obstruction. Patiently try again if initial attempts are unsuccessful. Once the ledge is bypassed, do not remove the instrument; rather, start circumferential instrumentation of the canal, filing the walls, and removing the ledge, before withdrawing the instrument from the canal. Repeat this procedure with sequentially larger instruments, and recapitulating with similar size instruments, until the ledge is filed away and the desired enlargement at the established working length is made.

If the ledge cannot be bypassed, clean, shape, and fill the root canal to the level of the obstruction. If the terminus of the filling is close to the canal apex, monitor the tooth for healing and repair. If the endodontic treatment is unsatisfactory and will probably fail, consider an alternate treatment procedure, such as retrograde-amalgam surgery, hemisection or radisectomy, intentional replantation, or extraction.

CHELATING AGENTS (CHEMICAL AIDS TO INSTRUMENTATION)

The chelating agent ethylenediaminotetraacetic acid, commonly called EDTA, was

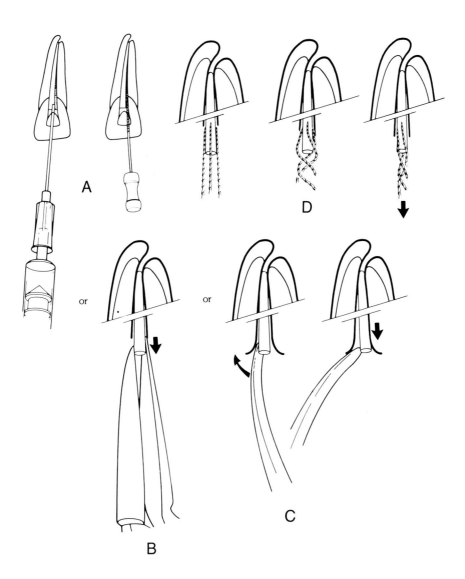

Fig. 11–44. Removal of silver cones. *A*, Silver cones can be loosened by softening the cementing media with chloroform or xylol, introducing a small file by the side of the silver cone to work the dissolving solution deeper into the cement, and vibrating the butt end of the silver cone with an ultrasonic scaler. The cone may then be removed with Stieglitz pliers (*B*), with Caufield silver point retrievers, or with endodontic spoon excavators (*C*). If the silver point butt is below the root canal orifice, twisting three Hedstroem files around the silver cone may produce enough grip to remove the silver cone (*D*).

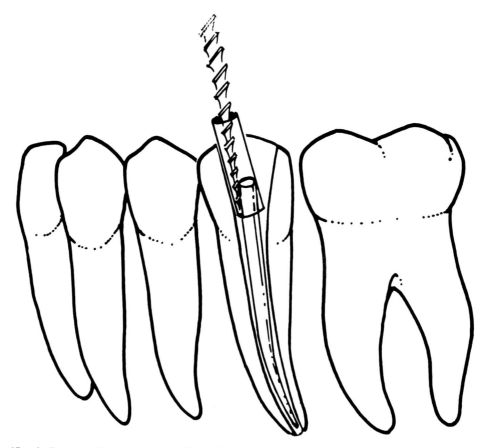

Fig. 11—45. A silver cone that is below the orifices of the root canal can be retrieved by making a sleeve out of a large-gauge hypodermic needle, placing it over the silver cone after removal of the cementing media around the butt end, vibrating the silver cone and sleeve with an ultrasonic scaler, wedging a Hedstroem file along the side of the silver cone and sleeve, and pulling the cone out.

introduced into endodontic practice by Nygaard-Østby.[102] It functions by forming a calcium-chelate solution with the calcium ion of dentin; the dentin thereby becomes more friable and easier to instrument. Many clinicians use some form of EDTA routinely during cleaning and shaping of the root canal and find it effective for achieving canal patency, enlargement, and, with additives, debridement and disinfection.

EDTA contains four acetic acid groups attached to ethylenediamine. The structural formula is as follows:

$$C_2H_3O_2 \diagdown \qquad\qquad \diagup C_2H_3O_2$$
$$N\!-\!CH_2\!-\!CH_2\!-\!N$$
$$C_2H_3O_2 \diagup \qquad\qquad \diagdown C_2H_3O_2$$

EDTA is relatively nontoxic and only slightly irritating in weak solutions. It forms highly stable, soluble, metal chelates in combination with heavy metals or alkaline earth ions.

Beause it is not metabolized, EDTA may be used to remove calcium from the body, to form a calcium chelate.[1]

$$C_2H_3O_2 \qquad\qquad\qquad C_2H_3O_2$$
$$N\!-\!CH_2\!-\!CH_2\!-\!N$$
$$CH_2 \qquad\qquad\qquad CH_2$$
$$CA$$
$$O\!=\!C \qquad\qquad\qquad C\!=\!O$$
$$O \qquad\qquad O$$

Salts of EDTA may be used to chelate the calcium ions of tooth structure and so decalcify dentin.[102] The formula is as follows:

disodium salt of EDTA ....17.0 g
distilled water .... 100.0 ml
5N sodium hydroxide ....9.25 ml

If desired, 0.84 g of the bactericide Cetavlon

may be added. This 15% solution of EDTA has a pH of about 7.3 and is commercially available under the name of EDTAC because it contains Cetavlon, a quaternary-ammonium compound added for its disinfecting properties. EDTA is also available commercially for medical use.*

The effects of EDTA have been studied both in vitro and in vivo, and the following conclusions had been reported: (1) EDTA is effective in softening dentin, as determined by a knoop indentor; (2) EDTA has distinct antimicrobial properties; (3) EDTA is capable of causing a moderate degree of irritation; (4) EDTA has no deleterious effect when used clinically as an irrigating solution;[109] (5) irrigation with EDTA removes the smear layer;[47] (6) the extent of demineralization of EDTA is proportional to the exposure time;[157] and (7) EDTA effects partial demineralization of dentin to a depth of 20 to 30 μ in 5 min.[41]

A combination of EDTA and urea peroxide (R-C Prep)† developed by Stewart and colleagues was an effective lubricating and cleaning agent for root canals and allowed deeper penetration of the medicament into the dentin.[136] Cook and associates, using a radioactive tracer, studied the permeability of dentin following the use of R-C Prep. They reported twice as much leakage in canals obturated with gutta-percha or silver cones following cleaning and shaping with R-C Prep and sodium hypochlorite than with sodium hypochlorite alone.[26]

EDTA is inserted by depositing a few drops in the pulp chamber with a syringe or plastic pipette and then carefully pumping the solution into the root canal with a fine root canal instrument. Instrumentation is continued, with the solution bathing the canal at all times until cleaning and shaping are completed. When it is difficult to introduce a file into the canal, one should try to force the EDTA ahead of the instrument. When the canal is patent except for the last 2 or 3 mm, the same technique should be used to reach the apical foramen. If the root canal of a posterior tooth is narrow and if one risks breaking a fine instrument, it is better to pump EDTA into the canal and wait 2 or 3 min before attempting instrumentation. Once the apical foramen has been reached and the

canal has been enlarged, the canal should be irrigated in the usual manner.

BIBLIOGRAPHY

1. Abington, R.B.: U.S. Armed Forces Med. J., *9*:987, 1958.
2. Adams, W.R., et al.: J. Endod., *5*:121, 1979.
3. Adrian, S.A.: Tufts Dent. Outlook, *35*:5, 1959.
4. Allison, D.A., et al.: J. Endod., *5*:298, 1979.
4a. American Dental Association and American Heart Association (joint report): J. Am. Dent. Assoc., *68*:333, 1964.
5. Baker, N.A., et al.: J. Endod., *1*:127, 1975.
6. Barnett, F., et al.: Endod. Dent. Traumatol., *1*:77, 1985.
7. Baumgartner, J.C., et al.: J. Endod.. *2*:135, 1976, and *3*:399, 1977.
8. Becker, G.H., et al.: Oral Surg., *38*:633, 1974.
9. Bence, R., et al.: Oral Surg., *35*:676, 1973.
10. Bender, I.B., et al.: Oral Surg., *16*:466, 1963.
11. Bhat, K.S.: Oral Surg., *38*:304, 1974.
12. Birchfield, J., and Rosenberg, P.A.: J. Endod., *1*:26, 1975.
13. Bjorndahl, A.M., et al.: Oral Surg., *38*:791, 1974.
14. Blank, L.W., et al.: J. Endod., *1*:141, 1975.
15. Blechman, H., and Cohen, M.: J. Dent. Res., *30*:503, 1951.
16. Bodnar, O., et al.: Prakt. Zub. Lek., *25*:84, 1977.
17. Burke, J.H.: U.S. Navy Med. Newsletter., *52*:16, 1968.
18. Busch, L.R., et al.: J. Endod., *2*:295, 1976.
19. Brown, R.D.: Br. Dent. J., *151*:47, 1981.
20. Braumante, C.M., and Berbert, A.: Oral Surg., *37*:463, 1974.
21. Cameron, J.A.: J. Endod., *8*:472, 1982.
22. Cash, P.W.: Texas Dent. J., *90*:21, 1972.
23. Clarke, J., and Holmes, G.: Dent. Pract., *10*:36, 1959.
24. Coffae, K.P., and Brilliant, J.D.: J. Endod., *1*:211, 1975.
25. Cohen, S.: Oral Surg., *29*:631, 1970.
26. Cook, H., et al.: J. Endod., *2*:312, 1976.
27. Coolidge, E.D., and Kesel, R.G.: Textbook of Endodontology, 2nd Ed. Philadelphia, Lea & Febiger, 1956, p. 200.
28. Costich, E. (quoting H. Sicher): J. Am. Dent. Assoc., *75*:799, 1967.
29. Costigan, S.M.: J. Bacteriol., *34*:1, 1937.
30. Cunningham, W.T., and Joseph, S.W.: Oral Surg., *50*:569, 1980.
31. Cunningham, W.T., et al.: Oral Surg., *54*:238, 1982.
32. Cunningham, W.T., et al.: Oral Surg., *53*:527, 1982.
33. Cunningham, W.T., et al.: Oral Surg., *53*:401, 1982.
34. Craig, R.G., and Payton, F.A.: Oral Surg., *15*:213, 1962 and *16*:217, 1963.
35. Craig, R.G., et al.: Oral Surg., *25*:239, 1968.
36. Crump, M.C., and Natkin, E.: J. Am. Dent. Assoc., *80*:1341, 1970.
37. Cvek, M., et al.: Odontol. Revy., *27*:1, 1976.
38. Ellerbruch, E.S., and Murphy, R.A.: J. Endod., *3*:189, 1977.
39. Endodontic System Technique. Milford, DE, L.D. Caulk Co., 1984.
40. Ether, S.S., et al.: Rev. Farmacol. Odontol., *45*:7, 1978.
41. Fehr, F., and Nygaard-Østby, B.: Oral Surg., *16*:199, 1963.
42. Fox, J., et al.: Oral Surg., *30*:123, 1970.
43. Fujita, M.: Shikwa Gakuho, *77*:773, 1977.

---

*Endrate, Abbott, Chicago, Illinois.

†Premier Dental Products, Norristown, Pennsylvania.

44. Frank, A.L.: Oral Surg., *24*:219, 1967.
45. Fraser, J.G.: Oral Surg., *37*:803, 1974.
46. Fraser, J.G., and Laws, A.J.: Oral Surg., *41*:534, 1976.
47. Goldman, L.B., et al.: Oral Surg., *52*:197, 1981.
48. Goldman, L.B., et al.: Oral Surg., *48*:79, 1979.
49. Göllmer, L.: Int. J. Orthod., *23*:101, 1937.
50. Goodman, A., et al.: J. Endod., *11*:249, 1985.
51. Gordon, T., D'Amato, D.F., and Christen, P.: Personal communication.
52. Gottlieb, B., et al.: Ondontologia (Madrid), *42*:345, 1933.
53. Grahnen, H., and Krasse, B.: Odontol. Revy, *14*:167, 1963.
54. Green, D.: Morphology of the Endodontic System, 1969.
55. Green, E.N.: Oral Surg., *10*:532, 1957.
56. Grossman, L.I.: Oral Surg., *28*:746, 1969.
57. Grossman, L.I.: J. Br. Endod. Soc., *2*:35, 1968.
58. Grossman, L.I.: J. Am. Dent. Assoc., *61*:671, 1960.
59. Grossman, L.I.: J. Am. Dent. Assoc., *30*:1915, 1943.
60. Grossman, L.I.: J. Dent. Res., *22*:487, 1943.
61. Grossman, L.I., and Meiman, J.: J. Am. Dent. Assoc., *28*:233, 1941.
62. Gutierrez, J.H., and Garcia, J.: Oral Surg., *25*:108, 1968.
63. Hadfield, W.A.: *In* Antiseptics, Disinfectants, Fungicides and Sterilization. Edited by C.W. Reddish. Philadelphia, Lea & Febiger, 1954, p. 465.
64. Haga, C.: Northwest Univ. Bull., *57*:11, 1967.
65. Hand, R.E., et al.: J. Endod., *4*:60, 1978.
66. Harris, M.: Oral Surg., *18*:16, 1964.
67. Harris, W.E.: J. Endod., *2*:126, 1976.
68. Harrison, J.W.: Dent. Clin. North. Am., *28*:797, 1984.
69. Harrison, J.W., et al.: J. Endod., *4*:6, 1978.
70. Harty, F.J., and Stock, C.J.: Br. Dent. J., *137*:239, 1974.
71. Heling, B., et al.: Oral Surg., *19*:531, 1965.
72. Heuer, M.A.: Instruments and Materials in Pathways of the Pulp, 3rd Ed. St. Louis, C.V. Mosby, 1984.
73. Hession, R.W.: Oral Surg., *44*:775, 1977.
74. Ingle, J.I., and LeVine, M.J.: *In* Transactions of the Second International Conference on Endodontics. Edited by L.I. Grossman. Philadelphia, University of Pennsylvania, 1958, p. 123.
75. Ingle, J.I., and Taintor, J.F.: Endodontics, 3rd Ed. Philadelphia, Lea & Febiger, 1985.
76. Inoue, N.: J. Can. Dent. Assoc., *39*:630, 1973.
77. Kaufman, E., et al.: J. Dent. Res., *63*:287, 1984. (abstract 1045)
78. Kaufman, H., et al.: J. Dent. Res., *56*:1232, 1977.
79. Klayman, S.M., and Brilliant, J.D.: J. Endod., *1*:334, 1975.
80. Krueger, L.F.: J. Can. Dent. Assoc., *1*:533, 1935.
81. Kuttler, Y.: J. Am. Dent. Assoc., *50*:544, 1955.
82. Lechner, H., and Kroncke, A.: Dtsch. Zahnartzl. Z., *28*:347, 1973.
83. Lentine, F.H.: J. Endod., *5*:181, 1979.
84. Leonardo, M.R., et al.: Oral Surg., *49*:441, 1980.
85. Lindström, G.: Svensk. Tandlaek. Tidskr., *57*:807, 1964.
86. McComb, D., and Smith, D.C.: J. Endod., *1*:238, 1975.
87. Magnin, J.: Rev. Mens. Suisse Odontol., *68*:437, 1958.
88. Malamed, S.F.: The Management of Pain and Anx-

iety in Pathways of the Pulp, 3rd Ed. St. Louis, C.V. Mosby, 1984.
89. Malamed, S.F.: Oral Surg., *51*:463, 1981.
90. Marshall, F.J., et al.: Oral Surg., *13*:208, 1960.
91. Martin, H.: Oral Surg., *42*:92, 1976.
92. Martin, H., and Cunningham, W.T.: Oral Surg., *54*:74, 1982.
93. Martin, H., and Cunningham, W.T.: Oral Surg., *53*:611, 1982.
94. Martin, H., et al.: Oral Surg., *50*:566, 1980.
95. Martin, H., et al.: Oral Surg., *49*:79, 1980.
96. Masterson, J.B.: Dent. Pract., *15*:162, 1965.
97. Mizrahi, S.J., et al.: J. Endod., *1*:324, 1975.
98. Molven, O.: Oral Surg., *35*:232, 1973.
99. Neuwirth, F.: Dtsch. Monatschr. Zahnkd., *48*:634, 1930.
100. Nicholls, E.: Br. Dent. J., *112*:167, 1962.
101. Nicholson, R.L., et al.: Oral Surg., *26*:563, 1968.
102. Nygaard-Østby, B.: Odontol. Tidskr., *65*:1, 1957.
103. O'Connell, D.T., and Brayton, S.M.: Oral Surg., *39*:298, 1975.
104. O'Keefe, E.M.: J. Endod., *2*:315, 1976.
105. Okuna, K., et al.: J. Osaka Odontol. Soc., *39*:83, 1976.
106. Oliet, S., and Sorin, S.: Oral Surg., *36*:243, 1973.
107. O'Neill, L.J.: Oral Surg., *38*:469, 1974.
108. Oswald, R.J., and Friedman, C.E.: Oral Surg., *49*:344, 1980.
109. Patterson, S.S.: Oral Surg., *16*:83, 1963.
110. Pearson, S.L.: Br. Dent. J., *105*:92, 1958.
111. Peters, D.D.: J. Endod., *6*:518, 1980.
112. Plant, J.J., and Newman, R.F.: J. Endod., *2*:215, 1976.
113. Prader, F.: Schweiz, Monatsschr. Zahnkd., *57*:383, 1947.
114. Ram, Z.: Oral Surg., *49*:64, 1980.
115. Ram, Z.: Oral Surg., *44*:306, 1977.
116. Rickles, W.H., and Joshi, B.A.: J. Am. Dent. Assoc., *67*:397, 1963.
117. Ring, A.L.: Zahnarztl. Mitt., *58*:1024, 1968.
118. Rood, J.P., and Pateromichelakis, S.: Br. J. Oral Surg., *19*:67, 1981.
119. Rosenfeld, E.J., et al.: J. Endod., *4*:140, 1978.
120. Rubin, L.M., et al.: J. Endod., *5*:328, 1979.
121. Salzgreber, R., and Brilliant, J.: J. Endod., *3*:394, 1977.
122. San Marcos, P., and Montgomery, S.: Oral Surg., *57*:308, 1984.
123. Schilder, H.: Dent. Clin. North Am., *18*:269, 288, 1974.
124. Schilder, H., and Yee, F.S.: Canal Debridement and Disinfection in Pathways of the Pulp, 3rd Ed. St. Louis, C.V. Mosby, 1984.
125. Seidberg, B.H., et al.: J. Am. Dent. Assoc., *90*:379, 1975.
126. Senia, E.S., et al.: Oral Surg., *31*:96, 1971.
127. Sherman, P., and Calman, C.: Oral Surg., *7*:1267, 1954.
128. Shih, M., et al.: Oral Surg., *29*:613, 1970.
129. Shovelton, D.S.: Br. Dent. J., *102*:125, 1958.
130. Sintenis, C.: Dtsch. Monatsschr. Zahnkd., *43*:609, 1925.
131. Smith, G.N., and Walton, R.E.: Oral Surg., *55*:232, 1983.
132. Smith, G.N., and Pashley, D.H.: Oral Surg., *56*:571, 1983.
133. Soltanoff, W.: J. Endod., *4*:278, 1978.
134. Spangberg, L.: *In* Transactions of the Fifth International Conference on Endodontics. Edited by L.I.

Grossman. Philadelphia, University of Pennsylvania, 1973, p. 117.

135. Stewart, G.G.: Oral Surg., *8*:993, 1935.
136. Stewart, G.G., et al.: J. Am. Dent. Assoc., *78*:335, 1969.
137. Stewart, G.G., et al.: J. Am. Dent. Assoc., *63*:33, 1961.
138. Sunada, I.: J. Dent. Res., *41*:375, 1962.
139. Suzuki, K.: Jpn. J. Stomatol., *16*:411, 1942.
140. Svec, T.A., and Harrison, J.W.: J. Endod., *3*:49, 1977.
141. Thé, S.D., et al.: Oral Surg., *49*:460, 1980.
142. Trepagnier, C.M., et al.: J. Endod., *3*:194, 1977.
143. Tronstad, L.: Oral Surg., *45*:297, 1978.
144. Tronstad, L., et al.: Endod. Dent. Traumatol., *1*:69, 1985.
145. Tübingen, N.S.: ZWR, 86:11, 1977.
146. Tucker, J., et al.: Paper presented at the meeting of the American Association of Endodontists, New York, April, 1975.
147. Vande Visse, J.E., and Brilliant, J.D.: J. Endod., *1*:243, 1975.
148. Vande Voorde, H.E., and Bjorndahl, A.M.: Oral Surg., *27*:106, 1969.
149. Vessey, R.A.: Oral Surg., *27*:543, 1969.
150. Walton, R.E.: J. Endod., *2*:304, 1976.
151. Walton, R.E., and Abbott, B.J.: J. Am. Dent. Assoc., *103*:571, 1981.
152. Walton, R.E., and Garnick, J.J.: J. Endod., *8*:22, 1982.
153. Wayman, B.A., et al.: J. Endod., *5*:258, 1979.
154. Weine, F.: Endodontic Therapy, 3rd Ed. St. Louis, C.V. Mosby, 1982.
155. Weine, F.: J. Endod., *2*:298, 1976.
156. Wolch, I.: J. Can. Dent. Assoc., *41*:613, 1975.
157. Wyman, T.P., et al.: J. Dent. Res., *57A*:161, 1978.
158. Zeldow, B.J., and Ingle, J.I.: J. Am. Dent. Assoc., *57*:471, 1958.
159. Zerosi, C., and Viotti, L.: Rass. Trimes. Odontol., *39*:683, 1958.

12 Disinfection of the Root Canal

Disinfection of the root canal, that is, destruction of pathogenic microorganisms, presupposes previous adequate removal of pulp tissue and debris, cleaning and enlarging of the canal by biochemical means, and clearing of its contents by irrigation. Disinfection of the root canal is accomplished by intracanal medication.

The need for intracanal medication has been questioned. Evidence is sufficient to indicate that disinfection of the root canal is an important phase of endodontic treatment. Microorganisms present in the canal can invade the periapical tissue and may not only give rise to pain, but also destroy the periodontium including bone. Akpata,[1] Bystrom and Sundqvist,[8] Holland and colleagues,[21] Pitt Ford,[29] and Zielke[45] have shown by experimental studies that intracanal medication reduces or eliminates the microbial flora in the root canal. According to a study by Bystrom and Sundqvist, when no intracanal medicament was used between appointments, pathogenic microorganisms increased in numbers.[7] The need for an intracanal medicament to destroy or reduce the number of microorganisms seems apparent. Bender and others are of the opinion that irrigation with 5% sodium hypochlorite and 3% hydrogen peroxide during biomechanical preparation of the root canal obviates the need for an intracanal medicament.[3]

ROOT CANAL FLORA

Before considering intracanal medication, we might ask the question: What microorganisms are we trying to destroy? In most cases, gram-positive organisms are present; in some cases, gram-negative organisms; in a few cases, yeasts. These organisms are found most often in various combinations rather than as a single species. Obligate anaerobes are often associated with teeth that have a periapical lesion (see Chap. 13).

The microbial flora of root canals is likely to comprise organisms that can survive on dead pulp tissue, that is, saprophytes, those that can grow in an environment of low oxygen tension, and those that can survive the rigors of a limited pabulum. The organisms reaching the root canal obviously have their origin in the mouth.[16] Although all varieties of microorganisms may have an equal chance of invading the pulp tissue or the root canal, only those best fit for survival in this environment do survive. A census of microorganisms recovered from pulp tissue or root canals shows that the commonest organisms of the mouth, streptococci, are also the most frequently found in root canals. The endodontic problem is primarily one of eliminating gram-positive organisms because they are the most abundant, consisting chiefly of streptococci and staphylococci. Among the streptococci is a small but resistant group of enterococci. In addition, a small percentage of gram-negative organisms and yeasts can be isolated from saliva and from root canals.

Recent reports on bacterial flora describe the presence of obligate and facultative anaerobes, a result related to the use of improved technology in sampling and culturing anaerobic microorganisms (see Chap. 13).

Four factors either predispose teeth to infection or counteract disinfection, whether it be of a wound or the root canal of a pulpless tooth. These factors may also delay healing. They are: (1) trauma; the tooth under treatment should be disoccluded if necessary; (2) devitalized tissue; if present in the root canal or periapical tissue, it will interfere with disinfection or with repair; (3) dead spaces; for maximum effect, the medicament should be in contact with the microorganisms in the root canal; and (4) accumulation of exudate; exudate should be allowed to drain or be removed as it accumulates. Root canal dressings should be changed at least once a week and more often in the case of an acute apical abscess under treatment.

INTRACANAL MEDICAMENTS

The requirements of a root canal disinfectant are as follows: (1) it should be an effective germicide and fungicide; (2) it should be nonirritating to the periapical tissues; (3) it should remain stable in solution; (4) it should have a prolonged antimicrobial effect; (5) it should be active in the presence of blood, serum, and protein derivatives of tissue; (6) it should have low surface tension; (7) it should not interfere with repair of periapical tissues; (8) it should not stain tooth structure; (9) it should be capable of inactivation in a culture medium, and (10) it should not induce a cell-mediated immune response. Root canal disinfectants may be grouped arbitrarily as essential oils, phenolic compounds, halogens, and antibiotics, for example.

Essential Oils

As a group, the essential oils are weak disinfectants.

Eugenol. This substance is the chemical essence of oil of clove and is related to phenol. It is slightly more irritating than oil of clove and is both an antiseptic and an anodyne. Trowbridge has shown that eugenol inhibited intradental nerve impulses.[39] A few reports of allergy to eugenol have been reported.

Phenolic Compounds

Phenol. This white crystalline substance has a characteristic odor derived from coal tar. Liquefied phenol (carbolic acid) consists of 9 parts of phenol and 1 part water. Phenol is a protoplasm poison and produces necrosis of soft tissue.

Para-chlorophenol. This compound is a substitution product of phenol in which chlorine replaces one of the hydrogen atoms (C_6H_4OHCl). On trituration with gum camphor, these substances combine to form an oily liquid. Harrison and Madonia have recommended a 1% aqueous solution of para-chlorophenol.[19] In tests in vitro, the aqueous solution destroyed a variety of microorganisms ordinarily found in infected root canals. Avny and associates,[2] as well as Taylor and colleagues,[37] have shown that the aqueous solution of para-chlorophenol penetrates deeper into the dentinal tubules than camphorated chlorophenol.

Camphorated Para-chlorophenol. This compound is composed of 2 parts para-chlorophenol and 3 parts gum camphor. It has enjoyed a high degree of popularity as an intracanal medicament for a century. The camphor serves as a vehicle and a diluent and reduces the irritating effect of pure para-chlorophenol. It also prolongs the antimicrobial effect, which has been compared to that of other root canal medicaments by Grossman,[15,17] as well as by Ostrander and Crowley.[27] Wantulok and Brown have shown that the vapors of camphorated chlorophenol (and also of Cresatin) pass through the apical foramen.[42]

Formocresol. This substance is a combination of formalin and cresol in the proportions of 1:2 or 1:1. Formalin is a strong disinfectant that combines with albumin to form an insoluble, indecomposable substance. Black,[4] Grossman,[18] and Schilder and Amsterdam[31] have demonstrated the irritating effect of formocresol. In every case in which the compound was tested against living tissue, necrosis was followed by a persistent inflammatory reaction. Straffon and Han,[36] as well as Loos and Han,[24] have recommended using low concentrations of formocresol. Block and associates have reported that formocresol-treated tissue produced a cell-mediated immune response.[6] According to Van Mullen and colleagues, formocresol did not produce an immune reaction in nonsensitized animals, but it did in presensitized animals.[40] Formocresol is a nonspecific bactericidal medicament most effective against aerobic and anaerobic organisms found in a root canal.

Glutaraldehyde. This colorless oil is slightly soluble in water and thereby has a slightly acidic reaction. Like formalin, it is a strong disinfectant and fixative. S'Gravenmade[32] and Dankert[10] have recommended it in low concentration (2%) as an intracanal medicament, and Wemes found little or no inflammation on histologic examination of human material.[44] Formaldehyde produced an immunologic reaction through the T cells, according to Van Velzen,[41] but glutaraldehyde did not.

Cresatin. Also known as metacresylacetate, this substance is a clear, stable, oily liquid of low volatility. It is claimed to have both antiseptic and obtundant properties. The antimicrobial effect of Cresatin is less than that of either formocresol or camphorated para-chlorophenol, as demonstrated by Grossman,[17] but it is less irritating.

Calcium Hydroxide

This compound has also been used as an intracranal medicament. A brief study in cats' teeth by Stevens and Grossman did not find calcium hydroxide as effective as camphorated chlorophenol.[35] Its antiseptic action probably relates to its high pH and its leaching action on necrotic pulp tissue.[26] Tronstad and associates have shown that calcium hydroxide causes a significant increase in the pH of circumpulpal dentin when the compound is placed in the root canal.[38] Calcium hydroxide paste is best used as an intracanal medicament when one anticipates an excessive delay between appointments because it is efficacious as long as it remains within the root canal. Bystrom, in a clinical study of more than 100 periapically involved teeth, has reported that calcium hydroxide is a very effective intracanal disinfectant.[8a]

N2

N2, a compound containing paraformaldehyde as its primary ingredient, is claimed to be both an intracanal medicament and a sealer. N2 contains eugenol and phenylmercuric borate, and at times, additional ingredients, including lead, corticosteroids, antibiotics, and perfume.[30] Claims that N2 has a permanent disinfectant action and unusual antimicrobial properties have been denied by the Council on Dental Therapeutics of the American Dental Association.[9] The antibacterial effect of N2 is short lived, and dissipated in about a week to 10 days.[14]

Halogens

Sodium Hypochlorite. This compound is sometimes used as an intracanal medicament. In general, the disinfectant action of the halogens is inversely proportional to their atomic weights. Chlorine, with the lowest atomic weight, has the greatest disinfectant action of the members of this group. Chlorine disinfectants are not stable compounds because they interact rapidly with organic matter. Ellerbruch and Murphy found that sodium hypochlorite vapors were bactericidal, whereas those of formocresol, aqueous para-chlorophenol, and camphorated chlorophenol were bacteriostatic.[11] Mentz found sodium hypochlorite an effective intracanal medicament as well as irrigant.[25] Because the activity of sodium hypochlorite is intense but of short duration, the compound should preferably be applied to the root canal every other day.

Iodides. These compounds have been used as antiseptics for more than a century. Iodine is highly reactive, combining with proteins in a loosely bound manner so its penetration

is not impeded. It probably destroys microorganisms by forming salts that are inimical to the life of the organism. Engström and Spangberg have recommended a 2% solution of iodine in potassium iodide as a root canal disinfectant.[13] This compound consists of iodine crystals, 2 parts, potassium iodide, 4 parts, and distilled water, 94 parts. As with chlorine compounds, the antibacterial effect is of short duration. Spangberg and colleagues evaluated the potassium iodide-iodine solution both in vitro and in vivo and found it to be one of the least irritating medicaments.[33,34]

Quaternary Ammonium Compounds

The "quats" are compounds that lower the surface tension of solutions. They are inactivated by anionic compounds. Because the quaternary ammonium compounds are positively charged and the microorganisms are negatively charged, a surface-active effect results in which the compound clings to the microorganism and reverses the charge.

The compound 9-aminoacridine belongs to the group of mild cationic antiseptics. A derivative of an acridine dye, 9-aminoacridine may stain tooth structure.

IRRITATION POTENTIAL OF MEDICAMENTS

The irritation potential of root canal medicaments was studied by Black, who found some of the essential oils and formocresol highly irritating, especially formocresol.[4] In a "blind" study, Grossman found that camphorated chlorophenol and Cresatin had a moderate irritating effect when applied to the shaved skin of the arm for 48 hours;[18] (Fig. 12–1); formocresol caused necrosis that lasted 2 to 3 months. Schilder and Amsterdam found that hydrogen peroxide and sodium hypochlorite were less irritating than most intracanal medicaments, formocresol produced a high degree of irritation, and Cresatin caused little or no inflammation.[31] Cytotoxic studies of root canal medicaments have been made by Engström[12] and by Spangberg and associates.[33,34]

FREQUENCY OF MEDICATION

In accordance with general principles of root canal management, disinfectant dressings should preferably be renewed in a week and not longer than 2 weeks because dressings become diluted by periapical exudate

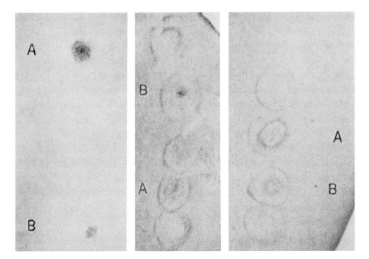

Fig. 12–1. Reactions to root canal medicaments after 48-hour application to the arm. *A* to *C*, the label A indicates pronounced inflammation and necrosis from formocresol, and the label B indicates slight inflammation from beechwood creosote. No reaction to chloroazodin, Cresatin, or camphorated chlorophenol was observed. *B* and *C*, The outer rings are pencil marks identifying the areas where medicaments had been applied.

and are decomposed by interaction with the microorganisms.

Traditionally, dressing a root canal, a short, blunt absorbent point moistened with the medicament is carried into the canal, a cotton pledget from which excess medicament has been expressed is placed in the pulp chamber, and the access cavity is sealed. In narrow canals, however, a moist absorbent point does not have sufficient stiffness to be introduced into the canal. In such cases, a dry absorbent is inserted, and a cotton pledget moistened with the medicament is placed against the absorbent point to moisten it. A dry cotton pledget is used to absorb the excess medicament, and the cavity is sealed.

Many endodontists prefer to dress a root canal with a medicated cotton pellet from which excess medicament has been removed. They depend on the vaporization of the medicament in the pulp chamber for antibacterial action, and they omit the placing of an absorbent point in the root canal. The vapors issuing from the medicament are sufficient to disinfect the pulp cavity.[42] The elimination of the absorbent point allows room in the canal for the accumulation of fluid exudate, reduces the possibility of periapical irritation from inadvertent extrusion of the medicament or absorbent point into the periapical tissue, eliminates the potential problem of removing a wedged, saturated absorbent point from the root canal during the succeeding visit, and reduces treatment time.

The canal is sealed after placing a second sterile dry cotton pellet over the medicated pellet, or placing a seal of temporary stopping over the medicated pellet, and completing the double seal with a temporary outer seal of Cavit, zinc oxide-eugenol cement, or IRM.

OUTLINE OF TREATMENT

The technique of treatment of infected teeth may be outlined as follows:

First Visit

1. Apply the rubber dam, and disinfect the field of operation. Prepare an access cavity.

2. Open into the pulp chamber with sterile burs until free access to all canals along straight lines is secured.

3. Without pressure, remove the contents of the pulp chamber with a sterile excavator. Identify the root canal orifices with the tip of long-bladed explorer or a D11 instrument. Apply sodium-hypochlorite solution at the orifices of the root canals.

4. Carefully explore the canal partway with a smooth broach, reamer, or file to determine patency. NOTE: All instruments used in the root canal should be prepared with instrument stops to confine instruments within the canal.

5. With an instrument stop or marker attached to a style "B" instrument at the provisional length of tooth minus 1 mm, insert the instrument into the canal, and take a ra-

diograph. Be careful not to traumatize the periapical tissue. Remove the instrument. Examine the radiograph. Reset the instrument stop if necessary.

6. Gradually enlarge the canal with files and reamers until the canal is prepared eventually to receive a gutta-percha filling.

7. Remove dentin shavings and organic debris in the canal by irrigating alternately with sodium-hypochlorite solution and hydrogen peroxide, with sodium hypochlorite as the final irrigating solution. Dry the canal. At this stage, access to the apical foramen throughout the entire length of the canal should be possible.

8. Seal the medicament in the canal. Remove the rubber dam.

Second Visit

1. Apply the rubber dam, and disinfect the field of operation.

2. Remove and discard the dressing and, if clinical conditions are satisfactory, take a culture as follows:

3. Culture Technique:

a. Swab the surface of the tooth with alcohol. Let it evaporate or dry it with a sterile cotton pellet.

b. With freshly sterilized cotton pliers, introduce a sterile absorbent point into the canal and with a wiping motion remove traces of the medicament. Repeat.

c. Introduce a dry, sterile absorbent point into the canal. Let the point remain for at least 1 min. On removal, if the tip of the absorbent point is moistened with exudate, remove the screw cap from the test tube, flame the lip of the tube, and drop the absorbent point into the tube of sterile culture medium. Replace the screw cap.

d. Apply a label to the culture tube, and place the tube in the incubator.

4. Seal the medicament.

5. Request the patient to return at the appointed time.

Third Visit

1. If the culture is negative and if no clinical contraindications exist, the root canal may be obturated. Otherwise, repeat the procedure.

2. Except in anticipation of immediate root resection, a root canal should not be obturated while infection is present, as shown by culture, or if the tooth is symptomatic.

Addendum. Predoctoral programs may vary the culturing technique outlined above in order to achieve different pedagogic objectives. Some culture the pulp chamber after completing the access opening, prior to irrigation, and compare that culture with those taken from the root canal at the beginning of each preceding appointment. These cultures are intended to monitor the student's aseptic technique, to develop expertise in taking cultures, and to determine the bacteriologic status of the root canal at different stages of treatment.

TEMPORARY FILLING MATERIAL

The adequacy of temporary filling materials in sealing root canal dressings is just as important as any other element in endodontic treatment. Leakage of the seal can counteract the most careful treatment. Temporary filling materials should meet certain requirements. The material should: (1) be impervious to fluids of the mouth and bacteria; (2) hermetically seal the access cavity peripherally; (3) not cause pressure on the dressing during insertion; (4) harden within a few minutes after insertion; (5) withstand the force of mastication; (6) be easy to manipulate and to remove; and (7) harmonize with the color of tooth structure. No material meets all these requirements satisfactorily. The zinc-oxide, quick-setting cements probably best meet these requirements, except for the setting time which can be accelerated by the addition of 0.5 to 1.0% zinc acetate. Cavit* and IRM† are also satisfactory temporary filling materials.

Parris and Kapsimalis found that Cavit maintained a leak-proof access cavity when tested with either a dye or a test microorganism.[28] Webber and associates have shown that a thickness of Cavit of at least 3.5 mm is necessary to prevent leakage,[43] and this finding has been confirmed by Lamers and colleagues,[23] who also found that long periods between appointments predisposed the tooth to leakage.

IRM becomes hard shortly after insertion in the access cavity, in contradistinction to Cavit, and showed no evidence of leakage when Proteus vulgaris was used as a test organism by Blaney and colleagues.[5] Keller and associates found no difference in sealing

---

*Premier Dental Products, Norristown, Pennsylvania.
†Intermediate Restorative Material, L.D. Caulk Co., Milford, Delaware.

properties between Cavit and IRM.[22] One may deduce that Cavit and IRM are suitable temporary filling materials when used properly.

BIBLIOGRAPHY

1. Akpata, E.S.: J. Endod., *2*:369, 1976.
2. Avny, W.Y., et al.: Oral Surg., *36*:80, 1973.
3. Bender, I.B.: Personal communication.
4. Black, G.V.: Special Dental Pathology, 2nd Ed. Chicago, Medical-Dental Publishing, 1920, p. 296.
5. Blaney, T.D., et al.: J. Endod., *7*:453, 1981.
6. Block, R., et al.: J. Endod., *3*:424, 1977.
7. Bystrom, A., and Sundqvist, G.: Int. Endod. J., *18*:35, 1985.
8. Bystrom, A., and Sundqvist, G.: Scand. J. Dent. Res., *89*:321, 1981.
8a. Bystrom, A.: Dissertation, University of Umea, Sweden, 1986.
9. Council on Dental Therapeutics, American Dental Association: J. Am. Dental Assoc., *64*:689, 1962.
10. Dankert, J.: J. Endod., *2*:42, 1976.
11. Ellerbruch, E.S., and Murphy, R.A.: J. Endod., *3*:189, 1977.
12. Engström, B.: Svensk. Tandpaek. Tidskr., *51*:1, 1958.
13. Engström, B., and Spangberg, L.: Acta Odontol. Scand., *25*:77, 1967.
14. Grossman, L.I.: J. Endod., *6*:594, 1980.
15. Grossman, L.I.: J. Am. Dent. Assoc., *85*:900, 1972.
16. Grossman, L.I.: J. Dent. Res., *46*:551, 1967.
17. Grossman, L.I.: J. Dent. Res., *42*:583, 1963.
18. Grossman, L.I.: Am. J. Orthod. Oral Surg., *30*:564, 1944.
19. Harrison, J.W., and Madonia, J.V.: Oral Surg., *30*:267, 1970, and *40*:670, 1975.
20. Heathersay, G.S.: Int. Endod. J. *18*:72, 1985.
21. Holland, R., et al.: Br. Endod. Soc., *12*:15, 1979.
22. Keller, D.L., et al.: J. Endod., *7*:413, 1981.
23. Lamers, A.C., et al.: Oral Surg., *49*:541, 1980.
24. Loos, P.J., and Han, S.S.: Oral Surg., *31*:571, 1971.
25. Mentz, T.C.F.: Int. Endod. J., *15*:132, 1982.
26. Nichols, E.: Endodontics, 3rd Ed. Bristol, England, Wright, 1984, p. 152.
27. Ostrander, F.D., and Crowley, M.C.: J. Endod., *3*:6, 1948.
28. Parris, L., and Kapsimalis, P.: Oral Surg., *18*:982, 1960, and *17*:771, 1964.
29. Pitt Ford, T.R.: Int. Endod. J., *15*:16, 1982.
30. Sargenti, H.G., and Richter, S.L.: Rationalized Root Canal Treatment. New York, AGSA Publishing, 1959.
31. Schilder, H., and Amsterdam, M.: Oral Surg., *12*:211, 1959.
32. S' Gravenmade, E.: J. Endod., *1*:233,1975.
33. Spangberg, L.: *In* Transactions of the Fifth International Conference on Endodontics. Edited by L.I. Grossman. Philadelphia, University of Pennsylvania Press, 1973, p. 108.
34. Spangberg, L., et al.: Oral Surg., *36*:856, 1973.
35. Stevens, R.H., and Grossman, L.I.: J. Endod., *9*:372, 1983.
36. Straffon, C.H., and Han, S.S.: Arch. Oral Biol., *13*:271, 1968, and Oral Surg., *29*:915, 1970.
37. Taylor, G.H., et al.: J. Endod., *2*:81, 1976.
38. Tronstad, L., et al.: J. Endod., *7*:17, 1981 and *5*:83, 1979.
39. Trowbridge, H.: J. Endod., *8*:403, 1982.
40. Van Mullen, P., et al.: J. Endod., *9*:25, 1983.
41. Van Velzen, S.K.: Ned. Tigdschr. Tand., *82*:23, 1975.
42. Wantulok, J.C., and Brown, J.I.: Oral Surg., *34*:653, 1972.
43. Webber, R.T., et al.: Oral Surg., *46*:123,1978.
44. Wemes, J.C., et al.: Oral Surg., *54*:329, 340, 1982.
45. Zielke, D.R., et al.: Oral Surg., *47*:83, 1979.

13 Microbiology

The role of microbiology in endodontic practice, although clearly important, has remained controversial through most of the twentieth century. Onderdenk suggested the need for bacteriologic examination of the root canal in 1901.[56] Shortly thereafter, in 1910, Hunter made his historic address in Montreal in which he condemned the "golden traps of sepsis," the ill-fitting crowns and bridgework of his day that inexplicably resulted in the extraction of countless numbers of treated pulpless teeth and the inception of the "focal infection theory."[36] Within 25 years, nearly 2000 papers on focal infection were published, many concerned with oral focal infection. During this period, a few voices were raised to stem the hysterical tide and to return endodontic care to its proper role in the healing arts. La Roche[42] and Coolidge[13] suggested that bacteriologic examination be used in treating the root canal. Histologic studies of repair were reported by Blayney in 1932,[6] by Coolidge in 1931,[12] by Kronfeld in 1939,[41] by Aisenberg in 1931,[2] by Hatton and associates in 1928,[33] by Orban in 1932,[57] by Gottlieb and colleagues in 1928,[25] and by others. Bacteriologic studies by Haden in 1928,[31] as well as by Burket in 1937,[9] examined the growth percentages of bacteria, probably aerobes, in cultures of vital and pulpless teeth. Another study was published in 1936 by Fish and MacLean,[19] who demonstrated that the pulp and periapical tissues of vital healthy teeth are invariably free of evidence of microorganisms when examined histologically, and that it is practically impossible to extract a tooth aseptically unless the crevicular gingiva is cauterized first. In 1935, Okell and Elliot reported a transient bacteremia following extraction,[53] and in 1936, Round and associates showed that a transient bacteremia occurred when a patient with a marked periodontal condition simply chewed candy.[60] Appleton suggested that without bacteria no need would exist for endodontic treatment,[3] a hypothesis supported by the study of Kakehashi and colleagues,[38] who reported that exposed pulps in gnoto-

biotic rats healed without treatment in a germ-free environment. Appleton maintained that the function of root canal therapy is to render the canal and periapical tissues sterile, and a bacteriologic examination was therefore necessary. Since 1901, the question of the validity of culturing remains, and the controversy continues.

Many have translated their rejection of bacteriologic examination into a rejection of any serious relationship between microbiology and endodontic treatment. Naidorf wrote, "the fatuous preoccupation with culturing technique has, unfortunately, diverted attention away from the basic biologic principles of host-parasite relationship."[51] Within the last decade, however, many reports have been published on the bacterial flora of the pulp and periapical and periodontal tissues, the pathways of infection, the immunologic reactions, and the inflammatory responses. Although treatment procedures have changed slowly, they reflect a better understanding of the host-parasite relationship and of the way in which such reactions are managed more effectively.

FLORA

The bacterial flora of the root canal has been studied over many years. Earlier papers described a flora consisting predominantly of aerobic and facultative anaerobic microorganisms. The differences in flora, as reported by different investigators over the past 5 years, are the result of improved technology in sampling, such as new anaerobic culturing techniques, new and improved culture media, and more sophisticated methods of isolation and identification of microorganisms. One obvious factor in the reports of changing flora is frequently overlooked; that is, the interest of the investigator. If one seeks to isolate and identify microorganisms from an environment substantially anaerobic, using anaerobic sampling techniques, and culturing in media and an environment that encourages growth of anaerobic types of microorganisms, it is not surprising to find a flora predominantly of anaerobes. The same is true of aerobic sampling.

In 1919, Henrici and Hartzell found a predominance of Streptococcus viridans (63%), followed by Staphylococcus albus (17%), diphtheroid bacilli (6.5%) and spore-bearing aerobes, Staphylococcus aureus, Bacillus proteus, Streptococcus hemolyticus, and B. coli, all in the pulps of pyorrhetic teeth.* Sommer and associates reported that the organisms most frequently isolated from a root canal were alpha-hemolytic streptococci, such as Streptococcus viridans.[65] Eighty-two percent of 357 cultures contained streptococci, 53% in pure cultures. Beta-hemolytic streptococci were found in fewer that 2% of cultures, and anhemolytic (gamma-group) streptococci, mostly enterococci (Lancefield group D), comprised about 9% of the total of isolates. Other microorganisms present in the original 357 cultures were staphylococci, lactobacilli, yeasts, actinomyces, gram-negative bacilli, and gram-negative cocci, among others.

Grossman, Slack, and others found similar organisms, but their frequency in the samples tested differed. Grossman found gas-producing organisms in 23 of 300 consecutive root canals cultured prior to treatment.[29] He wondered whether these organsims might be related to the unexpected flare-ups that periodically occur during endodontic treatment. Investigators who prepared smears of the root canals often found additional bacteria that did not grow in the culture media used, and they assumed that these were dead microorganisms. In fact, they were probably fastidious or obligate anaerobes requiring special conditions and media to survive and to grow.

Matusow reported alteration of the tissue oxidation-reduction potential as an etiologic factor in cellulitis exacerbation during endodontic treatment on 34 intact nonvital teeth.[45] He isolated 47 aerobic and facultative microbes, 80% of which were streptococci, primarily facultative, but no obligate anaerobes were isolated.

Naidorf compiled a list of generalizations regarding organisms isolated from root canals, as follows:[51]

1. Mixed infections are more common than single-organism isolates.

2. The wide variety of organisms found in root canals by different investigators can be partially related to the principal interests and culture techniques of these investigators.

3. The invasion of dentin from the pulp has been described, but the types of organism, growth rate, and viability are poorly understood.

4. Pulpal isolates are similar to oral flora, with gram-positive cocci predominating.

5. Approximately 25% of the isolated organisms are anaerobes.

6. Organisms associated with flare-ups do not differ from asymptomatic-canal isolates.

7. Organisms cultured from infected canals elaborate a variety of invasive enzymes, but this capability cannot always be equated with pathogenicity.

8. The present practice of treating the obvious source of infection, the root canal, and not the periapical tissue conforms to the findings of Hedman,[34] as well as those of Melville and Birch.[47]

ANAEROBIC BACTERIA

In an effort to sample microorganisms that were obligate and facultative anaerobes in root canals, several investigators examined the flora of intact teeth with necrotic pulps. Mazzarella and colleagues in 1955,[46] MacDonald and associates in 1957,[44] and Brown and Rudolph in 1957,[7] found minor differences in the number of microorganisms isolated from such teeth. Gram-positive organisms were found in approximately 75% of the samples; the most predominant were streptococci (28%), staphylococci (15%), corynebacteria (10 to 25%), yeasts (12%), and others. The gram-negative bacteria (24%) included spirochetes (9 to 12%), neisseria (4%), bacteroides (7%), fusobacterium (3%), pseudomonas (2%), coliform bacteria (1%), and others. Brown and Rudolph reported anaerobes in 24% of the isolates,[7] whereas MacDonald and associates found anaerobes in 32% of their samples.[44] Obligate anaerobes have been grown from root canals by Goodman,[24] by Kantz and Henry,[39] by Keudell and associates,[40] by Wittgow and Sebastian,[70] by Zielke and colleagues,[72] by Möller,[48] and by Sundqvist.[67]

Möller isolated anaerobes in 74% of his samples.[48] Sundqvist reported results obtained from 32 intact nonvital teeth;[67] he iso-

---

*The nomenclature of many bacteria listed in the reports cited in this paragraph has been changed since these reports were originally published.

lated 88 strains of organisms of which 90% were anaerobes. Only 5 strains grew in air. Most of these samples contained mixed strains and consisted of fusobacterium, bacteroides, eubacterium, peptococcus, peptostreptococcus, and campylobacter. Sundqvist found Bacteroides melaninogenicus in mixed infection in 7 patients with acute periapical inflammation. He concluded that periapical osteitis is connected with the presence of bacteria in the root canal, and acute periapical inflammation is generated by Bacteroides melaninogenicus in mixed flora. Stobberingh and Eggink found microaerophilic microorganisms in teeth with periapical radiolucencies and in those with "necrotic closed pulp," but they found no correlation between microaerophilic, anaerobic, or aerobic organisms and periapical radiolucency.[66]

BACTERIAL PATHWAYS INTO THE PULP

Bacteria enter the pulp in various ways: (1) through the crown or root following traumatic exposure of the pulp, through the dentinal tubules following carious invasion, restorative procedures including crown preparation, and leaking restorations,[4,11,63] and through external or internal resorption that can lead to pulp exposures; (2) from the periodontal tissue through exposed dentinal tubules, lateral and accessory canals, or apical and lateral foramina;[7,27,32,44] and (3) by the lymphatic or hematogenous route (anachoresis). Anachoresis is defined as the localization of transient bacteria in the blood into an inflamed area, such as a traumatized or inflamed pulp.

Both aerobic and anaerobic microorganisms, as well as facultative microorganisms, can be found in the root canal. A large portion of microorganisms isolated from intact nonvital teeth are anaerobes, especially of the genera bacteroides, peptococcus, peptostreptococcus, fusiform, bacilli and corynebacterium. The origin of most of these bacteria is the oral cavity of the infected periodontal pocket. Experiments by Csernyei,[14] by Robinson and Bolling,[59] by Burke and Knighton,[8] by Smith and Tappe,[64] and by Gier and Mitchell[23] have documented the anachoretic effect, but this mechanism was rejected by Delivanis and associates,[15] who were unable to induce anachoresis in their experiment on monkeys.

BACTERIOLOGIC EXAMINATION

Sterility of a canal or a reduction in the number of microorganisms in a root canal cannot be determined by sight and smell. Few organisms are chromogenic, and not all bacteria give off noxious odors; for example, pseudomonas has a pleasant odor. If one of the prime objectives of endodontic treatment is the elimination of infectious organisms, what folly it is to look at the dressing, to smell it, and so decide whether the root canal is sterile or not.

Evidence in favor of bacteriologic examination was furnished by Buchbinder, who showed that 10% more teeth had healed successfully on postoperative check-up if they had a negative culture before obturation.[10] Oliet evaluated 98 teeth, some of which yielded positive cultures and others negative cultures at the time of root canal filling and on check-up found that "a greater degree of success in healing occurred when teeth were filled with no evidence of microorganisms in the root canals."[54] In an additional 300 cases reported by Oliet and Sorin, "healing" occurred in 11% more cases when the culture was negative at the time of root canal filling than when it was positive.[55] Zeldow and Ingle have shown a 12% higher success rate under similar circumstances.[71] Frostell has presented data to show that the culture has clinical significance.[21] Heling and Shapiro evaluated 118 teeth 1 to 5 years after treatment and found that when negative cultures had been obtained prior to root canal obturation, the success rate was 10% higher than when canals had been filled without cultures or in the presence of a positive culture.[35]

Bender and colleagues, however, question the significance of a negative culture during endodontic treatment; these investigators noted an 82% healing response in teeth filled in the presence of positive or negative cultures.[4] They state, however, that "these results should not be interpreted to mean that attempts to reduce the numbers of microorganisms are unnecessary." Eggink found no difference in healing for up to 3 years, when root canals were obturated in the presence of positive or negative cultures from the time of filling.[16] Stobberingh and Eggink bacteriologically examined more than 1800 root canals and found a low incidence (28%) of positive cultures on opening canals of intact teeth without periapical rarefaction.[66] These investigators therefore advocate the omission of further bacteriologic tests in such cases.

Morse contended that the success rate is the same whether the root canal yields a positive or negative culture at the time of obturation.[50] Morse later stated, however, that "anaerobic microbes are becoming clinically important and with the adoption of simplified anaerobic culture techniques, it may once again become important to take cultures."[49]

Although the difference of approximately 10% in results obtained by most investigators does not appear to be great, it is nevertheless significant in that in 10% of all teeth treated and filled in the presence of a positive culture, success would not be likely. Endodontic treatment without the benefit of bacteriologic control is justified neither economically nor ethically. Table 13–1 gives endodontic success rates in terms of bacteriologic examination.

The question of the value of a negative culture has often been raised. Some concede that a positive culture is sufficient evidence that a root canal should not be filled, but uncertainty remains whether any living microbes are still present in the root canal after obtaining a negative culture. Although a negative culture is not invariably conclusive evidence that all microorganisms have been eliminated, it is still the best indicator of whether numbers of microorganisms are reduced during treatment. By means of culture technique, one monitors the effectiveness of the biomechanical and chemomechanical preparation of the root canals and the effectiveness of the interappointment medication

and seal; justifiably, culture is a valuable and important treatment tool in the hands of the clinician.

Culture Media

Although not all microorganisms present in a root canal grow in readily available culture media, especially obligate anaerobes, exposure to air during endodontic treatment or to the chemical agents used in the root canals, such as sodium hypochlorite, will destroy obligate anaerobes. In an in vitro study, Foley found that full-strength Clorox (5.2% chlorinated soda) or Gly-oxide* (carbamide peroxide 10% in flavored anhydrous glycerol) killed Bacteroides melaninogenicus in 15 sec, but even a dilution of 1:10,000 Clorox was effective in destroying the organism, whereas diluted Gly-oxide was not effective.[20]

It has also been stated that if the sample from the root canal is small, growth will not be sustained. It takes few organisms to sustain growth. Grossman has shown that a single organism of certain species of oral microorganisms is sufficient to initiate growth in a culture medium, and the maximum number of microorganisms needed is ten.[29] This finding has been confirmed by Palmer and associates, who found that fewer than ten microorganisms are needed for growth in a culture medium.[58]

Several media are satisfactory for culturing material from root canals, such as brain heart infusion broth with 0.1% agar, trypticase soy

---

*Marion Laboratories, Inc., Kansas City, Missouri.

Table 13–1. Percentage of Successful Cases in Relation to Bacteriologic Culture Results

	Number of Teeth	Teeth With Negative Cultures (%)	Teeth Without Negative Cultures (%)	Length of Time Observed (months)
Abramson[1]	124	95	84	1+
Bender, et al.[4]	706	84	82	24
Buchbinder[10]	245	92	82	20
Engström and Lundberg[18]	129	89	76	42–48
Frostell[21]		94	86	48–60
Heling and Shapiro[35]	118	80	70	12–60
Ingle[37]	89	94	83	6
Morse[50]	776	91	91	12
Oliet[54]	98	94	79	6
Oliet and Sorin[55]	352	92	81	6–12+
Zeldow and Ingle[71]	162	94	83	24

broth with 0.1% agar (TSA), thioglycollate, and glucose ascites broth. Leavitt and colleagues recommended the addition of 0.1% agar in TSA to facilitate growth of anaerobes.[43] Others have recommended the addition of 5% ascitic fluid or 10% horse serum to enable fastidious organisms to grow. Moreover, tall tubes, filled to a high level, should be used for culturing in preference to short tubes, to provide different degrees of oxygen tension at different levels in the culture medium.

Möller investigated the influence of water quality, various salts, organic materials, reducing agents, and different methods of obtaining an oxygen-free environment.[48] Viability medium for growth (VMG) and Stuart's transport medium were investigated; both equally effective for most species of organisms. The in vitro test included 156 strains of organisms of 27 species and 18 genera. Most strains survived better (longer) in VMG, especially streptococci and anaerobic nonsporulating organisms. VMG-stored samples showed 90% growth in 3 days.

Möller developed a base culture medium containing veal, veal heart, peptone products in an agar gel, and certain supplements. Better growth was obtained than with commercial dehydrated media. In sampling from root canals of 5000 human teeth, 90 to 95% of positive samples showed growth after 4 days, but incubation was continued for 2 weeks, to give slow growers time to produce a positive result. The predominant organisms were identified as alpha-hemolytic streptococci, lactobacilli, and anaerobes including gram-positive cocci, such as peptococci and streptopeptococci, and gram-positive rods, such as eubacteria, lactobacilli, and corynebacteria.

Sundqvist used prereduced media, prepared as described by Holdeman and Moore, and obtained his samples according to a procedure described by Möller.[67] Using an anaerobic glove box, Sundqvist grew and identified a predominant number of anaerobes (90%). Griffee and associates found prereduced thioglycollate medium twice as effective for growing microorganisms from root canals as unreduced trypticase soy broth.[26]

Some investigators believe that a culture medium that permits growth of all aerobes and anaerobes will never be found. They therefore conclude that all culture media currently available are useless. Not so, although currently available culture media and the techniques used to sample and to grow root canal microorganisms may not be perfect, they remain valuable tools that guide and suggest better pathways to more effective treatment of patients.

Taking the Culture

The technique of taking a culture is simple. If forgotten, it can be relearned by the practicing dentist in a matter of minutes. The details are as follows: The dressing from the previous visit is removed from the root canal and is discarded. A sterile absorbent point is inserted into the canal, with a wiping motion, to cleanse the canal surface of any trace of medicament. The point is removed and is discarded, although Garber suggested using this absorbent point to collect the sample for culturing.[22] The purpose of wiping the root canal is to prevent the transfer to the culture medium of any intracanal medicament, which could inhibit bacterial growth and could result in a false-negative culture.

A fresh, sterile absorbent point is now inserted in to the apical foramen and is allowed to remain there for at least 1 min, to absorb as much periapical exudate and microorganisms from the root canal as possible. The absorbent point is removed with sterilized cotton pliers held with the thumb, index, and middle fingers, while the plug or cap of the test tube is removed with the little finger and palm of the same hand. The test tube is held in the other hand and is tilted slightly to prevent air contamination. The absorbent point is dropped into the medium, the lip of the tube is flamed, and the plug or cap is replaced and the culture tube is incubated properly (Fig. 13–1).

Anaerobic Culturing: A Clinical Concept

Culturing obligate anaerobes is a fastidious process that requires special equipment and media used in a temperature-controlled oxygen-free environment. The following procedure should suffice for those clinicians who wish to culture anaerobic microorganisms from samples obtained from the root canal and periradicular tissue.

Periradicular Sample. Using an aseptic technique, insert the sterile needle of a Luer Lok syringe into the periradicular space (i.e., swelling), aspirate fluid, eject any air inside the syringe barrel immediately, insert the needle through the rubber septum stopper of

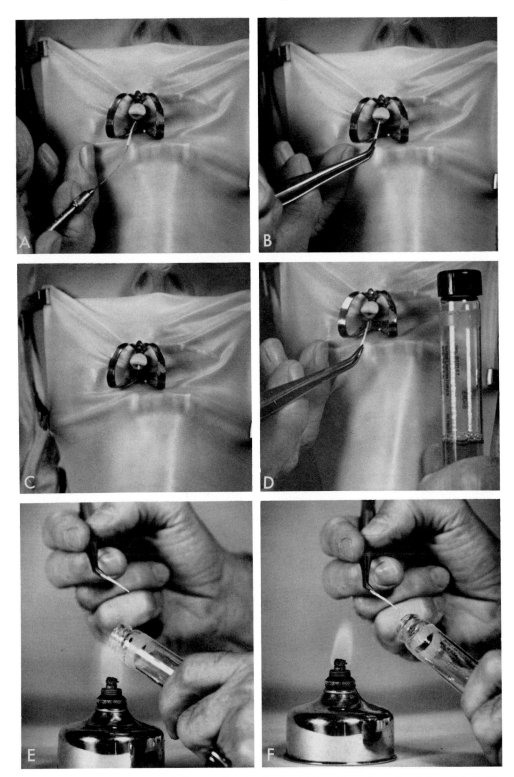

Fig. 13—1. Steps in taking a culture. *A,* Remove the absorbent point from the root canal and discard it. *B,* Wipe away residual antibiotic or antiseptic from the surface of the root canal; repeat twice or three times. *C,* Insert the absorbent point and let remain in the root canal for at least a minute, so the tip of the absorbent point will be moist when it is removed from the root canal. *D,* Remove the absorbent point from the root canal and examine the tip to make sure it is moist. *E,* Unscrew the cap by wrapping the little finger of the right hand around it and turning the culture tube counterclockwise with the left hand; flame the lip of the tube. *F,* Drop the absorbent point into the culture tube and replace the cap.

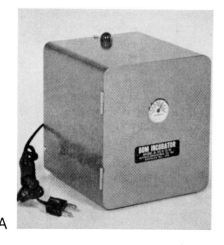 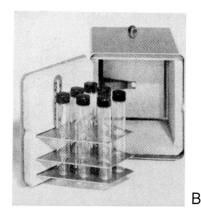

A   B

Fig. 13–2. *A* and *B*, Incubator for dental use. (Courtesy of Buffalo Dental Manufacturing Co., Brooklyn, New York.)

an Anaport vial,* and eject the fluid. The Anaport vial, a 10-ml vial with a rubber septum stopper from which the gas has been removed, should be transported to any anaerobic culturing depot, usually located in a hospital or health-care institution in most cities, within 4 hours after taking the sample.

Root Canal Sample. Aseptically prepare an access cavity into the pulp chamber. Inject a few drops of prereduced, anaerobically sterilized medium (chopped-meat glucose broth was used by Sundqvist) into the chamber, pump the medium into the root canal with a sterile endodontic file, aspirate the

---

*Scott Laboratories Inc., Fiskeville, RI

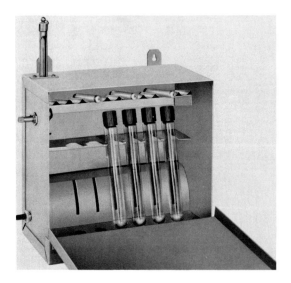

Fig. 13–3. Incubator for dental use. (Courtesy of Union Broach Co., Long Island City, New York.)

fluid with a Luer Lok syringe, eject any air from the syringe barrel immediately, insert the needle through the rubber stopper of an Anaport vial and eject the fluid. Transport the sample to an anaerobic culturing depot within 4 hours. If an exudate is present inside the root canal, the injection of additional medium is unnecessary for sampling.

Culture Reversal

Grossman examined approximately 1000 cases and found that 2% of the cultures were negative after 48 hours of incubation, but they turned positive when incubated for 10 days[30] (Fig. 13–2). It is advisable to allow more than 48 hours between taking the culture and filling the root canal, preferably 96 or more hours, and it is recommended that the culture tube be re-examined immediately before obturating a canal to make certain that no evidence of growth is present (Fig. 13–3).

The incidence of culture reversal, that is, a negative culture that becomes a positive culture by the time of obturation, varies with the investigator, as follows: Engström and Frostell, 14%;[17] Nicholls, 4%;[52] Seltzer and colleagues, 16%;[61] Serene and McDonald, approximately 10%;[62] Tsatsas and associates, 23% when taken by students;[68] and Winkler and van Amerongen, 3% when taken by experienced operators and 9% when taken by students.[69] This incidence seems to indicate that care in taking the culture, possible leakage between treatments, and the capability of the culture medium to sustain growth of the microorganisms all play a role in culture reversal.

BIBLIOGRAPHY

1. Abramson, I.I.: Lecture, American Association of Endodontists, Chicago, 1961.
2. Aisenberg, M.S.: J. Am. Dent. Assoc., *18*:136, 1931.
3. Appleton, J.L.T.: Bacterial Infection. Philadelphia, Lea & Febiger, 1933.
4. Bender, I.B., et al.: Oral Surg., *18*:527, 1964.
5. Bender, I.B., et al.: J. Am. Dent. Assoc., *59*:720, 1959.
6. Blayney, J.R.: Dent. Cosmos, *74*:635, 1932.
7. Brown, L.E., and Rudolph, C.E.: Oral Surg., *10*:1094, 1957.
8. Burke, G.W., and Knighton, H.T.: J. Dent. Res., *39*:205, 1960.
9. Burket, L.W.: Yale J. Biol. Med., *9*:271, 1937.
10. Buchbinder, M.: J. Dent. Res., *20*:92, 1941.
11. Chirnside, J.M.: N.Z. Dent. J., *54*:173, 1958.
12. Coolidge, E.D.: J. Am. Dent. Assoc., *18*:499, 1931.
13. Coolidge, E.D.: J. Natl. Dent. Assoc., *6*:337, 1919.
14. Csernyei, J.: J. Dent. Res., *18*:527, 1939.
15. Delivanis, P.D., et al.: Oral Surg., *52*:430, 1981.
16. Eggink, C.O.: Int. Endod. J., *15*:79, 1982.
17. Engström, B., and Frostell, G.: Acta Ondontol. Scand., *22*:43, 1961.
18. Engström, B., and Lundberg, M.: Odontol. Revy, *15*:257, 1964, and *74*:189, 1966.
19. Fish, E.W., and MacLean, I.: Br. Dent. J., *61*:336, 1936.
20. Foley, D.B.: J. Endod., *9*:236, 1983.
21. Frostell, G.: *In* Transactions of the Third International Conference on Endodontics. Edited by L.I. Grossman. Philadelphia, University of Pennsylvania Press, 1963, p. 112.
22. Garber, F.N.: Oral Surg., *16*:474, 1963.
23. Gier, R.E., and Mitchell, D.F.: J. Dent. Res., *47*:564, 1968.
24. Goodman, A.D.: Oral Surg., *44*:128, 1977.
25. Gottlieb, B., et al.: Z. Stomatol., *26*:1151, 1928.
26. Griffee, M.B., et al.: Oral Surg., *52*:433, 1981.
27. Grossman, L.I.: J. Dent. Res., *26*:551, 1967.
28. Grossman, L.I.: J. Dent. Res., *45*:81, 1966.
29. Grossman, L.I.: J. Dent. Res., *41*:495, 1962.
30. Grossman, L.I.: J. Dent. Res., *2*:57, 1933.
31. Haden, R.L.: Dental Infection and Systemic Disease. Philadelphia, Lea & Febiger, 1928.
32. Hampp, E.G.: Oral Surg., *10*:1100, 1957.
33. Hatton, E.H., et al.: J. Am. Dent. Assoc., *15*:56, 1928.
34. Hedman, W.J.: Oral Surg., *4*:1173, 1951.
35. Heling, B., and Shapiro, J.: Quint. Int., *11*:79, 1978.
36. Hunter, W.: Dent. Reg., *65*:579, 1911, and Dent. Brief, *16*:850, 1911.
37. Ingle, J.I.: Oral Surg., *14*:83, 1961.
38. Kakehashi, S., et al.: Oral Surg., *201*:340, 1965.
39. Kantz, W.E., and Henry, C.A.: Arch. Oral Biol., *19*:91, 1974.
40. Keudell, K., et al.: J. Endod., *2*:146, 1976.
41. Kronfeld, R.: Histopathology of Teeth. Philadelphia, Lea & Febiger, 1939.
42. La Roche, M.: J. Allied. Dent. Soc., *13*:155, 1918.
43. Leavitt, J.M., et al.: Oral Surg., *11*:302, 1958.
44. MacDonald, J.B., et al.: Oral Surg., *10*:318, 1957.
45. Matusow, R.J.: Oral Surg., *61*:90, 96, 1986.
46. Mazzarella, M.A., et al.: Classification of Microorganisms from the Pulp Canal of Non-Vital Teeth: Research Report. Bethesda, M.D., U.S. Naval Dental School, 1955.
47. Melville, T.H., and Birch, R.H.: Oral Surg., *23*:93, 1967.
48. Möller, A.J.R.: Microbiologic Examination of Root Canals and Periapical Tissues of Human Teeth. Goteborg, Akademiforlaget, 1966.
49. Morse, D.R.: Int. Dent. J., *14*:78, 1981.
50. Morse, D.R.: Dent. Clin. North Am., *15*:793, 1971.
51. Naidorf, I.J.: *In* The Biology of the Human Dental Pulp. Edited by M. Siskin. St. Louis, C.V. Mosby, 1973, p. 391.
52. Nicholls, E.: Br. Dent. J., *112*:167, 1962.
53. Okell, C.C., and Elliott, S.D.: Lancet, *2*:869, 1935.
54. Oliet, S.: Oral Surg., *15*:727, 1962.
55. Oliet, S., and Sorin, S.M.: J. Br. Endod. Soc., *3*:3, 1969.
56. Onderdenk, T.W.: Int. Dent. J., *22*:20, 1901.
57. Orban, B.: J. Am. Dent. Assoc., *19*:1348, 1932.
58. Palmer, G.R., et al.: Oral Surg., *42*:824, 1976.
59. Robinson, H.B.G., and Bolling, L.R.: J. Am. Dent. Assoc., *28*:268, 1941.
60. Round, S., et al.: Proc. R. Soc. Med., *29*:1552, 1936.
61. Seltzer, S., et al.: J. Am. Dent. Assoc., *67*:651, 1963.
62. Serene, T.P., and McDonald, E.P.: J. Am. Dent. Assoc., *78*:1013, 1969.
63. Shovelton, D.S.: Ala. Dent. Rev., *7*:7, 1959.
64. Smith, L.S., and Tappe, G.D.: J. Dent. Res., *41*:17, 1962.
65. Sommer, R.F., et al.: Clinical Endodontics, 2nd Ed. Philadelphia, W.B. Saunders, 1961, p. 374.
66. Stobberingh, E.E., and Eggink, C.D.: Int. Endod. J., *15*:87, 1982.
67. Sundqvist, G.: Bacteriological Studies of Necrotic Dental Pulps. Umeä, Sweden, University Odontology Dissertations, 1976.
68. Tsatsas, B., et al.: J. Br. Endod. Soc., *7*:78, 1974.
69. Winkler, K.C., and van Amerongen, J.: Oral Surg., *12*:857, 1959.
70. Wittgow, W.C., and Sebastian, C.B.: J. Endod., *1*:168, 1975.
71. Zeldow, B.J., and Ingle, J.: J. Am. Dent. Assoc., *66*:9, 1963.
72. Zielke, D.R., et al.: Oral Surg., *42*:830, 1976.

14 Obturation of the Root Canal

The function of a root canal filling is to obturate the canal and eliminate all portals of entry between the periodontium and the root canal. The better the seal, the better the prognosis of the tooth. Achieving the ideal seal, however, is as complex as the anatomy of the root canal system itself. Because all root canal fillings must seal all foramina leading into the periodontium, an ideal filling must be well condensed, must conform and adhere to the instrumented canal walls, and must end at the juncture of the root canal and the periodontium.

The objective of obturating the root canal is the substitution of an inert filling in the space previously occupied by the pulp tissue, to prevent recurrent infection by way of the circulation (anachoresis) or through a break in the integrity of the crown of the tooth. Naidorf has stated that inadequate obturation of the crown exposes it to periapical tissue fluids, which provide material for growth of microorganisms or localization of bacteria in such dead spaces by a transient bacteremia.[93] According to a study made by Ingle and Beveridge,[60] 58% of endodontic failures can be attributed to incomplete obturation of root canals (Fig. 14–1).

WHEN TO OBTURATE THE ROOT CANAL

A root canal may be obturated when the tooth is asymptomatic and the root canal is reasonably dry. Although other valid criteria, such as obturation after obtaining a negative culture and closure of an existing sinus tract, have been summarily dismissed as time consuming or impractical, studies have shown that the use of these criteria for obturation has raised the percentage of endodontic successes. Reduction in the number of microorganisms by canal preparation and medication (surgical sterility), even though bacteriologic sterility may not have been obtained as determined by culture, increases the probability of healing and a successful result in at least 10% of cases.[43] This subject is discussed in greater detail in Chapter 13. A root canal should not be obturated in the presence of a persistent sinus tract (fistula).

When seepage into the root canal is excessive, it can be treated and eliminated by irrigating the root canal with a 5% sodium-hypochlorite solution, reinstrumenting and enlarging the canal to its apical foramen, irrigating and drying the canal again with absorbent points, and sealing it with an intracanal medicament, such as calcium-hydroxide paste. Under no circumstances should a root canal be obturated if the tooth is tender.

REQUIREMENTS FOR AN IDEAL ROOT CANAL FILLING MATERIAL

The following requirements for an ideal root canal filling material have been suggested by Grossman:[43] (1) the material should be easily introduced into the root canal; (2) it should seal the canal laterally as well as apically; (3) it should not shrink after being inserted; (4) it should be impervious to moisture; (5) it should be bactericidal, or at least, should discourage growth; (6) it should be radiopaque; (7) it should not stain tooth structure; (8) it should not irritate periapical tissue or affect tooth structure; (9) it should be sterile, or easily and quickly sterilized immediately before insertion; and (10) it should be easily removable from the root canal if necessary.[44]

GUTTA-PERCHA

Over the years, many different filling materials have been used to seal root canals. None have proved to possess all the ideal characteristics. Currently, the material used most often as a solid-core filling is gutta-percha.

Properties and Composition

Introduced by Bowman in 1867,[14] gutta-percha is a desirable filling material because it does not shrink after insertion unless it is

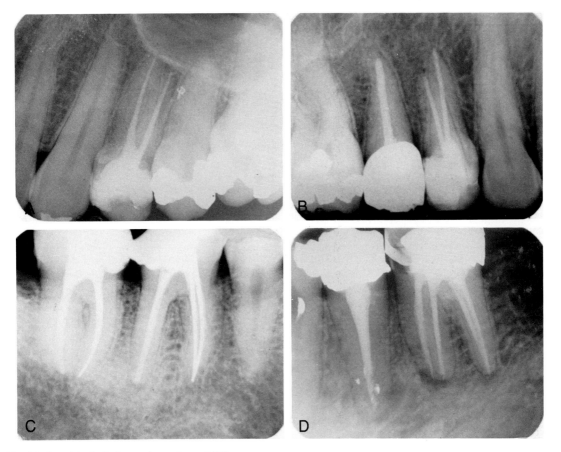

Fig. 14–1. *A* to *D*, Gutta-percha root canal fillings.

plasticized with a solvent or heat. It is easily sterilized prior to insertion and does not encourage bacterial growth. It is radiopaque, nonstaining, and impervious to moisture. Gutta-percha can be removed easily from the root canal if necessary. It is probably the least toxic and least irritating to periapical tissue of all root canal filling materials. Conversely, it is difficult to introduce into a narrow root canal, and it does not seal a canal apically or laterally unless it is combined with a root canal cement or sealer. Finally, gutta-percha has a limited shelf life. It becomes brittle with age, a process hastened with warmth and delayed when refrigerated. Sorin and Oliet described this aging process and introduced a technique to rejuvenate the aged brittle cone by momentary immersion in hot tap water (55° C) followed by instant cooling in cold tap water[118] (Fig. 14–2).

The composition of gutta-percha cones varies with each manufacturer. Friedman and associates[4] described the approximate composition as 20% gutta-percha (matrix), 66% zinc oxide (filler), 11% heavy-metal sulfates (radiopacifier), and 3% waxes or resins (plasticizer).[35] These investigators reported that the essential differences in the mechanical properties of the individual brands were a function of the gutta-percha and zinc-oxide concentrations. Because of the poor sealing property of gutta-percha, regardless of technique, it must be combined with a root canal cement or sealer, to ensure proper filling and sealing of the root canal.

Obturation Technique

Many methods of obturating a root canal with gutta-percha and a sealer are used. Some are old, tried, and tested; others new, innovative, and awaiting final judgment. These techniques include: (1) lateral condensation; (2) vertical condensation (warm gutta-percha); (3) sectional condensation; (4) compaction (McSpadden technique); (5) thermoplasticized gutta-percha technique; and (6) chemically plasticized gutta-percha (chloropercha, eucapercha) technique.

Basically, all methods use the physical characteristic of gutta-percha called the

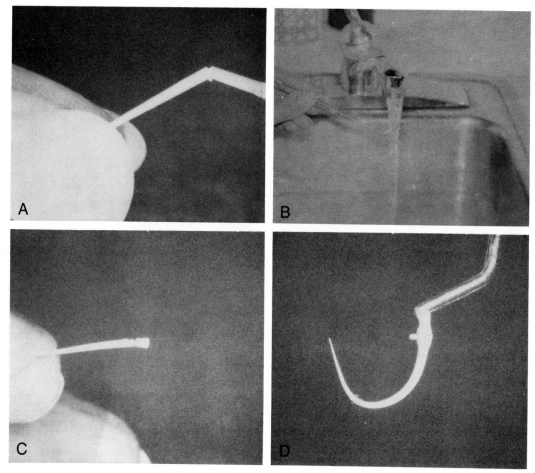

Fig. 14–2. Rejuvenation of brittle, aged gutta-percha. *A,* Brittle gutta-percha cone, easily broken and without flexibility. *B,* One should grasp the gutta-percha cone on the butt end and immerse in hot (approximately 55° C) tap water briefly until gentle pressure on cotton pliers compresses the gutta-percha; one should then rinse the cone in cold tap water. *C,* Compressed butt end of a rejuvenated gutta-percha cone after treatment with hot and cold water. *D,* Flexible, rejuvenated gutta-percha cone.

property of plasticity or flow. Plasticity is inversely related to viscosity and can be defined as the ability to deform and to flow away from a force directed at its mass.

Each technique is designed to force the gutta-percha filling to flow into the root canal, compress against its walls, fill fine tortuous canals, seal the various foramina exiting into the periodontium, and finally, condense into a solid core filling. The lateral-condensation method of filling uses spreaders and pluggers to force gutta-percha to flow by inserting these instruments alongside the filling material and compressing them laterally and apically. The vertical-condensation technique uses vertical force combined with applied heat to drive the gutta-percha apically and laterally. Thermoplastic techniques use more heat to increase the plastic-

ity of gutta-percha and thereby to enable the operator to fill the root canal by using less pressure. Chemical solvents, such as chloroform, eucalyptol, and xylol, decrease gutta-percha viscosity to a more fluid state and increase its plasticity beyond that of the thermoplasticized state. This change enables the gutta-percha filling to flow into small and tortuous canals. Unfortunately, the more gutta-percha is plasticized, the greater will be the shrinkage of the filling material as the filling cools or returns to a solid-core-state.

Lateral-Condensation Method

In the lateral-condensation technique of obturation, a gutta-percha cone, called the primary or master cone, is fitted to the instrumented main canal. The primary cone is inserted into the root canal to the established working length. It should fit snugly and should resist removal ("tug-back") (Fig. 14–3). A radiograph is taken to determine the apical and lateral fit of the primary cone. The gutta-percha cone is adjusted; if it protrudes through the apical foramen, the tip should be cut off so the reinserted primary cone fits snugly, has "tug-back," and seals the apical canal approximately 1 mm short of the pulpoperiapical juncture. If the initial fit of the primary cone is 2 or 3 mm short of the apex, a new primary cone should be measured or the canal should be reprepared to the corrected length and another primary cone fitted. Another radiograph is taken to verify the fit of the cone (Fig. 14–4).

The purpose of fitting the primary cone short of the canal apex is to avoid inadvertent overfilling of the root canal during condensation. In lateral condensation, when the primary cone is forced laterally against the canal wall to make room for the insertion of the accessory cones, one sees a component apical movement in the tip of the primary cone. Unless this movement is anticipated and compensated for in advance, the primary cone will be driven beyond the apical foramen into the periapical tissues.

Once the primary cone has been accurately seated in the root canal, it is removed, and the canal is dried again. The walls of the canal are coated with a thin layer of cement or sealer. The apical half of the primary cone is coated with cement and is carefully replaced in the canal. A spreader is inserted alongside the primary cone and is pressed apically. The spreader is disengaged from the cone by rotating it between the fingertips or, when using a long-handled spreader, by rotating the handle in an arc. Once disengaged, the spreader can be removed without disturbing the seated gutta-percha. An accessory cone is inserted in the space previously occupied by the spreader. This maneuver is done by positioning the (secondary, lateral) accessory cone parallel to the spreader blade and inserting it immediately into the opening created by the removal of the spreader. A cement coating is not necessary for secondary cones. This process is repeated until the entire canal is filled with a well-condensed gutta-percha filling. After verifying the fit of the obturated canal by radiograph, the butt end of the gutta-percha in the pulp chamber is cut off with a hot instrument, the chamber is cleaned, and a temporary restoration is placed in the access cavity.

The size of the spreader is determined by the width of the prepared canal and the lateral fit of the primary cone; the greater the space between the canal wall and the butt end of the gutta-percha, the larger (wider) the spreader used. The amount of force used for compression is determined by the apical fit of the primary cone and by the distance it must flow to seal the root canal to its apical juncture. Additional secondary cones are inserted until the spreader cannot be reinserted, an indication that the root canal is fully condensed laterally.

Several radiographs must be taken while one obturates the canal, to check the accuracy of the procedure. The fit of the primary cone is verified by radiograph. Another radiograph should be taken when two or three secondary cones have been condensed in the root canal, to determine the amount of flow and to avoid overfilling. Adjustment can still be made and the gutta-percha cone retrieved if overfilling occurs or if the primary cone does not flow to the apical foramen. A final

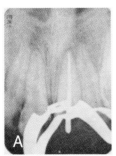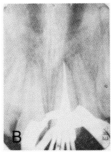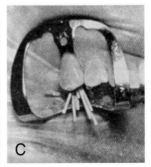

Fig. 14–3. Lateral-condensation method of filling a wide root canal. *A,* Primary gutta-percha cone in place to seal the apical foramen. *B,* Secondary gutta-percha cones inserted to fill the root canal laterally. *C,* Photograph of secondary gutta-percha cones used in filling the root canal by the lateral-condensation method.

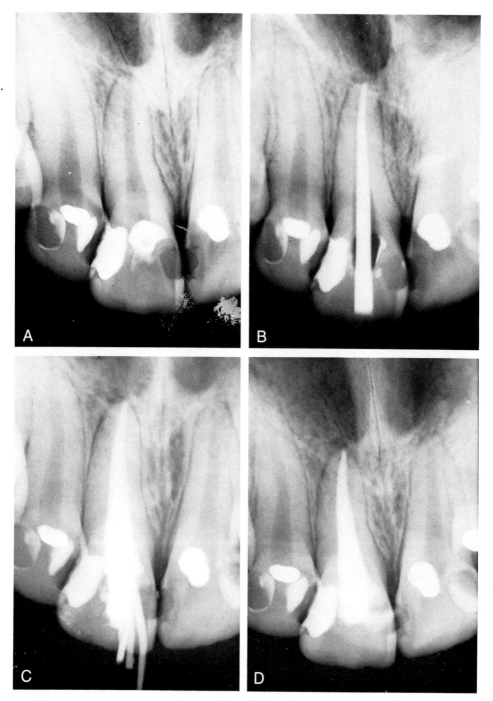

Fig. 14—4.   Lateral condensation. *A*, Preoperative radiograph. *B*, Fitting of a gutta-percha cone; about 1 mm of the cone's tip was removed to prevent the cone from being forced apically through the foramen during condensation. *C*, The cone has been cemented, and a number of secondary cones have been inserted between the primary cone and the wall of the root canal. *D*, Completed obturation of the root canal.

radiograph must be taken of the completed root canal filling (Fig. 14–5).

Vertical-Condensation Method (Warm Gutta-Percha)

The vertical-condensation or "warm gutta-percha" technique of filling root canals was introduced by Schilder with the object of filling lateral and accessory canals as well as the main root canal.[108] This method of vertical condensation is used with the step-back technique of root canal preparation. Using heated pluggers, one applies pressure in a vertical direction to the heat-softened gutta-percha and thereby causes it to flow and to fill the entire lumen of the canal (Fig. 14–6).

Schilder described the steps in cleansing and shaping of the root canal in preparation for obturation by the vertical condensation method.[108] Essentially, the requirements are that: (1) a continuous tapering funnel should be present from the root canal orifice to the root apex; (2) the root canal should be prepared so it flows with the shape of the original canal; (3) the shape of the apical foramen should not be changed or moved; and (4) the apical foramen should be small, so excess gutta-percha will not be forced through it during vertical condensation.

The steps in vertical condensation are as follows:

1. A primary gutta-perch cone corresponding to the last instrument used is fitted in the canal in the usual manner.
2. The canal wall is coated with a thin layer of root canal cement.
3. The cone is cemented.
4. The coronal end of the cone is cut off with a hot instrument.
5. A "heat carrier," such as a root canal plugger, is heated to redness and is immediately forced into the coronal third of the gutta-percha. Some of the coronal gutta-percha is seared off by the plugger as it is removed from the canal.
6. A vertical condenser of suitable size is inserted, and vertical pressure is applied to the heated gutta-percha, to force the plasticized material apically.
7. This alternate application of heat carrier and condenser is repeated until the plasticized gutta-percha seals the larger accessory canals and fills the lumen of the canal in three dimensions up to the apical foramen. The remaining portion of the canal is plugged with warm sections of additional pieces of gutta-percha.

Lifshitz and colleagues used the scanning electron microscope to determine the effectiveness of the vertical-condensation method of sealing root canals in conjunction with a sealer.[76] These investigators found a wall-to-wall adaptation of the gutta-percha in the apical area, as demonstrated by a solid interface among dentin sealer, and gutta-percha. In an in vitro study, Goodman and associates have shown that the maximum regional temperature to which gutta-percha is subjected during the vertical condensation method is 80° C, and the temperature in the apical region is between 40 and 42° C.[39]

The advantages of this technique are the excellent seal of the canal, apically and laterally, and the obturation of the larger lateral and accessory canals. The disadvantages of this technique are the amount of time it takes, the risk of vertical root fracture resulting from undue force, and periodic overfilling with gutta percha or cement that cannot be retrieved from the periapical tissue.

Sectional Method

The sectional method of filling a root canal derives its name from the technique of using a section of a gutta-percha cone to fill a section of the root canal. The canal wall is coated with cement. A root canal plugger that can be inserted in the canal to within 3 or 4 mm of the apex is heated in the hot-salt sterilizer for 10 sec. A gutta-percha cone of approximately the size of the prepared canal is cut into sections, each 3 or 4 mm long. The apical section is mounted on the heated plugger, is carried into the canal to the previously measured depth, and is pressed vertically. The plugger is disengaged carefully, to prevent dislodging of the inserted section of gutta-percha. A radiograph is taken to check the position and fit of the condensed section. The next section is dipped in eucalyptol, is warmed high over a flame, and is added to the previous section under vertical pressure, to condense the filling. The entire canal is filled in this manner. If a post-type crown is to be made, only the first or apical section is used to obturate the canal.

The advantage of this filling is that it seals the canal apically and laterally. The disadvantages of this technique are that it is time consuming, it is difficult to retrieve the section of gutta-percha if the canal is overfilled,

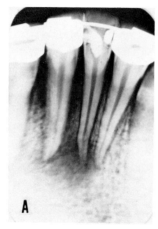

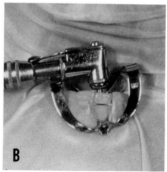

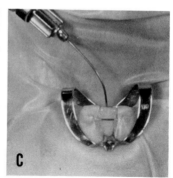

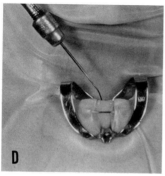

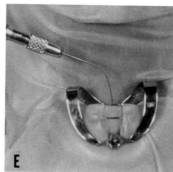

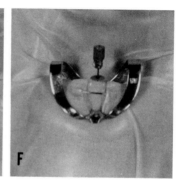

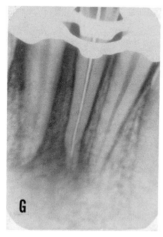

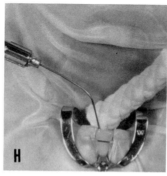

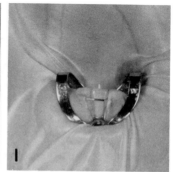

Fig. 14–5. *A,* Preoperative radiograph. *B,* Rubber dam applied; preparation of the access cavity. *C,* Irrigation with sodium-hypochlorite solution. *D,* Exploration with a smooth broach; note that the broach has been bent to conform to the approximate length of the tooth. *E,* Barbed broach about to be inserted; note the bend in the broach conforming to the approximate length of the tooth. *F,* Reamer with rubber disc attached is level with the incisal surface of the tooth and is ready for a radiograph, to determine the exact length of the tooth. *G,* Radiograph shows that the instrument is 1 mm short of the root apex. *H,* Following enlargement of the root canal with sequential sizes of instruments, the root canal is irrigated alternately with hydrogen peroxide and sodium hypochlorite. *I,* Root canal is dried with absorbent points.

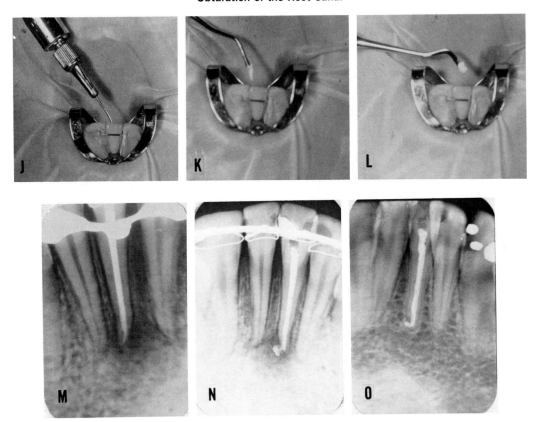

Fig. 14–5 Continued. *J,* Insertion of an antimicrobial agent into the root canal, followed by a short absorbent point. *K,* Placement of an inner seal. *L,* Placement of an outer seal. *M,* When a negative culture has been obtained, the gutta-percha cone is fitted in the root canal. *N,* Gutta-percha cone is cemented; note the surplus root canal cement beyond the apex, most of which will become resorbed in time. *O,* Check-up radiograph taken a year later shows complete repair of the periapical area; the cement is being resorbed, but it is well tolerated.

and it is difficult to condense the gutta-percha sections into a homogenous mass, often with resulting voids between sections.

Compaction Method (McSpadden)

The compaction method, introduced by McSpadden,[84] uses heat to decrease gutta-percha viscosity and to increase its plasticity. The heat is created by rotating a compacting instrument in a slow-speed contra-angle handpiece at 8,000 to 10,000 r.p.m. alongside gutta-percha cones inside the root canal. The compactor, whose spiraled 90° flutes are similar to the flutes on a Hedstroem file, but in reverse, forces the softened gutta-percha apically and laterally.

Because the compactor blade breaks easily if it binds, this method should be used to fill straight canals only. Using the step-back method, the canal should be enlarged to at least the size of a No. 45 instrument. Gutta-percha cones are inserted in the prepared canal short of the root apex, and a compactor blade, selected according to the width and length of the prepared canal, is inserted between the gutta-percha and the canal wall. With a rubber-dam stop on the compactor blade, the rotating tip of the blade is guided to within 1.5 mm of the root apex. Restriction of the blade within the canal prevents the forcing of thermoplasticized gutta-percha through the root apex. The plastic gutta-percha moves laterally and apically because the reversed flutes on the computer blade push the softened gutta-percha forward and sideways even when one is withdrawing the rotating blade from the canal.

The advantages of the compaction method are ease of selection and insertion of gutta-percha cones, economy of time, and rapid filling of canals apically and laterally, including irregular spaces within the canal if one uses a sealer. The disadvantages are the inability to use the technique in narrow canals, frequent breakage of compactor blades, frequent overfilling of the canal, and shrinkage of the cooled, set filling.

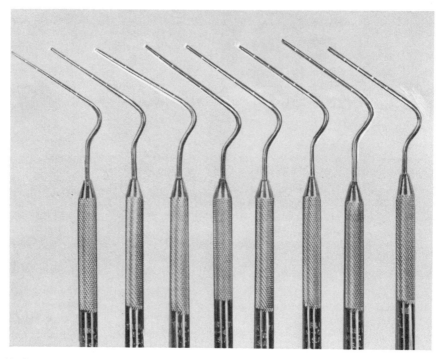

Fig. 14–6. Vertical condensers (Schilder) for vertical-condensation (warm gutta-percha) technique. The condensers are graduated in size and have markings 5 mm apart, to judge the depth of penetration into the root canal. (Courtesy of Star Dental Co, Valley Forge, Pennsylvania.)

Chemically Plasticized Gutta-Percha (Eucapercha, Chloropercha)

Gutta-percha can be plasticized by chemical solvents such as chloroform, eucalyptol, or xylol. The resulting slightly viscous and highly plastic gutta-percha can be forced into fine, tortuous canals, where other solid-core fillings cannot be inserted satisfactorily (Fig. 14–7).

Eucapercha has replaced chloropercha because chloroform has been designated a potential carcinogen.[88] Eucapercha is a paste made by softening the surface of gutta-percha in warm oil of eucalyptus (eucalyptol). Because this oil does not dissolve gutta-percha rapidly, as does chloroform, the softened gutta-percha cone can be used to coat the canal wall with a thin film of eucapercha. Then the same cone can be inserted and compressed with pluggers to the apical juncture, to seal the root canal and accessory canals.

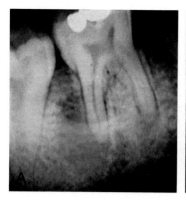
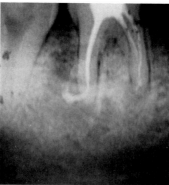
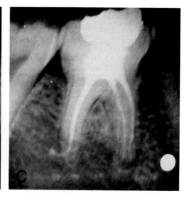

Fig. 14–7. Chloropercha obturation. *A*, Diagnostic radiograph. *B*, Postobturation radiograph; excess filling material was extruded inadvertently. *C*, Recall radiograph at 6 months; bone regeneration is evident, and the excess filling material is being resorbed (the white dot is the rubber-dam punch hole used to indicate a recall radiograph).

Unfortunately, it is difficult to avoid over-filling the canal. Excess eucapercha, expressed through the apical foramen, is usu-ally absorbed within a year. Initially, it can act as an irritant, but it does not interfere with repair of the periapical tissues.

The disadvantages of using a chemical-solvent filling material are the inability to control overfilling, with resultant periapical tissue reaction and shrinkage of the filling after set-ting, resulting in a poor apical and lateral seal (Fig. 14–8).

METAL-CORE OBTURATION

Metal-core obturation includes obturating the root canal with a silver cone, a sectioned silver cone, stainless steel (instrument blade), or amalgam. Only the metallic fillings of silver cone and stainless steel are pre-sented in this chapter; the retrograde amal-gam filling is discussed in Chapter 17.

Silver-Cone Method

Silver cones have been used to fill root canals successfully for over 50 years (Fig. 14–9). Generally, their use is restricted to teeth with fine, tortuous canals that cannot be filled properly with gutta-percha cones. Although silver cones are machined to pre-cise measurements corresponding to the instruments used for canal preparation, they require the addition of a root canal cement to compensate for their poor adaptation to the canal walls and poor sealing qualities. Once a primary silver cone is cemented, however, gutta-percha is laterally condensed around the cone to ensure a proper lateral seal. Silver cones are contraindicated in fill-ing a root canal if the tooth is to be restored with a post and core. The use of engine-dri-

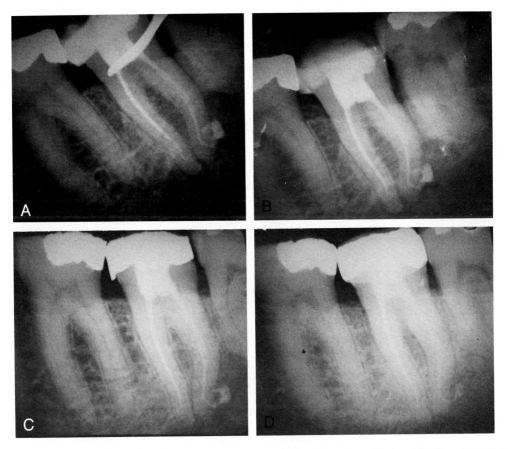

Fig. 14–8.   Chloropercha obturation. *A*, Radiograph shows the distal root canal overfilled and the fine, tortuous mesial root canals filled to the apex. *B*, Postobturation radiograph shows that the mesial root canal filling appears to be short of the apex. *C*, Recall radiograph at 6 months; the excess filling appears to be resorbing. *D*, Recall radiograph at 12 months; the mesial root canal filling appears to be several millimeters short of the apex, the excess filling material is being resorbed, and bone regeneration is evident.

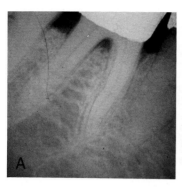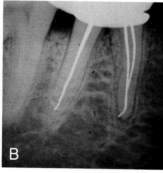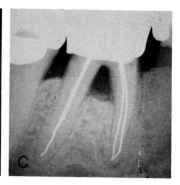

Fig. 14—9. Silver-cone obturation. *A,* Diagnostic radiograph. *B,* Radiograph showing silver cones inserted several millimeters short of the root apex; the root canals were instrumented to a corrected length, and the silver cones were cemented to the root apex. *C,* Recall radiograph at 10 years.

ven burs to cut the butt end of a silver cone deep enough for placement of a post can dislodge the cone, with loss of the apical seal, or can perforate a root.

When filling a root canal with a silver cone and cement, select a cone corresponding in size to the largest instrument used in the preparation of the canal. Sterilize the cone by alcohol flaming three times or by passing it through an open flame two or three times. Insert the cone in the canal using silver-cone pliers or Stieglitz forceps, and press it apically (Fig. 14–10). The cone should fit snugly and should bind at the apical foramen because it corresponds to the diameter and taper of the prepared canal. A canal instrumented for silver cone obturation should have tapered converging walls differing in shape from a canal prepared using the stepback technique. Take a radiograph to check the fit of the cone in the canal. If it protrudes beyond the apex, cut off the excess at the tip so the final fit will terminate 0.5 mm short of the root apex. If the silver cone is too short, either select another that fits or reprepare the canal so the selected cone seats properly. Coat the canal with cement and insert the

sterilized silver cone with slight pressure to the measured length. Take another radiograph to ensure that the filling is properly positioned. Laterally condense secondary gutta-percha cones around the primary silver cone (Fig. 14–11).

To complete the filling of a canal with a silver cone and gutta-percha, sear away the excess gutta-percha in the chamber, wipe the walls clean with chloroform or alcohol, and fill the crown with zinc-phosphate cement, which may serve as a temporary restoration. If a permanent restoration is desired, then, as soon as the cement has hardened, cut away the cement and cone 3 or 4 mm below the occlusal surface with an inverted cone bur in a high-speed handpiece, and reseal the access cavity with a permanent restoration.

The sectional or split-cone method of filling a canal with a silver cone is designed for a tooth whose restoration may require a post and core. The method consists of fitting the cone snugly, as described earlier. The cone is notched approximately 6 mm from the apical tip, it is sterilized, and it is cemented in the root canal. The wedged cemented cone is rotated until it breaks at the notch, and the

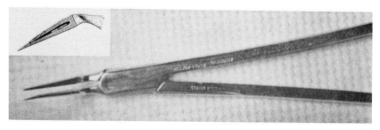

Fig. 14—10. Fine beaks of Steiglitz forceps. The forceps are useful for carrying silver cones into root canals and for bending over the butt ends of the silver cones prior to cementing them in the root canals. The forceps are also useful for conveying root canal instruments into root canals that are not readily accessible.

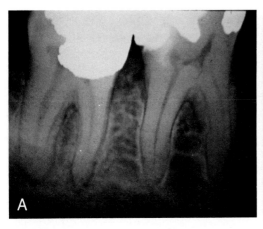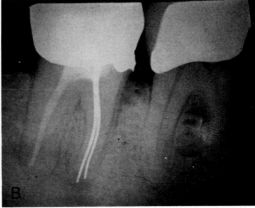

Fig. 14–11. Silver-cone and gutta-percha obturation. *A,* Diagnostic radiograph. *B,* Recall radiograph at 5 years; the distal root canal is filled with laterally condensed gutta-percha, and the mesial root canals were filled with cemented silver cones.

free end is removed, to leave enough space for preparation of a post.

The primary advantage of filling a canal with a silver cone is that silver is stiffer than gutta-percha and is therefore easier to insert into a fine, tortuous canal. The disadvantages are a poor lateral seal unless the filling is combined with laterally condensed gutta-percha, difficulty in retrieving the silver cone if retreatment becomes necessary, and a lower success rate than with gutta-percha.

Stainless Steel File Method

Stainless steel files can be used to fill fine, tortuous canals (Fig. 14–12). Originally suggested by Sampeck,[106] they have been used instead of silver cones. Because steel files are much more rigid than silver cones, they can be inserted into a canal with greater ease. Once the file has been cemented, its handle must be cut off with a high-speed bur, 3 or 4 mm below the occlusal surface, to allow space for a restoration. Fox and colleagues have reported only a 6 to 7% failure rate in 304 root canals filled by this method.[32]

Timpawat and associates found that silver cones or stainless steel files, when used with a sealer for obturation, leaked less than gutta-percha and sealer in severely curved canals.[131]

INJECTION TECHNIQUE OF OBTURATING CANALS

The concept of injecting a filling material into a root canal remains a novel idea although it is not new. Greenberg suggested the use of a pressure syringe to extrude cement into a canal,[40] and Krakow and Berk popularized the idea of sealing a root canal with cement by means of a pressure syringe.[69] Goldman and colleagues introduced Hydron as an injectable filling material,[36] and Torabinajed and Marlin and their associates described new methods of injecting thermoplasticized gutta-percha into a root canal.[81,133]

Hydron

Hydron is a rapid-setting hydrophilic plastic material used as a root canal sealer without the use of a core. According to Goldman and colleagues,[36] Hydron is a polymer of hydroxy-ethyl-methacrylate and is considered to be a biocompatible material that conforms to the shape of the root canal because of its plasticity.

The instructions for using Hydron state that the canal must be dry, and it sets in the root canal in 10 min. Injecting Hydron into a root canal requires the use of a special syringe and needle. Rising and associates,[104] as well as Benkel and co-workers,[7] found Hydron to be a biocompatible material for filling root canals. Nevertheless, one should proceed cautiously when using Hydron because it is injected as an unset material, and the polymers that hasten its set can cause tissue toxicity resulting in inflammation with macrophage activity, according to Langeland and colleagues.[74] Pyner reported a case of paresthesia resulting from overfilling of a lower molar.[102]

Thermoplasticized Gutta-Percha Method

The thermoplasticized gutta-percha method has been described by Torabinajed and associates,[133] Marlin and colleagues,[81]

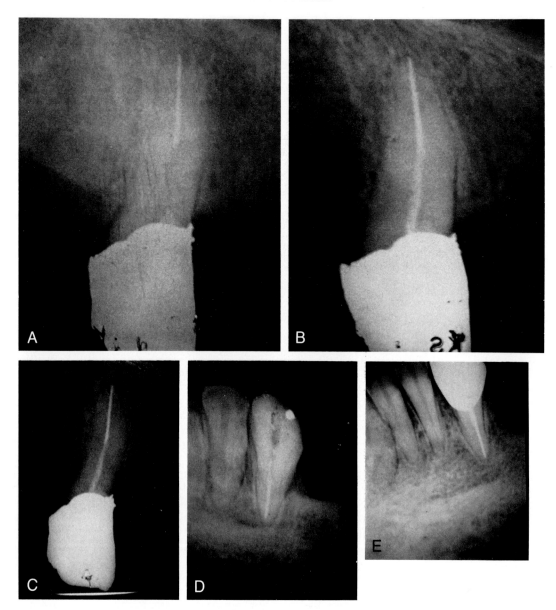

Fig. 14–12. Stainless steel file obturation. *A*, Diagnostic radiograph showing the stainless steel file broken during instrumentation sealing the root canal at the apex. *B*, Postobturation radiograph; gutta-percha is condensed in the remainder of the root canal. *C*, Recall radiograph at 1 year. *D*, Diagnostic radiograph; the root canal is sealed at the apex by a broken stainless steel file. *E*, Recall radiograph at 2 years.

and Yee and co-workers.[140] The pressure apparatus consists of an electrically heated syringe barrel, which is insulated, and a selection of needles ranging in size from 18 to 25 gauge (Fig. 14–13). The plunger is designed to prevent backward flow of the gutta-percha. The degree of heat is regulated to provide proper extrusion of the gutta-percha according to the size of the needle.

For the injection method, the canal preparation needs to be restricted apically with flaring of the body of the canal toward the access opening (step-back preparation). Torabinajed and colleagues found injection of plasticized gutta-percha from a pressure syringe produced obturation that was as satisfactory as from lateral or vertical condensation.[133] In a clinical follow-up of 125 teeth

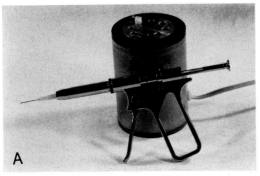
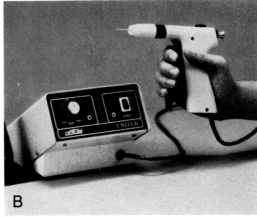

Fig. 14–13. Thermoplasticized gutta-percha filling. *A*, ULTRAFIL unit developed by Dr. A. Michanowicz and co-workers. (Courtesy of Hygenic Co., Akron, Ohio.) *B*, Obtura unit developed by Dr. J. Marlin and associates. (Courtesy of Unitek, Monrovia, California.)

from 6 months to a year, about half of which had periapical lesions, Marlin and associates found partial or complete healing in 94% of cases.[81]

Another thermoplasticized method has been described by Michanowicz and Czonsatkowsky.[86] This method involves the use of a carpule containing a low-temperature (70° C) gutta-percha formulation. A special heater warms the gutta-percha sufficiently to flow under pressure, and it is discharged through a needle of suitable gauge directly into the root canal.

Schilder and colleagues have cautioned that the thermoplasticized method of obturation that uses gutta-percha above 45° C predisposes the filling to shrinkage as the gutta-percha cools unless it is compacted with instruments toward the apex.[109] (Note: Thermoplasticized gutta-percha is heated from 70° to 160° C, depending on the method or material used.)

The thermoplasticed method has one defect in common with all injection techniques, namely, lack of precision in delivering the gutta-percha near the apical foramen and not beyond, even though it may fill the canal laterally in all its interstices. The injection technique relies on the heated and plasticized gutta-percha to flow apically with minimal apical compression, when compared to the forces or pressures used in lateral and vertical condensation. Unless vertical pressure is combined with the injection method of obturation, the interface seal between the gutta-percha and the canal walls is weakened, and voids can occur in the final set filling.

ROOT CANAL CEMENTS

The ideal root canal cement should: (1) provide an excellent seal when set; (2) produce adequate adhesion among it, the canal walls, and the filling material; (3) be radiopaque; (4) be nonstaining; (5) be dimensionally stable; (6) be easily mixed and introduced into the canals; (7) be easily removed if necessary; (8) be insoluble in tissue fluids; (9) be bactericidal or discourage bacterial growth; (10) be nonirritating to periapical tissue; and (11) be slow setting, to ensure sufficient working time.

Zinc-Oxide-Resin Cements

Most of the cements in common use contain zinc-oxide resin as a base ingredient of the powder. Included in this group are Grossman's cement, Kerr Root Canal Sealer,* Kerr Tubli-Seal,* Kloroperka N-O,† N_2 normal, Wachs Cement,‡ and Endomethasone.§ The liquid usually consists of eugenol alone or in combination with other liquids such as Canada balsam, eucalyptol, beechwood creosote, or oil of sweet almond in varying amounts. Kloroperka N-O and chloropercha are mixed with chloroform.

Grossman developed a nonstaining cement

---

*Kerr Manufacturing Co., Romulus, Michigan.
†Union Broach Co., Long Island, New York.
‡Not manufactured; formulated by pharmacists.
§Spécialités Septodont, Paris, France.

that meets most of the ideal requirements for a root canal cement.[46] The formula is as follows:

Powder	Parts
Zinc oxide, reagent	42
Staybelite resin	27
Bismuth subcarbonate	15
Barium sulfate	15
Sodium borate, anhydrous	1

Liquid
Eugenol or oil of pimenta leaf

Grossman's cement hardens in approximately 2 hours at 37° C and 100% relative humidity. Its setting time in a canal is less. It begins to set in the root canal within 10 to 30 min because of the moisture present in dentin. The setting time is also influenced by the quality of the zinc oxide and the pH of the resin used,[44] the care and technique in mixing the cement to its proper consistency, the amount of humidity in the atmosphere, and the temperature and dryness of the mixing slab and spatula.

Root canal cement is mixed on a sterile glass slab with a sterile spatula. The slab is sterilized by an alcohol scrub and is dried, and the spatula is passed through an open flame two or three times. Depending on the number of canals to be filled, one uses two or three drops of root canal cement liquid. Slowly, small increments of cement powder are added to the liquid while one spatulates it to a smooth, creamy mix. The spatulation time depends on the number of drops of liquid used, a minute per drop.

The completed mix can be tested for proper consistency by raising the flat blade of the spatula up from the mixed mass. The cement should "string out" for at least an inch before breaking (Fig. 14–14). Another test for consistency is that the suspended mix should cling to the inverted spatula blade for 10 to 15 sec before dropping from the spatula. The cement is now inserted into the dried root canal. (Afterward, the glass slab and spatula can be wiped clean with alcohol or chloroform.)

Because moisture accelerates the set of the cement, the pulp chamber and canals should be thoroughly dried before inserting the cement. Using a smooth broach, reamer, or file with an instrument stop attached, carry small amounts of cement into the canal. This procedure prevents air bubbles from becoming trapped in the cement. Coat the walls of the canal with a thin layer of cement by means

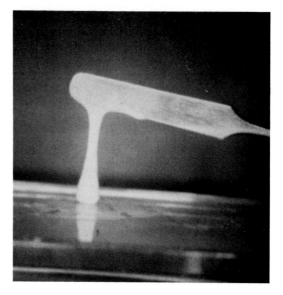

Fig. 14–14. Consistency. Cement, when mixed, should adhere to the spatula blade and should "string out" from the cement slab an inch before falling.

of a lateral or rotary motion. Avoid forcing any cement into the periapical tissue.

Chaisrisookumporn and Rabinowitz found that the use of Grossman's sealer reduced leakage nearly 50% when they compared the lateral-condensation and compaction methods with and without the use of the sealer.[20] Tagger and associates confirmed the finding of others that with the compactor method, when the procedure is done without sealer, one often fails to fill the canal adequately, and a cement must be used to ensure an adequate seal.[126]

The liquid vehicle in the root canal cement mix is an important factor in the properties of the mix. In an investigation of the tissue tolerance of 26 essential oils, Grossman and Lally found that oil of pimenta leaf was less irritating than eugenol, and when properly mixed, the cement set within a reasonable time.[47] Barnett and colleagues confirmed that oil of pimenta leaf is less irritating than eugenol.[5] Morse and co-workers found eugenol more irritating than either eucalyptol or chloroform in a biologic test in rats.[89]

Frauenhofer and Branstetter studied the physical properties of a noneugenol cement (Nogenol*) and 2 eugenol-containing cements.[34] They found that Nogenol did not set hard, but remained rubbery, and its water

---

*Coe Laboratories, Inc., Chicago, Illinois.

sorption was high. Crane and associates have demonstrated that Nogenol is more biocompatible than 2 other zinc-oxide-eugenol cements when examined after 6 months.[24] Using an electrochemical method for determining leakage, Mattison and Frauenhofer found Procosol* (Grossman's cement) the "material of choice" among 5 commonly used root canal sealers.[84] Beyer-Olen and colleagues found that Procosol cement and N_2 had the least amount of leakage, whereas Kloroperka had the most, according to their method of testing;[10] these reports indicate that the method of obturation and the method of testing for leakage may give variable results.

In other studies, Brodin and colleagues found that Procosol had a reversibly inhibited effect on nerve tissue;[16] AH 26† and Diaket‡ had a partially reversible inhibited effect; and that N_2 and Endomethasone have an irreversibly inhibiting effect.

At times, a small bead of cement may be extruded inadvertently through the apical foramen (Fig. 14–15). Toxicity studies in animals have shown that a small amount of extruded cement at first may cause an inflammatory reaction; nevertheless, it is well tolerated by the periapical tissue. Spangberg is of the opinion that when a periapical lesion is present, a transient toxic effect of a medicament is permissible because healing continues longer than toxicity.[119] Often, the excess cement is removed from the periapical tissue by phagocytosis.

Radioactive-isotope seepage studies by Kapsimalis and Evans have shown that Grossman's cement prevented penetration of isotopes into root canals.[63] Comparative tests on the marginal seals of AH 26, amalgam, and Grossman's cement showed no differences, according to Motta and collegues.[90] Wenger and associates implanted polyethylene tubes in rat tibias filled either flush or 1 mm short with Grossman's cement.[135] Tissue tolerance of the material was satisfactory, with little inflammation and no inhibition of repair. Langeland and co-workers have stated that all root canal cements are irritating in their freshly mixed state, but on setting, most become relatively inert.[75] The sealing properties of several root canal cements have been studied by Fogel,[30] Grieve,[41] Kapsimalis and

Evans,[63] Marshall and Massler,[82] Messing,[85] and Yates and Hembree.[139]

Calcium-Hydroxide Cement

Some zinc-oxide-eugenol cements have been modified by incorporating calcium hydroxide. Sealapex,* a product of Kerr Manufacturing Company, has been described as noneugenol, calcium-hydroxide polymeric-resin root canal sealer. Hovland and Dumsha reported approximately the same amount of microleakage of Sealapex, Procosol, and Tubli-Seal when these materials were used in filling root canals.[58] Cox and associates reported healing at the root apices of teeth of monkeys 6 months after sealing of the canals with Sealapex.[23] When these investigators compared postoperative results with AH 26, Rickert's sealer,† and Sealapex, healing was more advanced with Sealapex. Another zinc-oxide-type cement containing calcium hydroxide is CRCS,‡ a product of the Hygenic Corporation, which reported that set CRCS contains 14% by weight of calcium hydroxide. Additional in vivo reports are necessary to determine whether calcium-hydroxide-type sealers are superior to existing zinc-oxide-eugenol cements.

Paraformaldehyde Cement

Although the basic ingredient of the paraformaldehyde cements is zinc oxide, they usually contain other ingredients, including paraformaldehyde, that are objectionable. N_2 normal contains lead tetroxide and a corticosteroid, whereas Endomethasone contains a corticosteroid. Lead is toxic to the human organism and adds little benefit to the properties of the cement. Paraformaldehyde is highly irritating and destructive to tissue. Corticosteroids are supposed to reduce postoperative pain, but that claim is still unproved. The Council on Dental Therapeutics of the American Dental Association has issued a report on N_2 to refute claims that N_2 has a permanent disinfectant action; the report states that "none of the tests showed unusual antiseptic properties of the material."[22]

AH 26

AH 26 is an epoxy resin containing a nontoxic hardener. Its radiopacity is imparted to

---

*Star Dental Co., Valley Forge, Pennsylvania.
†L.D. Caulk Co., Milford, Delaware.
‡Premier Dental Products, Norristown, Pennsylvania.

*Kerr Manufacturing Co., Romulus, Michigan.
†Kerr Manufacturing Co., Romulus, Michigan.
‡Hygenic Corp., Akron, Ohio.

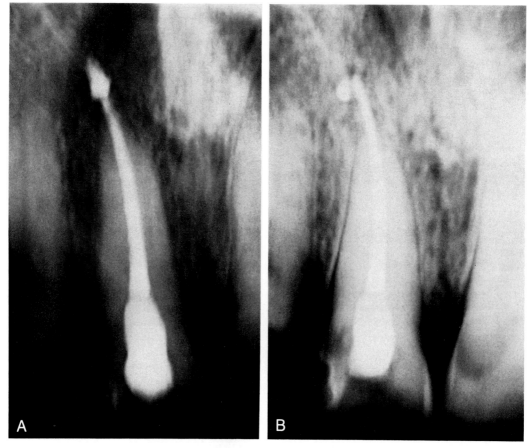

Fig. 14–15. Cement extruded beyond the root apex. *A*, Postobturation radiograph; excess cement has extruded into the periapical tissue. *B*, Recall radiograph at 6 months; excess cement is being resorbed, and bone regeneration is evident.

it by bismuth oxide. It has strong adhesive properties and contracts slightly while hardening. Schroeder has shown that AH 26 is well tolerated by the periapical tissues.[110] When material was embedded subcutaneously or intramuscularly in rats, local inflammation and encapsulation ensued. The inflammation subsided in several weeks.

AH 26 hardens slowly at body temperature in 36 to 48 hours. Fogel tested marginal leakage around gutta-percha and silver cones cemented with AH 26, Cavit, and zinc-oxide-eugenol cement.[30] AH 26 had the least amount of leakage, but all gave satisfactory results under conditions of the tests.

Hörsted and Söholm reported a case of sensitivity to AH 26 liquid.[57] Block and associates found an antibody reaction to AH 26 in dogs.[13] Torabinejad and co-workers found no evidence of either an antibody reaction or a delayed sensitivity reaction.[132]

Tamse and colleagues have reported 2 cases of paresthesia following the use of AH 26, with partial recovery in 1 to 2 years.[128]

Diaket

Diaket is a polyvinyl resin (polyketone) introduced in Europe by Scheufele in 1952.[107] Diaket consists of a fine, pure white powder and a viscous, honey-colored liquid. Two drops of liquid are mixed with one scoop of powder. Changing the ratio of powder to liquid affects the hardness of the final set and radiopacity.

Stewart found Diaket superior to other sealers when comparing tensile strength and resistance to permeability.[121] Muruzabal and Erausquin studied the reaction of rat molars to AH 26 and Diaket.[92] In preliminary observations, these investigators found a mild inflammatory reaction when the canals were overfilled. When gross overfilling was present, "modification of apical cementum and alveolar bone occurred." Diaket showed a greater tendency toward fibrous encapsulation, whereas AH 26 tended to disintegrate into fine granules, which were phagocytosed.

Pastes

Resorbable pastes, which are intended to be carried to or through the apical foramen to influence the healing or repair of a periapical lesion, consist of a base of zinc oxide-eugenol and various chemical agents such as iodoform, thymol iodide, camphorated phenol, and paraformaldehyde. They were used at a time when the dental profession correlated a periapical lesion with infection. No support now exists for the belief that such pastes favorably influence repair of periapical bone.

SYNOPSIS OF OBTURATING ROOT CANALS

Lateral-Condensation Technique

1. Apply the rubber dam, and sterilize the field of operation. Dry the canal thoroughly with absorbent points.
2. Consult the radiograph, and select a standardized gutta-percha cone of the same number as the last reamer or file used in the root canal. Cut to the length of the tooth. Sterilize it in sodium hypochlorite for at least 1 min, then wash in alcohol.
3. Place the cone in the dry root canal. The butt end should be even with the incisal or occlusal surface of tooth. Take a radiograph to determine whether it satisfactorily fills the canal, apically and laterally, within 1 mm of apex.
4. Remove the cone and place it in alcohol.
5. Examine the radiograph, and if the gutta-percha cone does not fit satisfactorily, adjust it or select another and take a radiograph.
6. Mix root canal cement on a freshly sterilized slab with a sterile spatula. Test for proper consistency. Remove the absorbent point. Pick up a small amount of cement on a smooth broach, file, or reamer and coat the surface of the root canal. Repeat.
7. Air dry the gutta-percha cone, and coat the apical half with cement. Insert in the canal to a previously measured level.
8. Take a radiograph. If the cone does not fit to the root apex, ease it to its original location with a canal plugger.

9. Using spreaders, such as a Star D11 instrument or finger pluggers, fill the canal with additional gutta-percha points (lateral condensation).
10. Cut off the butt ends of gutta-percha with a hot instrument, and remove the excess from the pulp chamber. Wipe the pulp chamber with a cotton pledget moistened with chloroform, to complete the toilette. Seal the pulp chamber and cavity of the tooth with a temporary filling.

Technique With Silver Cones

1. Apply the rubber dam, sterilize the field of operation. Dry the canal thoroughly with absorbent points (Fig. 14–16).
2. Select a silver cone of the same size as the widest reamer or file used, and cut off the butt end, to give it proper length. Sterilize it over an alcohol flame. Insert it in canal to the apex until it binds, to make sure the cone is properly seated. The butt end of the cone should be at the level of the incisal or occlusal surface.
3. Take a radiograph. If the silver cone does not fit satisfactorily, reprepare the canal or select another size silver cone that will fit better. Take another radiograph.
4. Dry the canal, and insert a sterile absorbent point in the canal until ready for obturation.
5. Mix root canal cement to the proper consistency, and coat the wall of the canal.
6. Sterilize a silver cone over an alcohol lamp, and when cool, roll it back and forth in the cement until it is well coated.
7. Carry the cone into the canal with sterile cotton pliers or Stieglitz forceps until it fits snugly. Take a radiograph. If satisfactory, laterally condense accessory gutta-percha cones alongside the silver cone.
8. In posterior teeth, the butt end may be folded against the floor of the pulp chamber. A layer of baseplate gutta-percha is applied to facilitate removal of the silver cone, should it become necessary later.
9. Remove excess cement in the pulp chamber with a cotton pellet slightly moistened with chloroform. Seal the

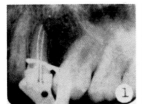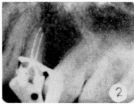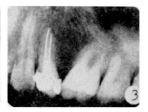

Fig. 14–16. Obturation of an upper premolar with silver cones. *1.* Silver cones corresponding in size to the largest instruments used in root canals are tried. The cones fit snugly and reach the apical foramina. *2.* The butt ends of the silver cones are cut off, and the cones are cemented with root canal cement. The cones are positioned in the apical foramina. Any necessary corrections may be made at this time. *3.* When the pulp chamber and cavity have been filled with zinc phosphate cement, and the rubber dam has been removed, a postoperative radiograph is taken to complete the records.

pulp chamber and cavity with zinc-phosphate cement.

10. Take a final radiograph after removing the rubber dam.

REACTIONS TO FILLING MATERIALS

The reaction of connective tissue to root canal cements and filling materials has been studied by many investigators. No root canal cementing medium or core is entirely innocuous. In fact, any foreign body, such as cement or core, extruded into the periapical tissue can be highly irritating and may reduce the probability of healing by as much as 25%.[96] The zinc-oxide-eugenol type of cements are probably irritating because of the eugenol; epoxy-resin cements because of the accelerator; polyvinyl resin because of the ketones; and resorbable cements because of the iodoform, for example. Fortunately, the irritation caused by overfilling is generally mild for most filling materials. Nevertheless, all filling materials should be confined within the root canal.

OVERFILLING AND UNDERFILLING

Although it may be desirable to fill root canals at a level even with the apical foramen, we cannot always attain this goal (Fig. 14–17). Boysen and colleagues,[15] as well as Oliet,[96] found that overfilled canals had a reduced potential for healing than those filled to the apex. Klevant and Eggink found that healing in teeth with periapical lesions was better after 2 years in those that were underfilled, or flush filled, than in teeth with overfilled root canals.[68] Blayney,[12] Grove,[50] Kuttler,[72] and Strindberg[122] have indicated that slight underfilling is preferable to filling to the apex. Morse and co-workers, in an evaluation of 220 obturated teeth, found that the rate of success was higher when teeth whose pulps were vital at extirpation were underfilled than when teeth with nonvital pulps were underfilled.[89]

The reaction to overfilling and underfilling was studied by Muruzabal and Erausquin.[91] These investigators found that the reaction to overfilling depended partly on the physical properties of the cement, that is, when it was hard it was encapsulated, but when the material did not harden (paste), it disintegrated and provoked an intense tissue reaction. They also found that "underfilled or filled flush with the apex showed less periapical reaction than overfilled canals."

Nitzan described several cases of overfilling with AH 26, Diaket, or N_2 resulting in paresthesia requiring a surgical procedure for removal of the extruded sealer (Fig. 14–18).[95] Lead, derived from N_2 root filling material, has been disseminated in the circulation and has been found in visceral organs by Chong and Senzer,[21] Harndt and Kaul,[51] Oswald and Cohn,[98] Shapiro and colleagues,[115] and West and associates.[136] Paresthesia from overfilling the root canal with N_2 has been reported by Ehrmann,[28] Forman and Rood,[31] Grossman,[45] Grossman and Tatoian,[48] Kaufman and Rosenberg,[64] Montgomery,[87] and Serene and colleagues.[114] Bernhoft and associates made a 6-year evaluation of teeth overfilled with N_2 alone and those overfilled with gutta-percha and sealer; failure rates were 100% with N_2 and 22% with gutta-percha.[9]

The general opinion that overfilling predisposes periradicular tissue to epithelial proliferation, chronic inflammation, and impaired repair of periapical tissue is based on research studies by Binnie and Rowe,[11] Brynolf,[18] Eggink,[27] Heling and Kischinovsky,[56] Malooly and colleagues,[79] Pritz,[101] Seltzer,[112] and others.

The dentinoenamel junction, where the

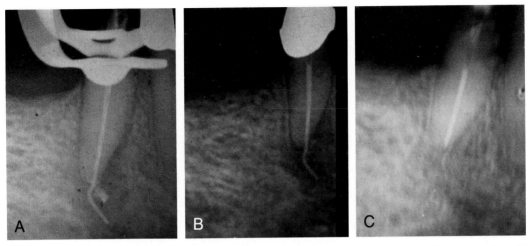

Fig. 14—17. Extruded gutta-percha and cement beyond the root apex. *A,* Radiograph showing the root canal overfilled with gutta-percha and cement that cannot be retrieved. *B,* Recall radiograph at 6 months. *C,* Recall radiograph at 8 years; one sees bone regenerations with probable encapsulation of the extruded gutta-percha cone.

pulp ends and the periapical tissue begins, and where the root canal filling should terminate, is within the root canal, usually within a millimeter from the root apex. Root canal fillings should extend up to, or should be slightly short of, the apex so as not to impinge on periapical tissue, and they should tightly seal all apical foramina. Overfilling should be avoided if possible, although in many successful cases slight overfilling of the canal has occurred.

LEAKAGE AND OTHER PROBLEMS IN OBTURATION

Leakage between the root canal and periapical tissue at the interface of the root canal filling can adversely affect healing and repair. Many studies have been published on such leakage, the determination of its occurrence

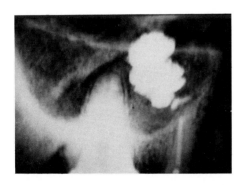

Fig. 14—18. Paste filling material has extruded into the maxillary sinus (Donor unknown).

and extent, and techniques of obturation for effective prevention.

Matloff and associates compared the use of three different radioisotopes and methylene blue as indicators of leakage after obturation with gutta-percha and sealant; they found methylene blue a more sensitive indicator of leakage than radioisotopes.[83]

In a comparative study of vertical- and lateral-condensation methods of obturation, Brothman found twice as many accessory canals filled by the vertical-condensation method in the apical third of the canal.[17] Histologically, no statistical difference in the quality of obturation was found when the two methods were compared. Benner and co-workers used a radioactive tracer to compare the apical seal of lateral condensation, vertical condensation (with and without a sealer), and the thermoplastic (compaction) method of obturating canals.[8] The differences were not significant. Wong and colleagues used an in vitro method to determine the sealing properties of gutta-percha when manipulated by the lateral-condensation, vertical-condensation, and compaction techniques; they found no significant changes in volume among the three techniques, but the replication of the compaction technique was better than the lateral-condensation and inferior to the vertical-condensation methods.[138]

Lugassy and Yee, using extracted teeth, compared the vertical-condensation method of obturation with the compaction method; they concluded that both methods filled the canals completely, and the compaction method is quicker.[77] Defects were found in both methods, such as deformation and the presence of residual pools of sealer. Tagger and associates confirmed the finding of others that the compaction method, when no sealer is used, does not fill the canal adequately and results in leakage if stratification occurs.[126] Harris and co-workers found the lateral-condensation method superior to the compaction technique when compaction was done without cement, with a resulting higher incidence of leakage.[52] Ishley and El Deeb used methylene blue dye followed by a spectrometric method to assess leakage after obturating root canals by lateral condensation or by the compactor method with sealer; they found no statistical difference between either method.[61]

In an in vitro study using India ink as an indicator, O'Neill and colleagues found less apical leakage when the canals were filled with gutta-percha and Grossman's cement than with a chloroform-softened primary cone and the McSpadden compactor; they also observed the following disadvantages of the compaction method: (1) gouged walls; (2) vertical root fracture; and (3) instrument breakage.[97] Kerekes and Rowe found the compaction method of obturation superior to lateral condensation in irregularly shaped root canals.[66] Tagger and associates described a hybrid method in which the primary gutta-percha cone was cemented, and a finger plugger was used to make enough space for the insertion of a compactor.[125] The engine-operated compactor was then inserted 5 mm into the canal and was operated for 1 sec or until resistance was met. Leakage with this method was slightly less than with lateral condensation.

Harris reported that a silver cone will show evidence of disintegration over a long period of time.[53] In an evaluation of more than 1000 teeth after 1 to 10 years, Swartz and colleagues found a lower success rate when obturation was by silver cones (88.4%) compared to gutta-percha (91.2%).[124]

Zakariasen and Stadem found that laterally condensed gutta-percha and sealer leaked less apically than either eucapercha or chloropercha.[141] Beatty and Zakariasen compared leakage after lateral condensation and found no difference between using a primary cone that was momentarily dipped in chloroform and one that was not dipped.[6] Keane and Harrington have shown that when chloroform is used to soften the tip of the primary

gutta-percha cone for no more than 1 sec and is inserted with sealer, it improves the seal of the canal.[65] Russin and associates compared leakage following obturation in vitro of 72 teeth filled either with gutta-percha and sealer or laterally condensed gutta-percha softened with chloroform.[105] Dye penetration was less pronounced with gutta-percha and sealer. Wong and associates evaluated the volumetric changes of chloropercha, Kloroperka, and chloroform-dipped gutta-percha and found a decrease in volume of 12.4, 4.86, and 1.40%, respectively.[137]

Rhome and co-workers used a radioactive tracer and found greater leakage of canals filled with Hydron than those filled with gutta-percha and cement, either by lateral or vertical condensation.[103] Langeland and associates found that Hydron interfered with repair of tissue because of its toxicity.[74] Tanzilli and colleagues compared the histologic reaction to Hydron and gutta-percha in overfilled and underfilled canals; there was less of an inflammatory reaction to gutta-percha than to Hydron in the overfilled canals, but no difference between them was noted in the underfilled canals.[130] These same investigators questioned the use of Hydron in endodontics because of its dimensional instability; in a subcutaneous-implant study in rats, they found it to be inferior to gutta-percha and sealer.[129]

REMOVAL OF ROOT CANAL FILLINGS

Gutta-Percha

The removal of a gutta-percha filling is a simple operation. The objective is to remove it without forcing the filling material into the periapical tissue. Remove the gutta-percha from the chamber by searing it with a heated excavator, or grind it out with a slowly revolving round bur. Flood the pulp chamber with chloroform or xylol to soften the gutta-percha. Insert a No. 25 or 30 reamer or file into the canal alongside the gutta-percha, and remove the softened filling, piece by piece. Repeat the process of softening the filling and instrumenting pieces out of the canal until all the gutta-percha has been removed. As the apical third of the canal is approached, smaller instruments may be used to conform to the decreasing diameter of the canal. This procedure allows continued removal of the gutta-percha without enlarging the canal or binding the instrument. If an instrument binds excessively, withdraw it carefully to avoid breakage, deposit another few drops of solvent to soften the gutta-percha, and continue the procedure. As the apex is approached, insert and rotate a heated instrument so its tip is embedded in the remaining gutta-percha, allow it to cool, and withdraw the remaining filling from the canal. If the gutta-percha does not fill the canal laterally, it may be possible to insinuate a Hedstroem file alongside the gutta-percha as close to the apex as possible and remove it entirely after softening it with chloroform or xylol. A radiograph is taken to determine whether the gutta-percha has been completely removed from the canal.

Silver Cones

A silver cone is not removed as easily as a gutta-percha filling unless the butt end extends into the pulp chamber (Fig. 14–19). In such cases, chloroform or xylol is used to soften the cement and gutta-percha surrounding the butt end of the silver cone. An explorer tip can be used to free the silver cone of gutta-percha and cement around the canal orifice. This precautionary technique frees the butt end without breaking it below the chamber floor. First, flood the pulp chamber with chloroform, to help to dissolve the cement around the cone. Grasp the projecting section of silver cone with a pair of narrow beak pliers (Stieglitz) and remove it from the canal. If this cannot be done, then clear and free the butt end with solvent again, insert an excavator blade alongside the cone, and

pry it out with an elevating motion. Be careful not to sever the butt end of the silver cone during this procedure. When the silver cone is completely in the root canal, an end-cutting bur or Masserann instrument can be rotated alongside the cone to channel the dentin around the cone so it can be grasped or elevated out of the canal. Another technique for retrieving a silver cone was suggested by Krell and associates,[70] who inserted a Hedstroem file alongside the cone and dislodged it with the assistance of an ultrasonic device. Obviously, a well-fitted silver cone is not easily removed from a root canal (Fig. 14–20).

Paste

Pastes are seldom encountered today, but most root canal pastes are soluble in chloroform or xylol. The use of a file facilitates the removal of the paste.

REPAIR FOLLOWING ENDODONTIC TREATMENT

The periapical tissue of a pulpless tooth without an area of rarefaction prior to treatment should remain normal after treatment. Occasionally, immediately after treatment, the radiograph shows a slight amount of bone destroyed, indicating a response to previous irritation, whether mechanical, chemical, or bacterial. This clearing up of destroyed periapical tissue is generally considered a prelude to repair. Repair begins as soon as infection is controlled.

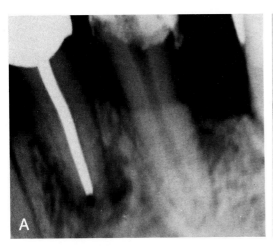 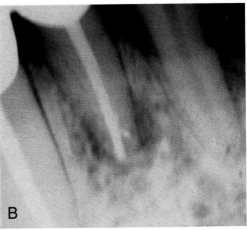

Fig. 14—19. Replacement of a silver-cone filling with laterally condensed gutta-percha. *A*, Radiograph taken 6 months after obturation with a cemented silver cone; a periapical radiolucency has developed. *B*, After removal of the silver cone, the tooth was reinstrumented, and a laterally condensed gutta-percha filling was placed; note the apical accessory canal sealed with gutta-percha and cement.

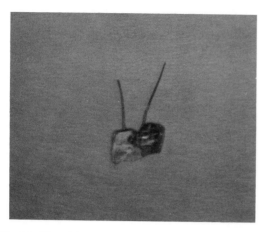

Fig. 14–20. Failure after obturation with silver cones. The butt ends of cemented silver cones protruded into the tooth chamber and were embedded in the zinc phosphate cement used to cement the crown restoration. When the restoration broke loose, the silver cones were extracted from the root canals.

The stages of repair may be described in simplified form as follows: after organization of the blood clot comes formation of granulation tissue. During this stage, the endothelial loops become canalized, probably by the pressure of the blood, and so open new channels for circulation of blood. Anastomosis of these loops now occurs, forming a rich network of small blood vessels. When an area of rarefaction is present, this stage has already occurred in most cases.

In soft tissue, the next stage is the development of scar tissue. Fibroblasts grow along fibrin strands and help to form the protein matrix by laying down collagen fibers. Both the fibroblasts and the capillaries become fewer in number, and avascular fibrous tissue or scar tissue is formed.

In bone, the process is not materially different, but is more complicated because soft tissue must be converted to hard tissue. Bone is composed of a protein matrix infiltrated with calcium salts, probably calcium phosphate and calcium carbonate. The protein matrix is formed by the osteoblasts, which are specialized fibroblastic cells. Bathing the matrix is a fluid subsaturated with calcium salts. The osteoblasts produce an enzyme, alkaline phosphatase, which splits off inorganic phosphorus from organically bound phosphorus. The increase in phosphate ions forms a saturated solution of calcium phosphate that is precipitated into the matrix. These areas or islands in which the calcium phosphate is precipitated unite to form spongy trabeculae.

Osteoblastic activity is stimulated by stresses and strains, such as exercise of long bones or mastication, in the case of the jaws. If a pulpless tooth is already completely out of occlusion, the potential for repair of the periapical tissue is reduced. Moreover, corticosteroids, if given for a prolonged period, as in arthritis, inhibit fibroblastic activity during repair of tissue and delay the development of granulation tissue, thus retarding or interfering with complete repair.

A chronic inflammatory reaction of the periapical tissue is common in the presence of an infected root canal. Shortly after the root canal has been sterilized, the inflammatory reaction subsides, and fibroblasts and osteoblasts become more prominent. Minute areas of new bone develop and, in time, replace the lost alveolar bone. Even though some periodontal fibers have become detached, reattachment occurs once the source of infection is removed. Meanwhile, if areas of resorption have developed on the root surface in the region of the destroyed bone, they will be repaired by cementoblasts, and these areas will become anchor points for attachment of new periodontal fibers running to the newly laid bone. Resorption and deposition of bone may occur simultaneously. In fact, new bone may even be deposited on old, as can be seen in new lamellae interwoven with old lamellae.

Suzuki found that when the radiographic examination showed repair, the accuracy of the radiographic interpretation agreed with the histopathologic findings in almost 84% of cases.[123] He also observed that a reduction in periapical radiolucency and reappearance of bone trabeculae are dependable signs of repair.

The question is often asked whether incompletely developed young teeth will continue to erupt after root canal treatment. It has been our observation that endodontic treatment seldom interferes with tooth eruption. Whether to do root canal treatment before or during orthodontic movement is also a question occasionally propounded. We have treated teeth both prior to and during orthodontic treatment without interfering with the work of the orthodontist or with the movement of the teeth. In most cases, the bands were left on the teeth because they did not interfere with endodontic treatment. Heuttner and Whitman have shown that when vital teeth are moved with gentle pressure, the pulp remains normal, and repair processes are not disturbed in any way.[59] The periodontal ligament is even less likely to be disturbed following endodontic treatment, except when inflammation occurred during treatment; in such cases, at least a week should elapse before continuing orthodontic movement.

Following endodontic treatment, repair generally occurs in 6 months to a year, depending on the original degree of damage to the periapical tissue. In some cases, repair may take longer. Strindberg observed stabilization of healing after 3 years, but in some cases, the area of rarefaction did not disappear completely until 8 or 9 years after endodontic treatment; he therefore doubted whether "it is possible to establish a practicable upper limit for the observation period beyond which disappearance of rarefaction can be regarded as unlikely."[122]

A diminishing but persistent small area of rarefaction following endodontic treatment is not necessarily indicative of infection. Repair may be effected by connective tissue rather than by bone regeneration. Repair always proceeds from the periphery toward the center. Granulation tissue develops, and loose fibrous connective tissue proliferates, to provide a matrix for formation of bone. In some cases, the connective tissue matures into dense fibrous tissue instead of bone. Once this occurs trabeculated bone will not be formed. Penick[99] and Kukidome[71] have described clinical cases in which an area of rarefaction was present, but histologic examination showed dense avascular fibrous connective tissue.

RESTORATION OF TOOTH FOLLOWING OBTURATION

The question is often asked, how soon after obturation of the root canal may a permanent restoration of the crown be made or may the tooth be used as a bridge abutment? No definite rule exists, but it is judicious to wait at least a week before placing a permanent restoration. Although slight discomfort is occasionally felt by the patient for a few hours following obturation of the canal (in about 1 to 2% of cases), no drastic reaction or "flare-up" should occur. If a reaction does occur, it will generally be within the first 24 hours after obturation. If a questionable prognosis still exists after completion of endodontic treatment, it might be well to wait half a year or even longer until some radiographic evidence suggests that healing is occurring. Meanwhile, the tooth should be restored properly, albeit temporarily, to prevent cusp fracture. When periapical bone is normal, however, as in the case of pulpectomy, no period of observation is necessary before proceeding with the restoration. When pulpless teeth are to be used for bridge abutments, the entire occlusal surface should preferably be covered with metal, such as gold inlay or crown, to prevent cusp fracture because of the reduced amount of moisture in the dentinal tubules of pulpless teeth and because of weakening of the crown of the tooth from loss of dentin overlying the roof of the pulp chamber, as well as from enlarging of the pulp cavity to obtain direct access. Helfer and associates found that pulpless teeth have about 9% less moisture than vital teeth.[55] The principal reason that pulpless teeth fracture, however, is that they are weakened structurally when one gains access to the pulp chamber and root canals. Posterior teeth should therefore have adequate occlusal coverage to prevent crown fracture. Complete coverage is recommended in all such cases.

Post and Core Preparation

Preparing an obturated tooth for a post and core can be a major problem. Deciding how wide and deep the post preparation should be, how much of the root canal filling should remain, what kind of post should be used, how the dentin of the walls surrounding the post preparation should be prepared for cementation, and what kind of cement should be used can directly affect the healing, function, and retention of the tooth.

Dickey and colleagues found evidence of leakage when the post space was prepared immediately after obturation, but not when the space was made a week after obturation.[25] Apparently, Kwan and Harrington disagreed when they reported that post spaces prepared with Gates Glidden reamers immediately after obturation of the canal had no effect on the apical seal of that canal.[73] Portell and associates found that a delay of 2 weeks after obturation increased the likelihood of leakage if only 3 mm of filling remained in the canal apex, whereas immediate removal of gutta-percha with a hot instrument and leaving 7 mm of apical obturation decreased peripheral leakage.[100]

Goldman and co-workers have shown that

removing the smear layer by irrigating the canal with ethylenediaminotetra-acetate (EDTA) followed by sodium hypochlorite increased the tensile strength of posts cemented with an unfilled resin; these investigators suggested that this method permitted the use of smaller posts in shallower preparations without loss of retention.[37] Sörensen and Martinoff, in a retrospective review, found that posts in endodontally treated teeth did not cause a significant increase in the success rate in reinforcing the tooth; coronal coverage of anterior teeth did not help either, but coronal coverage of posterior teeth effectively prolonged the life of the teeth.[117]

In an examination of 66 post-crowned teeth 5 years after endodontic treatment, Turner found 7.7% of periapical bone loss.[134] The restoration of pulpless teeth following endodontic treatment has been discussed by Baraban,[3] Frank,[33] Healey,[54] Markley,[80] Shillingburg,[116] and Spasser.[120]

SUCCESS AND FAILURE IN ENDODONTICS

When root canal treatment is unsuccessful, we are apt to blame the technique, the antiseptic dressing, the filling material, the radiographic interpretation, the tooth, or even the patient. In fact, we blame everyone and everything except ourselves. As often as not, no one is to blame but ourselves for poor judgment in accepting the tooth for treatment, for careless preparatory cleansing of the canal, for inadequate instrumental enlargement of the canal, for the slips that occur in the chain of asepsis, for failure to determine whether the canal was clean before obturation, for an inadequately filled root canal, for lack of judgment in determining whether endodontic treatment should have been followed by root resection. Treatment of pulpless teeth with areas of rarefaction is not always successful, although a successful result may be expected in more than 90% of cases if the endodontic operation has been properly performed.

The percentage of successfully treated cases naturally varies with judgment in selection of cases for treatment, with the method of therapy, with the skill of the operator with the technical difficulties, with whether resection or root canal treatment alone was carried out, and with other factors. Nevertheless, some idea of the probability of suc-

cess can be gained from published reports, as listed in Table 14–1.

In a "blind" study, Goldman and associates have shown that a high percentage of error can occur in interpreting postoperative radiographs of endodontally treated teeth.[38] In examining and evaluating check-up films, 5 of 6 examiners agreed only 67% of the time. This finding compares with a 76% agreement in an evaluation of radiographs made by Eggink.[27]

Some of the possible causes of failure are: (1) lack of judgment in accepting a tooth for treatment either because of operative difficulties or poor health of the patient; (2) lack of adequate debridement during canal preparation; (3) traumatic injury of periapical tissue during canal instrumentation; (4) irritating irrigants or antiseptics passed beyond the apical foramen; (5) failure to disinfect the root canal; many pulpless teeth are still treated without a bacteriologic examination; (6) infection in accessory canals with failure to sterilize them; this comprises a small percentage of cases; (7) imperfect root canal obturation failing to seal off the apical foramen; (8) action of an overfilled canal as an irritant; (9) excessive amount of cement in periapical tissue. A poorly functioning tooth, that is one out of occlusion or in traumatic occlusion, this may also contribute to slow healing of the periapical tissues. In addition, a general systemic condition may contribute to poor healing of the periapical tissues, such as failure to lay down collagen by the fibroblasts because of vitamin C deficiency, hormone imbalance, uncontrolled diabetes, nephritis, and long-term corticosteroid intake.

An excellent evaluation of failures following endodontic treatment has been published by Andreasen and Rud.[1] They found bacteria in the dentinal tubules and root canals, but not usually in the cementum. No correlation was found between the presence of bacteria in the tubules and the degree of periapical inflammation. The reasons for failure were: (1) inaccessible canal in a multirooted tooth; (2) inaccessible lateral (accessory) canal; (3) broken instrument or other cause of blockage of canal; (4) perforation; (5) inadequate instrumentation; (6) inadequate sterilization; (7) inadequate obturation; and (8) severe periodontal involvement communicating with a root canal.

In an evaluation of nearly 300 endodontally treated roots by Nelson after 2 to 30

Table 14—1. Incidence of Successes and Failures in Endodontic Treatment

	Number of Teeth or Roots*	Percentage of Success (%)	Percentage of Doubtful Cases	Percentage of Failure (%)	Follow-up (Years)
Auerbach[2]	299 (t)	83	—	17	.5—3
Barbakow, et al.[4]	335 (t)	87	6	7	1+
Castagnola and Orlay[19]	1,000 (t)	78	9	13	2+
Fechter[29]	8,886 (r)	65	—	—	1.25
Grahnén and Hansson[39a]	763 (t)	83	5	12	4—5
Grossman, et al.[49]	432 (t)	90	1	9	1—5
Ingle and Beveridge[60]	162 (t)	94	—	6	2
Jokinen, et al.[62]	1,304 (r)	53	13	34	2—7
Kerekes and Tronstad[67]	501 (r)	91	4	5	3—5
Morse, et al.[89]	220 (t)	94	—	—	1—3
Selden[111]	355 (t)	93	—	7	1.5
Strindberg[122]	529 (t)	83	3	14	6
Swartz, et al.[124]	1,007 (t)	89	—	—	1—10
Tamse and Heling[127]	122 (t)	85	—	15	1—6

*t, Teeth; r, roots.

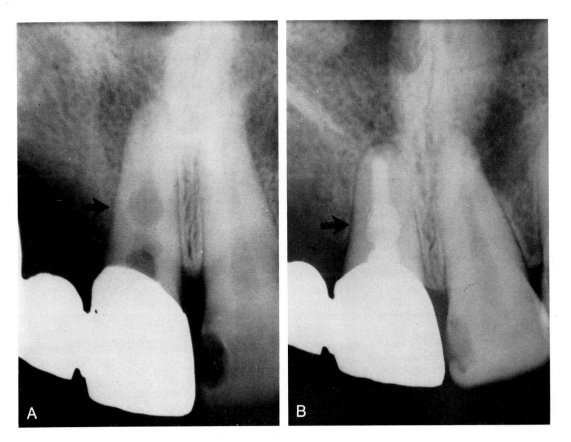

Fig. 14—21. Vertical-condensation method. *A,* Arrow points to an area of internal resorption. *B,* Root canal, including resorbed area, obturated with warm gutta-percha.

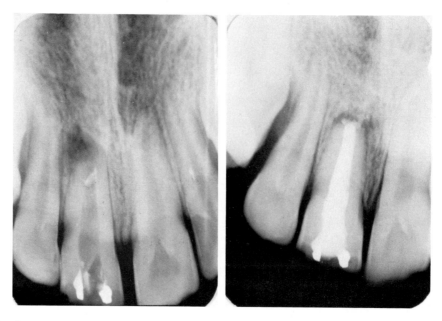

Fig. 14–22. Rolled cone. *A*, Preoperative radiograph showing wide root canal. *B*, Completed root canal filling.

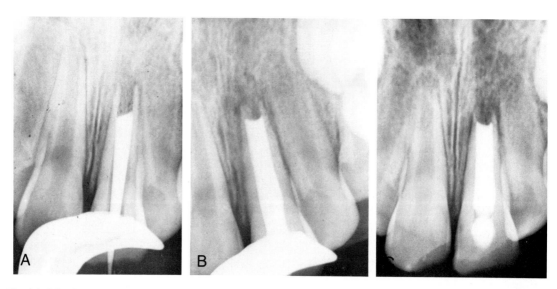

Fig. 14–23. Inverted-cone method. *A*, Butt end of a gutta-percha cone is fitted into the root canal. *B*, Primary cone is cemented, and secondary cones are packed around it. *C*, Completed root canal filling.

years, it was found that early diagnosis and treatment before a periapical lesion developed were associated with a greater degree of success; adequate adaptation and condensation of the gutta-percha filling also contributed to success; and raw data indicated a lower degree of success in molar teeth.[94] Swartz and associates reported a success rate of 89.6% in 1000 teeth treated in the endodontic department of the University of West Virginia.[124] Grossman and colleagues reported a similar success rate in teeth treated in the endodontic department of the University of Pennsylvania[49] (Figs. 14–21 to 14–23).

BIBLIOGRAPHY

1. Andreason, J.O., and Rud, J.: Int. J. Oral Surg., *1*:225, 1972.
2. Auerbach, M.: J. Am. Dent Assoc., *25*:939, 1938.
3. Baraban, D.J.: Dent. Clin. North Am., Nov.: 633, 1967.
4. Barbakow, F.H., et al.: J. Endod., *6*:485, 1980.
5. Barnett, F., et al.: Oral Surg., *58*:605, 1984.

6. Beatty, R.G., and Zakariasen, K.L.: Int. Endod. J., *17*:67, 1984.
7. Benkel, B.H., et al.: J. Endod., *2*:196, 1976.
8. Benner, M.D., et al.: J. Endod., *7*:500, 1981.
9. Bernhoft, J., et al.: Dtsch. Zahnarztl. Z., *36*:222, 1981.
10. Beyer-Olen, E.M, et al.: Int. Endod. J., *16*:51, 1983.
11. Binnie, W.H., and Rowe, A.H.: Br. Dent. J., *137*:56, 1974.
12. Blayney, J.R.: J. Dent. Res., *9*:221, 1929.
13. Block, R.M., et al.: Oral Surg., *48*:169, 1979.
14. Bowman, G.A.: *In* History of Dentistry in Missouri. Fulton, MO, Ovid Bell Press, 1938, p. 423.
15. Boysen, H., et al.: Tandl. Bladet., *76*:425, 1972.
16. Brodin, P., et al.: J. Dent. Res., *6*:1020, 1982.
17. Brothman, P.J.: J. Endod., *7*:27, 1981.
18. Brynolf, L.: Odontol. Revy., *18*:128, 1967.
19. Castagnola, L., and Orlay, H.: Br. Dent. J., *93*:29, 1952.
20. Chaisrisookumporn, S., and Rabinowitz, J.: J. Endod., *8*:493, 1982.
21. Chong, R., and Senzer, J.: J. Endod., *2*:381, 1976.
22. Council of Dental Therapeutics, American Dental Association: J. Am. Dent. Assoc., *64*:689, 1962.
23. Cox, C.F., et al.: University of Michigan (Kerr Prospectus) 1985.
24. Crane, E., et al.: J. Endod., *6*:438, 1980.
25. Dickey, D.J., et al.: J. Endod., *8*:355, 1982.
26. Director, R.C., et al.: J. Endod., *8*:149, 1982.
27. Eggink, C.O.: Results of Treatment Based on a Standardized Evaluation. Utrecht. Schotemus en Jens, 1964, p. 212.
28. Ehrmann, E.H.: Aust. Dent. J., *18*:434, 1963.
29. Fechter, B.: Int. Endod. J., *8*:235, 1958.
30. Fogel, B.B.: Oral Surg., *43*:284, 1977.
31. Forman, G.H., and Rood, J.P.: J. Dent., *5*:47, 1977.
32. Fox, J., et al.: N.Y. State Dent. J., *38*:154, 1972.
33. Frank, A.L.: J. Am. Dent. Assoc., *59*:895, 1959.
34. Frauenhofer, J.A., and Branstetter, J.: J. Endod., *8*:126, 1982.
35. Friedman, C.E., et al.: J. Endod., *3*:304, 1977.
36. Goldman, L.B., et al.: J. Dent. Res., abstract No. 349, 1978.
37. Goldman, M.: J. Dent. Res., *51*:544, 1983.
38. Goldman, M., et al.: Oral. Surg., *33*:431, 1972.
39. Goodman, A., et al.: Oral Surg., *51*:544, 1981.
39a.Grahnén, H., and Hansson, L.: Odontol. Revy, *12*:146, 1961.
40. Greenberg, M.: Dent. Dig., *67*:574, 1961, and *71*:544, 1965.
41. Grieve, A.R.: Br. Dent. J., *132*:19, 1958.
42. Grossman, L.I.: J. Endod., *8*:326, 1982.
43. Grossman, L.I.: Endodontic Practice, 10th Ed. Philadelphia, Lea & Febiger, 1980, p. 321.
44. Grossman, L.I.: Endodontic Practice, 10th Ed. Philadelphia, Lea & Febiger, 1980, p. 279.
45. Grossman, L.I.: Oral Surg., *43*:114, 1978.
46. Grossman, L.I.: J. Am. Dent. Assoc., *56*:381, 1958.
47. Grossman, L.I., and Lally, E.T.: J. Endod., *8*:208, 1982.
48. Grossman, L.I., and Tatoian, J.: Oral Surg., *46*:700, 1978.
49. Grossman, L.I., et al.: Oral Surg., *17*:368, 1964.
50. Grove, C.J.: Dent. Cosmos, *63*:968, 1921.
51. Harndt, R., and Kaul, A.: Dtsch. Zahnarztl. Z., *28*:580, 1973.
52. Harris, G.Z., et al.: J. Endod., *8*:273, 1982.
53. Harris, W.E.: J. Endod., *7*:426, 1981.
54. Healey, H.: J. Prosthet. Dent., *4*:842, 1954, and

Transactions of the Third International Conference on Endodontics. Philadelphia, University of Pennsylvania Press, 1963, p. 205.
55. Helfer, A.R., et al.: Oral Surg., *34*:661, 1972.
56. Heling, B., and Kischinovsky, D.: J. Br. Endod. Soc. *12*:93, 1979.
57. Hörsted, P., and Söholm, B.: Tandläg., *80*:194, 1976.
58. Hovland, E.J., and Dumsha, T.C: University of Maryland Report (Kerr Prospectus) 1985.
59. Huettner, R.J., and Whitman, C.L.: Am. J. Orthod., *44*:328, 1958.
60. Ingle, J.I., and Beveridge, E.E.: Endodontics, Philadelphia, 3rd Ed., Lea & Febiger, 1985, p. 37.
61. Ishley, B.J., and El Deeb, M.E.: J. Endod., *9*:242, 1983.
62. Jokinen, M.A., et al.: Scand. J. Dent. Res., *86*:366, 1978.
63. Kapsimalis, P., and Evans, R.: Oral Surg., *22*:386, 1966.
64. Kaufman, A., and Rosenberg, L.: J. Endod., *6*:529, 1980.
65. Keane, K.M., and Harrington, G.W.: J. Endod., *10*:57, 1984.
66. Kerekes, K., and Rowe, A.H.R., Int. Endod. J., *16*:68, 1983.
67. Kerekes, K., and Tronstad, L.: J. Endod., *5*:82, 1979.
68. Klevant, F.J., and Eggink, C.O.: Int. Endod. J., *16*:68, 1983.
69. Krakow, A.A., and Berk, H.: Dent. Clin. North Am., *July*:387, 1965.
70. Krell, K.V., et al.: J. Endod., *10*:269, 1984.
71. Kukidome, K.: Bull. Oral Pathol., *2*:65, 1957.
72. Kuttler, Y.: J. Am. Dent. Assoc., *56*:38, 1958.
73. Kwan, E.H., and Harrington, G.W.: J. Endod., *7*:325, 1981.
74. Langeland, K., et al.: J. Endod., *7*:196, 1981.
75. Langeland, K., et al.: Dent. Clin. North Am., *18*:309, 1974.
76. Lifshitz, J., et al.: J. Endod., *9*:17, 1983.
77. Lugassy, A.A., and Yee, F.J.: J. Endod., *8*:120, 1982.
78. McSpadden, J.T.: Presentation at the American Association of Endodontists, Atlanta, 1979.
79. Malooly, J., et al.: Oral Surg., *47*:545, 1979.
80. Markley, M.: J. Am. Dent. Assoc., *73*:1275, 1966, and Dent. Clin. North. Am., *Nov*:229, 1967.
81. Marlin, J.: J. Endod., *7*:277, 1981.
82. Marshall, F.J., and Massler, M.: J. Dent. Med., *16*:172, 1961.
83. Matloff, I.R., et al.: Oral Surg., *33*:203, 1982.
84. Mattison, G.D., and Frauenhofer, J.A.: Oral Surg., *55*:402, 1983.
85. Messing, J.J.: J. Br. Endod. Soc., *4*:18, 1970, and Br. Dent. J., *148*:41, 1980.
86. Michanowicz, A.E., and Czonsatkowsky, M.J.: J. Endod., *10*:563, 1984.
87. Montgomery, S.: J. Endod., *2*:345, 1976.
88. Morse, D., et al.: Oral Surg., *56*:190, 1983.
89. Morse, D., et al.: Oral Surg., *55*:607, 1983.
90. Motta, A., et al.: Rev. Bras. Odontol., *34*:17, 1977.
91. Muruzabal, M., and Erausquin, J.: Arch. Oral Biol., *11*:373, 1966.
92. Muruzabal, M., and Erausquin, J.: Oral Surg., *21*:786, 1966.
93. Naidorf, I.J.: Dent. Clin. North Am., *18*:329, 1974.
94. Nelson, I.: Int. Endod. J., *15*:168, 1982.
95. Nitzan, D.W.: J. Endod., *9*:81, 1983.
96. Oliet, S.: J. Endod., *9*:147, 1983.
97. O'Neill, E., et al.: J. Endod., *9*:190, 1983.

98. Oswald, R.J., and Cohn, S.A.: J. Endod., *1*:59, 1975.

99. Penick, E.C.: Oral Surg., *14*:239, 1961.

100. Portell, F.R., et al.: J. Endod., *8*:154, 1982.

101. Pritz, W.: Oesterr. Z. Stomatol., *71*:242, 1974.

102. Pyner, D.A.: J. Endod., *6*:527, 1974.

103. Rhome, B., et al.: J. Endod., *7*:458, 1981.

104. Rising, D.W., et al.: J. Endod., *1*:172, 1975.

105. Russin, T.P., et al.: J. Endod., *6*:678, 1980.

106. Sampeck, A.: Thesis, University of Michigan, Ann Arbor, 1961.

107. Scheufele, J.: Dtsch. Zahnarztl. Z., *7*:913, 1952.

108. Schilder, H.: Dent. Clin. North Am., *4*:269, 1974.

109. Schilder, H., et al.: Oral Surg., *59*:285, 1985.

110. Schroeder, A.: Zahnarztl. Welt Reform, *58*:531, 1957.

111. Selden, H.S.: Oral Surg., *37*:271, 1974.

112. Seltzer, S., et al.: Oral Surg., *33*:589, 1972, and *36*:725, 1973.

113. Senia, E.S., et al.: J. Endod., *1*:136, 1975.

114. Serene, T.P., et al.: J. Am. Dent. Assoc., *96*:101, 1978.

115. Shapiro, I., et al.: J. Endod., *1*:294, 1975.

116. Shillingburg, H.T., et al.: J. Prosthet. Dent., *24*:401, 1970.

117. Sörensen, J.A., and Martinoff, J.: J. Dent. Res., *62*:263, 1983.

118. Sorin, S., and Oliet, S.: J. Endod., *5*:233, 1979.

119. Spangberg, L.: Odontol. Tidskr., *77*:11, 133, 1969.

120. Spasser, H.F.: N.Y. State Dent. J., *29*:247, 1963.

121. Stewart, G.G.: Oral Surg., *11*:1029, 1174, 1958.

122. Strindberg, L.Z.: Acta Odontol. Scand., *14(Suppl. 21)*:101, 1956.

123. Suzuki, A.: Shikwa Gakuho, *60*:37, 1960.

124. Swartz, B.B., et al.: J. Endod., *9*:198, 1983.

125. Tagger, M., et al.: J. Endod., *10*:299, 1984.

126. Tagger, M., et al.: Oral Surg., *56*:641, 1983.

127. Tamse, A., and Heling, B.: Ann. Dent., *32*:20, 1973.

128. Tamse, A., et al.: J. Endod., *8*:88, 1982.

129. Tanzilli, J.P., et al.: Oral Surg., *55*:507, 1983.

130. Tanzilli, J.P., et al.: J. Endod., *7*:396, 1981.

131. Timpawat, S., et al.: Oral Surg., *55*:180, 1983.

132. Torabinajed, M., et al.: J. Endod., *10*:304, 1984.

133. Torabinajed, M., et al.: J. Endod., *4*:245, 1978.

134. Turner, C.: J. Dent., *9*:109, 1981.

135. Wenger, J.S., et al.: Oral Surg., *46*:88, 1978.

136. West, N.M., et al.: J. Endod., *6*:598, 1978.

137. Wong, M., et al.: J. Endod., *8*:4, 1982.

138. Wong, M., et al.: J. Endod., *7*:551, 1981.

139. Yates, J.L., and Hembree, J.H.: J. Endod., *6*:591, 1975.

140. Yee, F.S., et al.: J. Endod., *1*:145, 1975.

141. Zakariasen, K.I., and Stadem, P.S.: Int. Endod. J., *15*:67, 1982.

15 Bleaching of Discolored Teeth

Esthetics is an important factor in a patient's decision to undergo endodontic treatment. A frequent question is, "Will my tooth turn black?" The usual response is a "qualified no," with the explanation that modern treatment procedures are designed to avoid crown staining and tooth discoloration. Nevertheless, teeth can and do discolor, sometimes before endodontic treatment, sometimes afterward, in spite of all precautions taken to prevent color changes. When teeth discolor, bleaching should be considered as a means of restoring tooth esthetics.

The normal color of primary teeth is bluish white. The color of permanent teeth is grayish yellow, grayish white, or yellowish white. The color of the teeth is determined by the translucency and thickness of the enamel, the thickness and color of the underlying dentin, and the color of the pulp. Alterations in the color may be physiologic or pathologic and endogenous or exogenous in nature.

With age, the enamel becomes thinner because of abrasion and erosion, and the dentin becomes thicker because of the deposition of secondary and reparative dentin, which produce color changes in teeth during one's life. Teeth of elderly persons are usually more yellow or grayish yellow than those of younger persons.

Classification of Tooth Discoloration

Tooth discoloration can be classified as either extrinsic or intrinsic.

Extrinsic Discoloration

Extrinsic discolorations are found on the outer surface of the teeth and are usually of local origin, such as tobacco stains. Some extrinsic discoloration, such as the green discoloration associated with the Nasmyth's membrane in children, and tea and tobacco stains, can be removed by scaling and polishing during tooth prophylaxis. Other types of extrinsic discoloration, such as silver nitrate stains, are almost impossible to eliminate without grinding because the stains penetrate the surface of the crowns and are difficult to remove by chemical means alone.

Intrinsic Discolorations

Intrinsic discolorations are stains within the enamel and dentin caused by the deposition or incorporation of substances within these structures, such as tetracycline stains. If incorporated into the dentin, they become visible because of the translucency of the enamel. They can be related to periods of tooth development, as in dentinogenesis imperfecta, or they may be acquired after completion of tooth development, as in pulp necrosis. Intrinsic discolorations such as those occurring with amelogenesis imperfecta or dentinogenesis imperfecta are impossible to eliminate because they originate from developmental defects of the enamel and dentin. Stains that result from pulp necrosis, however, can usually be removed by bleaching procedures.

CAUSES OF TOOTH DISCOLORATION

The principal causes of discoloration are: (1) decomposition of pulp tissue; (2) excessive hemorrhage following pulp removal; (3) trauma; (4) medicaments; and (5) filling materials. In addition to these causes, teeth may be discolored because of general systemic conditions, for example, red or purple discoloration as in congenital porphyria, violaceous as in hereditary opalescent dentin, mottled brown as in endemic fluorosis, grayish brown as in erythroblastosis fetalis, and brown as in jaundice. The tetracycline group of antibiotics causes irreversible discoloration of tooth structure by forming a bound complex with dentin that stains the tooth in gradations from yellow to gray or brown. Discoloration from systemic causes occurs only during developmental stages of the teeth.

The prognosis for bleaching of a discolored pulpless tooth is good when the discoloration is due to products of pulp decomposition, food debris, or chromogenic bacteria that gain access to the dentinal tubules. When the discoloration is due to metallic salts, bleaching is less successful.

Decomposition of pulp tissue is probably the most common cause of tooth discoloration, particularly if the pulp is necrotic. It often goes unnoticed for some time, perhaps several months after death of the pulp or treatment of the tooth, because of the slow formation of color-producing compounds.

Traumatic injury of a tooth may cause the blood vessels in the pulp to rupture, with diffusion of blood into the dentinal tubules. Such teeth have a dark pinkish hue almost immediately after the accident and turn pinkish brown some days afterward. The discoloration persists even after the pulp is removed or if the pulp recovers. Particularly in young people, the pigment resulting from the breakdown of the erythrocytes in the dentinal tubules persists, causing discoloration of the crown. Usually, however, the pulp succumbs to trauma, and as a result, the hemoglobin breaks down, with formation of various colored compounds such as hemin, hematin, hematoidin, hematoporphyrin, and hemosiderin. At times, hydrogen sulfide produced by bacteria combines with the hemoglobin to darken the tooth.

Discoloration of the tooth may occur if hemorrhage is excessive during pulp extirpation. Staining of the crown of the tooth through the pulp chamber following profuse pulpal bleeding is common. When hemorrhage persists, it usually indicates that a vital pulp fragment is still present in the root canal. Hemorrhage ceases on removal of the pulp remnant. The pulp chamber and root canal should be thoroughly irrigated, to prevent discoloration, by removing blood elements from the dentinal tubules.

Certain root canal medicaments may cause discoloration. Some stain the tooth directly, whereas others stain only on decomposing or combining with some other agent used in endodontic treatment; for example, essential oils form resinous substances that discolor tooth structure. Although some medicaments stain almost immediately, the effect of others may not be apparent for some time.

Discoloration from filling materials depends on the kind of filling used. Silver amalgam produces a stain ranging from slate gray to dark gray, copper amalgam produces a bluish black to black stain, and gold, which seldom causes discoloration, may combine with the products of decay to produce a dark brown stain. Stains from amalgam are likely to occur when the dentinal wall is thin, and the filling material almost shimmers through the enamel. Fewer discolorations from amalgam fillings are seen nowadays because the dentinal walls are covered with liners and because improvements in the refining process of silver alloy and mercury have produced materials of greater purity. Discoloration from direct gold fillings is uncommon today because this technique is infrequently used. Metallic stains are difficult to remove.

Fewer than 5% of treated pulpless teeth become noticeably discolored because of dehydration of tooth substance with subsequent loss of translucency. Of these, most respond satisfactorily to bleaching. This concept is borne out by evaluation of bleached teeth observed over a 1- to 5-year period.[6]

PREVENTION OF TOOTH DISCOLORATION

Discoloration of pulpless teeth can be prevented by detailed attention to various aspects of treatment, especially debridement. Proper access cavity preparations that permit removal of all pulpal tissue, particularly in the pulp horns, are critical. All traces of blood should be removed by thorough irrigation with sodium hypochlorite. All strands of pulp tissue that will cause hemorrhage should be removed before the medicated dressing is placed in the pulp chamber. Any defective restorations should be replaced. Nonstaining medicaments and materials should be used. Root canal sealer and obturating materials should be removed from the pulp chamber beyond a level 1 to 3 mm apical to the free gingival margin. The pulp chamber should be filled with a translucent material, such as a silicate cement, with a composite resin obturating the access cavity.[9]

The goal of bleaching procedures is the restoration of normal color to a tooth by decolorizing the stain with a powerful oxidizing or reducing agent. The oxidizing agents generally used are Superoxol* (hydrogen peroxide 30%) and sodium perborate.

BLEACHING AGENTS

Superoxol is a 30% solution of hydrogen peroxide by weight, and 100% by volume in

---

*Merck and Co., Rahway, New Jersey.

pure distilled water. It is a clear, colorless, odorless liquid, stored in lightproof amber bottles. It is unstable and should be kept away from heat, which could cause it to explode. Superoxol should be stored in sealed refrigerated containers where it retains sufficient potency for approximately 3 to 4 months, but it decomposes readily in an open container and in the presence of organic debris. Care should be exercised when handling Superoxol because its ischemic effect on skin and mucous membrane resembles a chemical burn. It is especially painful if it comes in contact with the nail bed or the soft tissue under the fingernail. Because the amount needed for a bleaching operation is about 1 to 2 ml, the solution can be dispensed into a clean dappen dish. Once treatment has been completed, any remaining solution should be discarded. Superoxol can be used alone or mixed with sodium perborate into a paste for use in the "walking bleach."

Sodium perborate is a stable, white powder, normally supplied in a granular form, that has to be ground into a powder before using. The powder is water soluble and decomposes into sodium metaborate and hydrogen peroxide, releasing oxygen.[23] When mixed into a paste with Superoxol, this paste decomposes into sodium metaborate, water and oxygen. When sealed into the pulp chamber, it oxidizes and discolors the stain slowly, continuing its activity over a longer period of time. This procedure is called the "walking bleach."[19]

TECHNIQUE FOR BLEACHING PULPLESS TEETH

Preparation

Prior to bleaching a tooth, one should examine and evaluate the condition of its crown and the status of its obturated root. The crowns of teeth to be bleached should be relatively intact. Crowns weakened by an access preparation and with large or multiple restorations or large carious lesions are not amenable to bleaching. These teeth should be restored with a post and core and a full-veneer porcelain crown for the best functional and esthetic result.

The root canal filling should be well condensed, radiopaque, with no voids, and it should be well adapted to the root canal walls, to prevent percolation of the bleaching solution into the periapical tissues that will cause an acute apical periodontitis. If the canal is obturated with a silver cone; the cone should be replaced with a well-condensed gutta-percha filling, if possible, before bleaching is attempted. If one is unable to replace the silver cone, the orifice of the root canal should be obturated with Cavit, to prevent percolation of the bleaching solution into the periradicular area.

Walking Bleach

1. Prepare the tooth for bleaching by polishing the enamel surface with a prophylaxis paste to remove any gross surface debris or discolorations.

2. Apply petroleum jelly to the gingival tissues around the tooth to be bleached, for protection against tissue irritation. Superoxol, in contact with the skin or mucous membrane, may cause severe discomfort.

3. Adapt the rubber dam, invert it, ligate it with wax dental floss, and hold it securely in place with a clamp on the tooth to be bleached.

4. Re-establish the access cavity.

5. Remove any gutta-percha root canal filling that extends into the pulp chamber with a hot Weichman No. 1 instrument to the level of the crest of the alveolar bone. The remaining root canal filling should be vertically condensed with finger pluggers.

6. Examine the pulp chamber, and remove any residual debris or stains in the pulp horns and along the incisal edge of the pulp cavity with a small, round bur in a slow-speed contra-angle (Fig. 15–1).

7. Seal the orifice of the root canal with at least 1 mm Cavit over the gutta-percha, to prevent percolation of the bleaching agent into the apical area. A bead of Cavit is placed at the end of a finger plugger, is packed over the orifice, and is condensed with a damp cotton pellet held in Merriam pliers. Because Cavit from a freshly opened tube is difficult to handle, one should use Cavit from a tube that has been opened previously. The level of the root canal obturation should be about 1 mm below the free gingival margin. This level of obturation is important, to confine the bleaching agents to the crown of the tooth above the level of the bone. Because cervical root resorption has been reported following bleaching,[13,16,18] we believe that keeping the bleaching agents from the cervical area of the root canal may prevent cervical resorption (Fig. 15–2).

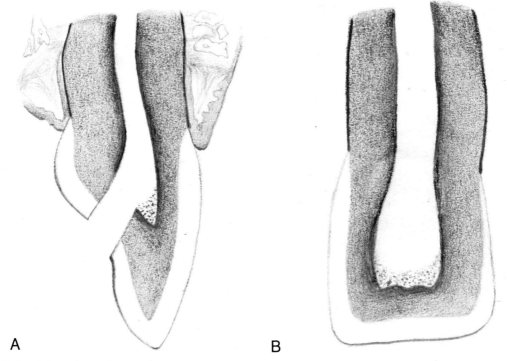

A   **B**

Fig. 15–1. Schematic drawing showing the area where pulp debris is likely to escape removal if access to the pulp chamber is inadequate. *A,* Debris along the incisal edge of the pulp cavity. *B,* Debris in pulp horns and along the incisal edge of the pulp cavity.

8. Remove the smear layer, and open the tubuli by applying a 25% solution of citric acid or a 30% solution of orthophosphoric acid to the dentinal surface of the pulp chamber.[15] Flush the surface with sodium hypochlorite or water to remove the acid. The smear layer may also be removed by flushing the chamber with alternate solutions of ethylenediaminotetra-acetate (EDTA) and sodium hypochlorite. Dry the tooth with suction.

9. Flush the pulp chamber with 95% alcohol, and dry with air to desiccate the dentin.

10. Protect the exposed areas of the patient's face by draping it and cover the patient's eyes with glasses. The patient's clothing should be covered with a plastic apron. The operator should wear gloves to protect his hands.

11. Mix sodium perborate powder with Superoxol to a thick paste in a clean dappen dish.

12. Carry the thick paste into the pulp chamber with a plastic instrument. Make sure the entire facial surface of the pulp chamber is covered with the paste.

13. Place a small cotton pellet, slightly moistened with Superoxol, over the bleaching paste.

14. Seal the access cavity with IRM* or zinc phosphate cement. Because the oxygen generated may dislodge the filling, apply pressure with the gloved finger against the tooth until the filling has set.

The maximum bleaching effect is attained about 24-hours after treatment (Fig. 15–3). The patient should return in 3 to 7 days, for evaluation of the result. If the shade is too dark, additional bleaching is necessary. If the shade is too light, the tooth should be permanently restored. Teeth that are bleached a shade too light seem to revert to their former color shortly after bleaching. This phenomenon may be associated with the ingress of pigmenting substances from the saliva into the dentin by way of the enamel, whose permeability may have been increased by the bleaching process. Generally, 2 treatments, performed about a week apart, are necessary to attain the desired shade, although in some cases a single treatment is sufficient.

Through the years, other techniques have

---

*L.D. Caulk Co., Milford, Delaware.

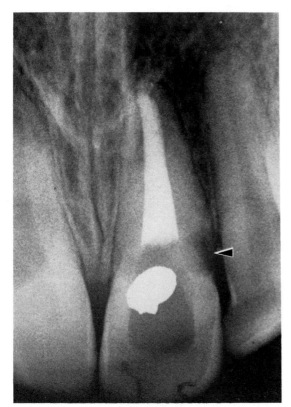

Fig. 15–2. External cervical resorption (arrow) in a maxillary left central incisor after internal bleaching 2 years previously. (From Montgomery, S.: Oral Surg., 57:203, 1984.)

been used to bleach pulpless teeth. These techniques differ only in the method used to activate the Superoxol to liberate the bleaching agent, oxygen. Whereas the walking bleach uses the reaction of sodium perborate with Superoxol to liberate the bleaching agent, the other techniques use heat and light.

Heat and Light Bleaching

After preparation of the tooth as previously described, a loose mat of cotton is placed on the labial surface and another is placed in the pulp chamber of the tooth to be bleached. The loose cotton mats are saturated with Superoxol. The solution is activated by exposing it to light and heat from a powerful light. The tooth is subject to several, usually 6, 5-min exposures, and one replenishes the bleaching solution at frequent intervals. On completion of the bleaching, a pellet of cotton moistened with Superoxol, or Superoxol and sodium perborate, is sealed in the pulp chamber until the following appointment.

An alternative to activate the Superoxol is the application of a thermostatically controlled electric heating instrument or a stainless steel instrument, such as a Woodson No. 2, heated over a flame. Heat and light from a photoflood light aimed directly on the tooth from a distance of 2 ft or more also activate Superoxol. Wisps of cotton, moistened with Superoxol, hold the bleaching agent inside the tooth chamber and on the labial and lingual surfaces of the crown. Superoxol is added to the cotton every 5 min during the bleaching process. The techniques can be used by themselves or in combination with the walking bleach.

An in vitro study comparing the bleaching of teeth with Superoxol and heat for 12 min to packing a paste of Superoxol and sodium perborate for 7 days, or a combination of the 2 techniques, showed no significant differences in bleaching efficacy.[10] Because the clinical results of these techniques do not appear to differ, the walking bleach, which is easy to perform, consumes the least time,

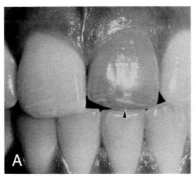

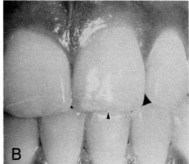

Fig. 15–3. Before (A) and after (B) bleaching of discolored pulpless teeth by the "walking-bleach" method. Arrows indicate the affected tooth. (Courtesy of Dr. T. L. Walker, San Antonio, Texas.)

and requires no special equipment, is the method of choice.

Bleaching of Vital Teeth

Teeth that have been discolored as a result of ingestion of a high amount of fluoride, such as 5 ppm in natural drinking water, or consuming tetracycline continuously for a long period of time as for the treatment of cystic fibrosis or other infections during the formative period of the teeth do not respond well to ordinary methods of bleaching.

In cases of endemic fluorosis (mottled enamel), a solution of anesthetic ether, hydrochloric acid, and Superoxol is used for bleaching.[2,4,17] The solution is prepared in a clean dappen dish, as follows:

1 part anesthetic ether	0.2 ml
5 parts hydrochloric acid (36%)	1.0 ml
5 parts hydrogen peroxide (30%)	1.0 ml

The anesthetic ether removes surface debris, the hydrochloric acid etches the enamel, and the hydrogen peroxide bleaches the enamel.

The technique of vital bleaching is as follows: Polish the crown with a prophylactic paste, protect the gingiva with petroleum jelly, and isolate the teeth to be bleached with a rubber dam that is carefully inverted and ligated. Protect the patient and operator as previously described. The solution should be freshly mixed and applied directly to the enamel surface for 5 min at 1-min intervals. On completion of the bleaching, the solution is neutralized with a baking soda solution and copious irrigation with water. The bleached surface should be polished with cuttle discs and a prophylactic paste. This procedure may have to be repeated 2 or 3 times before the desired shade is obtained (Fig. 15—4). Fluoride-stained teeth are difficult to bleach and require longer and repeated sessions to decolorize them.[21]

Little or no pulpal reaction was reported in a study that used an 18% hydrochloric-acid solution for 5 min and disc polishing for 15 sec.[5] In another study, the solution of ether, hydrochloric acid, and Superoxol was used; the solution etched the enamel, but did not penetrate it.[12] Tooth structure is not damaged, nor is any sensitivity of the teeth noted following this bleaching operation if it is done carefully.

Teeth discolored by tetracycline may also be bleached to some extent with Superoxol but the bleaching effect leaves something to be desired, with regard to both decoloration and permanency, because the chemical cannot reach the real cause of the discoloration, which is the incorporation of tetracycline into the dentin.[25] The degree of staining depends on the stage of tooth development at the time when medication is begun; the greater the amount of crown developed, the less severe the stain, and vice versa. Destaining of the yellow color is most successful, whereas brownish teeth are least successfully bleached.[21]

The use of Superoxol and a thermostatically controlled heat source for bleaching tetracycline-stained teeth has been described.[3,8] Unfortunately, the decoloration is only superficial and does not affect the stained dentin. Another method of bleaching tetracycline stain has been described.[1,11,14] In this method, the pulps of the teeth are intentionally extirpated, the root canals are cleaned, shaped and obturated, and the teeth are internally bleached as previously described. The result in humans,[1,11] as well as in dogs,[24] has been successful. We believe that labial veneers with composite resins or even porcelain-veneer full-crown restorations are indicated instead of intentional devitalization of a tooth with a normal pulp.

The application of heat to the tooth during bleaching procedures may cause some transitory reaction in the pulp. Although in one study the application of heat in the range of 115 to 124° F produced a slight superficial inflammation;[20] in another study, tempera-

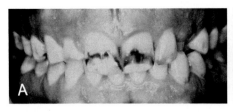 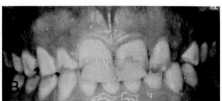

Fig. 15—4.   Before (A) and after (B) bleaching of tetracycline-stained teeth with a solution of anesthetic ether, hydrochloric acid, and hydrogen peroxide 30%.

tures of 114° F had no effect on the pulp.[22] In this second study, the use of Superoxol caused hemorrhage, inflammation, and destruction of the odontoblast layer of the pulp, but the reaction was reversible, and healing occurred within 60 days.[22]

RESTORATION OF THE PULPLESS TOOTH

To prevent discoloration from returning, any defective restoration should be replaced, and the access cavity should be restored. Restorative materials have been evaluated as to their property of preserving the normal translucency of the tooth.[9] Silicate cement, condensed in the pulp chamber with a restoration of composite sealing the access cavity, preserves the natural translucency of the tooth.

BIBLIOGRAPHY

1. Abou-Rass, M.: J. Endod., *8*:101, 1982.
2. Amess, J.W.: J. Am. Dent. Assoc., *24*:1674, 1937.
3. Arens, D.E., et al.: Oral Surg., *34*:812, 1972.
4. Bailey, R.W., and Christen, A.G.: Oral Surg., *26*:871, 1968.
5. Baumgartner, J.C., et al.: J. Endod., *9*:527, 1983.
6. Brown, G.: Oral Surg., *20*:238, 1965.
7. Cohen, S.C.: J. Endod., *5*:134, 1979.
8. Cohen, S.C., and Parkin, F.M.: Oral Surg., *29*:465, 1970.
9. Freccia, W.F., et al.: J. Endod., *8*:265, 1982.
10. Freccia, W.F., et al.: J. Endod., *8*:70, 1982.
11. Fields, J.P.: J. Endod., *8*:512, 1982.
12. Griffin, R.E., et al.: J. Endod., *3*:139, 1977.
13. Harrington, G.W., and Natkin, E.: J. Endod., *5*:344, 1979.
14. Hayashi, K., et al.: Dent. Surg., *56*:17, 1980.
15. Howell, R.A.: Br. Dent. J., *148*:159, 1980.
16. Lado, E.A., et al.: Oral Surg., *55*:78, 1983.
17. McInnes, J.: Ariz. Dent. J., *12*:13, 1966.
18. Montgomery, S.: Oral.Surg., *57*:203, 1984.
19. Nutting, E.B., and Poe, G.S.: J. South Calif. Dent. Soc., *31*:289, 1963, and Dent. Clin. North Am., *Nov.*:655, 1967.
20. Robertson, W.D., and Melfi, R.C.: J. Endod., *6*:645, 1980.
21. Seale, N.S., and Thrash, W.J.: J. Dent. Res., *64*:457, 1985.
22. Seale, N.S., et al.: J. Dent. Res., *60*:948, 1981.
23. Spasser, H.F.: N.Y. State Dent. J., *27*:332, 1961.
24. Walton, R.E.: J. Endod., *9*:416, 1983.
25. Walton, R.E., et al.: J. Endod., *8*:536, 1982.
26. Younger, H.B.: Tex. Dent. J., *57*:380, 1939.

16 Treatment of Traumatized Teeth

Trauma to the teeth may result either in injury of the pulp, with or without damage to the crown or root, or in displacement of the tooth from its socket. When the crown or root is fractured, the pulp may recover and survive the injury, it may succumb immediately, or it may undergo progressive degeneration and ultimately die. Sweet estimated that a large percentage of fractured anterior teeth are in the maxilla, and 90% of these teeth protrude so much that they are inadequately covered by the lips.[44] When luxation of a tooth occurs, the pulp may survive, depending on the violence of the blow and the degree of dislocation. Luxation of teeth occurs less often than fracture.

CAUSES AND INCIDENCE

Traumatic injuries to the teeth can occur at any age. Young children learning to walk or falling from a chair are subject to anterior tooth injuries. Frequently, child abuse results in facial and dental trauma. Bakland reported that children 8 to 12 years of age are most prone to dental accidents.[7] Sports accidents and fights affect teenagers and young adults, whereas auto accidents affect all age groups. It has been estimated that tooth injuries affect up to a quarter of the population of the United States and other countries.

The incidence of fractures is about 5%; Ellis reports an incidence of 4.2%,[17] and Grundy, 5.1%.[22] Boys have about 2 to 3 times as many fractured teeth as girls. Because so many dental accidents are sports related, every safeguard should be taken to protect the teeth of children from such accidents by using educational programs in addition to mouthguards.

CLASSIFICATION OF FRACTURED TEETH

Many classifications have been suggested for fractured anterior teeth. The Ellis Classification consists of six basic groups: (1) enamel fracture; (2) dentine fracture without pulp exposure; (3) crown fracture with pulp exposure; (4) root fracture; (5) tooth luxation; and (6) tooth intrusion.[17] Heithersay and Morile recommended a classification of subgingival fractures based on the level of the tooth fracture in relation to various horizontal planes of the periodontium, as follows: class 1, in which the fracture line does not extend below the level of the attached gingiva; class 2, in which the fracture line extends below the level of the attached gingiva, but not below the level of the alveolar crest; class 3, in which the fracture line extends below the level of the alveolar crest; and class 4, in which the fracture line is within the coronal third of the root, but below the level of the alveolar crest.[24]

The World Health Organization (WHO) adopted the following classification in 1978 with a code number corresponding to the International Classification of Diseases: 873.60, enamel fracture; 873.61, crown fracture involving enamel and dentin without pulp exposure; 873.62, crown fracture with pulp exposure; 873.63, root fracture; 873.64, crown-root fracture; 873.66, luxation; 873.67, intrusion or extrusion; 873.68, avulsion; and 873.69, other injuries, such as soft tissue laceration.[47] This classification was modified by Andreasen according to the following examples: (873.64) uncomplicated crown-root fracture without pulp exposure; (873.64) complicated crown-root fractures with pulp exposure; (873.66) concussion, an injury to the tooth-supporting structures without abnormal loosening or displacement of a tooth that reacts to percussion; (873.66) subluxation, an injury to the tooth-supporting structures with abnormal loosening but without displacement of the tooth; (873.66) lateral luxation, displacement of a tooth in a direction other than axially, accompanied by fracture of the alveolar socket.[3] Andreasen also classified injuries to the supporting bone and injuries to the oral mucosa.

FRACTURED TEETH

Fractures of the crowns of teeth are generally diagonal, involving a corner of the tooth, frequently the mesial. Fractures of the roots of teeth are more commonly horizontal, although diagonal and vertical fractures also occur. When the root fractures near the apical third of the tooth, the prognosis is better than when it fractures nearer the middle or cervical third because the middle or cervical third has less alveolar support for the fragment, and mobility of the tooth is greater.

Traumatic injuries that do not cause fracture of the crown or root are just as often responsible for pulp injury as those in which the crown or root is fractured. In injuries that do not fracture the crown or root, the impact of the blow is transmitted head-on to the pulp, which receives the full force of the blow, whereas in injuries that cause fracture, the impact is broken as the crown or root fractures, and the unexposed pulp is less likely to be injured seriously.

Ritchie reported 2 cases of root fracture with repair and continued vitality of the pulp more than 10 years after injury.[40] Oliet reported a case of horizontal root fracture in a youngster's permanent maxillary incisor with incomplete root development.[37] Ligation alone resulted in the formation of an anatomically normal root and canal, containing a vital pulp, including complete dentinal reattachment of the fractured fragments that obliterated any signs of the previous fracture. Sinai reported a case in a 7-year-old patient of compound root fracture of a maxillary anterior tooth with a sinus tract that was treated with a paste of calcium hydroxide and camphorated chlorophenol. Eight years later, repair was complete, with no evidence of a sinus tract.[41]

Concussion of a tooth, with and without fracture, may damage the blood vessels of the pulp, with resultant hemorrhage and extravasation of erythrocytes into the dentinal tubules. In most cases, the crown becomes discolored, and the pulp eventually dies, but in rare cases, the pulp remains vital even though the crown is discolored. A similar condition can arise, although infrequently, from the trauma created during the preparation of a tooth for a crown restoration.

Symptoms

The symptoms depend on whether the pulp is exposed, the degree of damage to the pulp, the age of the patient, and other factors. In a young person, even though the pulp is not exposed, if the break has bared the dentin, the tooth will become sensitive to temperature changes, and to sweet and sour, because the pulp chamber is large, the pulp horns are still extensive, and the dentinal tubules are relatively large containing tissue and fluids that are susceptible to noxious stimuli. When the pulp has become exposed, pain may occur with every breath, or it may be present almost constantly. In some cases, surprisingly, the patient is free of pain. In an older person, sufficient pulp recession may already have occurred to protect the pulp against irritation from external stimuli, and the tooth may be practically symptomless.

Calcification of the root canal from trauma has a small but ponderable incidence, considering the number of teeth traumatized in children and young people. If two adjacent teeth are traumatized at the same time, it is possible for the pulp of one tooth to be stimulated and to lay down dentin, ultimately resulting in calcification and partial or complete obliteration of the root canal; in the adjacent tooth, the pulp succumbs and becomes necrotic, resulting in a wide, open apical foramen (Fig. 16–1). At times, pulp pathosis is accompanied by internal or external resorption.

Anehill observed obliteration of the root canal in 27 of 181 traumatized teeth (15%).[1] Andreasen observed 189 traumatized teeth from 1 to 12 years and found that 45% developed variable degrees of pulp obliteration.[5] Jacobsen and Kerekes evaluated 122 traumatically injured teeth over a period of 10 to 23 years and found 36% of root canals partially calcified and 64% completely calcified.[26] Teeth with calcified root canals usually remain symptomless for many years, except for their radiographic appearance and some discoloration of their crown.

In cases of root fracture, the tooth may be entirely comfortable, or it may be tender on mastication only, depending on the location and severity of the break and on the status of the surrounding bone and mucosa. In severe cases, the tooth may be loose, and the patient may be tempted to wiggle it with his tongue or lip. In such cases, the prognosis is poor.

Diagnosis

Diagnosis is made from the patient's history, visual examination, radiographs, electric pulp test, and thermal tests. Following fracture of the root, the reaction to tests of pulp vitality may be negative for as long as 6 to 8 weeks; that is, the pulp is "stunned."

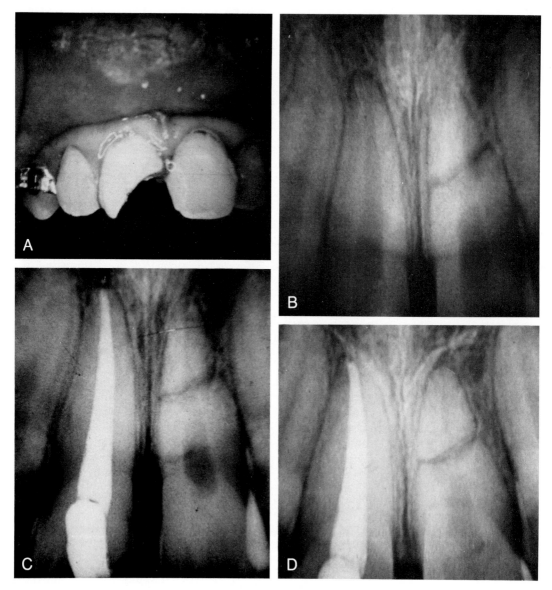

Fig. 16–1. Fractured central incisor (tooth No. 8). *A*, Labial view of fractured tooth No. 8. *B*, Diagnostic radiograph; the apical third of the root of tooth No. 9 is fractured. *C*, Recall radiograph 6 months after completion of endodontic treatment of tooth No. 8, in which pulp died; tooth No. 9 had been ligated only after the pulp tested vital to electric and cold stimuli. *D*, Recall radiograph at 1 year.

At first, the injured nerve bundles are paralyzed and do not respond, the blood vessels are torn, and hemorrhage may even be evident by a slight discoloration of the tooth (pinkish hue, "blushing" appearance) that gradually disappears as the tooth returns to its normal color. In time, *restituto ad integra* is accomplished, and the pulp responds to the electric pulp test, sparingly at first, but with an increasing response with the passage of time.

Although fracture of the crown is generally visible, the fracture may extend diagonally far under the gum. The radiograph is not always helpful in such cases because the fragment may be in close approximation to the root portion of the tooth and the alveolus. Removal of the fragment may be necessary to determine the extent of tissue damage. Horizontal and diagonal root fractures are best determined by radiograph, elongating the tooth image to accentuate the line of fracture.

Bacteriologic Features

The bacteriologic status of the pulp tissue or root canal of intact but traumatized teeth has been studied by MacDonald and colleagues,[30] as well as by Brown and Ruduloph.[12] Both groups found microorganisms, including anaerobic forms, in a higher percentage of cases than had previously been reported. MacDonald and associates found growth in 38 of 46 (82%) teeth studied, with anaerobic cocci constituting the third-largest group of microorganisms (32%).[30] Brown and Rudolph observed microbial forms in 90% of the 70 teeth studied, usually in a mixed infection with streptococci predominating; anaerobes constituted 23.9% of the microorganisms.[12] Engstrom and Frostell studied the bacteriologic status of 36 pulpless teeth with intact crowns, of teeth with enamel chips, or of those with small cavities.[18] Microorganisms were found in 26 teeth, of which 22 had areas of rarefaction. Eleven of the 26 infected and 8 of the uninfected teeth had intact crowns. Most of the organisms isolated were anaerobic, principally fusobacteria and streptococci. The root canals of 50 intact, traumatized, nonvital teeth were examined bacteriologically by Taklan.[45] He isolated microorganisms from all the teeth, mostly streptococci. Bacterial growth was obtained from intact pulp chambers, but not intact crowns, in 64% of 84 teeth by Bergenholtz.[10] Anaerobic organisms were isolated from 45% of 24 intact traumatized teeth by Kantz and Henry, who used the anaerobic glove-box method.[27] Wittgow and Sabistan obtained 31 obligate anaerobes from the root canals of 40 intact teeth with necrotic pulps using the VPI (Virginia Polytechnic Institute) method,[49] and Keudell and colleagues, using the same method, found 64% of necrotic pulps contained strict anaerobes, but none were found in vital pulps.[28] Sundqvist isolated microorganisms in 18 of 19 teeth with periapical lesions, but none in teeth without periapical rarefactions.[43] *Bacteroides melaninogenicus*, in combination with other microorganisms, was present in all teeth with painful symptoms. Grossman has shown that the source of the microorganisms in traumatized teeth is the gingival sulcus[20] (see Chap. 13).

Treatment

Treatment depends on the degree and type of pulp involvement, on whether it is exposed, and on other factors, as discussed in the following sections.

Fractured Crown without Pulp Exposure

The objective in treating a tooth with a fractured crown without pulp exposure is three-fold: (1) elimination of discomfort; (2) preservation of the vital pulp; and (3) restoration of the fractured crown. The tooth should be tested with the electric pulp tester or with ice or ethyl-chloride spray. If the pulp tests vital and the tooth is comfortable, it should be checked again within a week, month, 3 months, 6 months, and a year. Radiographs should be taken at 6-month intervals. If the pulp continues to respond normally during this time, the pulp can be assumed to have recovered. If progressively more current is necessary to elicit a vitality response, the pulpal prognosis is unfavorable, and the pulp will probably become necrotic necessitating endodontic treatment.

The exposed dentin should be protected by a sedative cement such as zinc-oxide-eugenol cement held in a crown form as soon after the fracture as possible. Vitality tests of the tooth can be conducted with ethyl-chloride spray or ice around the crown margins. If necessary, a cavity can be prepared lingually through the crown form until the enamel is reached, and an electric pulp test can be done in the usual manner. In a month, if the response continues to be within the normal range, a permanent restoration may be constructed for the tooth.

Zadek and associates reported a 2-year follow-up of 123 traumatized teeth in children.[51] Pathologic changes in the pulp usually occurred in 4 to 6 months. Of the 123 teeth, 109 reacted vital to the electric and cold tests after 1 to 2 years, but 12 required endodontic treatment, and the pulpal prognosis for the other 2 remained questionable.

Fractured Crown with Pulp Exposure

For a tooth with a fractured crown with pulp exposure, four kinds of treatment are possible: (1) pulpotomy (pulp is vital); (2) apexification (pulp is necrotic); (3) pulpectomy; endodontic treatment; and (4) root resection.

Pulpotomy. Pulpotomy is the operation of choice, rather than pulp capping, when the pulp exposure is 1 mm or more in diameter, when the pulp has been exposed less than 24 hours, when the pulp responds to vitality tests within normal limits, and when it does not appear to be grossly infected. Pulpotomy is particularly indicated if the root apex is not yet completely developed because maintaining the vitality of the pulp in the root enhances apexogenesis.

Generally speaking, the prognosis for the

continued vitality of the pulp is better following pulpotomy than following pulp capping. A tooth in which pulpotomy is performed also offers better support and retention of a restoration than one in which pulp capping was done. Cvek and colleagues have shown experimentally in monkeys that, in fracture of the crown of a vital tooth after 7 days, only about 2 mm of the pulp needs to be removed for a successful partial pulpotomy, using calcium hydroxide.[14]

The traumatized tooth with an incompletely formed root apex requires special consideration. The incompletely developed root end is funnel-shaped and, when examined microscopically, looks jagged and rough as a circular saw. In many respects, it suggests the root end of an exfoliated deciduous tooth. To fill such a canal properly is almost impossible, and every effort should be made to provide conditions that will permit complete formation of the apical end of the root. As long as some vital pulp tissue is left in the apical portion of the canal, the root end will continue to develop. Removal of the entire pulp tissue in the canal is contraindicated because apical development ceases, and one is confronted with a difficult task of both treating and filling the canal.

Apexification. Treatment by apexification should be tried when the pulp has died in a developing tooth with incomplete root formation. The presence or absence of an area of rarefaction surrounding the root has no significance in determining whether to use the apexification technique to induce completion of apexogenesis. An attempt should be made to encourage the development of hard tissue by inserting a calcium-hydroxide paste (made with a vehicle such as anesthetic solution or camphorated chlorophenol) throughout the entire canal, to facilitate obturation of the root canal after the formation of an apical "calcific barrier." The osteodentin or osteocementum cap that forms at the root apex serves as a stop for the gutta-percha filling and ensures an adequate seal. This procedure may be done even when an area of rarefaction has gradually developed.

Endodontic Treatment. When apical closure has not been achieved by apexification, endodontic treatment is often difficult. At this early age, the dentinal tubules are wide and permeable and provide recesses for growth of microorganisms. In many cases, the canal is wider than the largest size of root canal instruments available, and a satisfac-

tory job of cleansing the canal is not as readily done as in an adult tooth. To the difficulty in cleansing the canal properly may be added the further complication of considerable seepage into the root canal and the difficulty of obturating the canal because of its wide, flaring apical foramen.

The difficulty of seepage, that is, excessive periapical exudate flowing into the canal, is sometimes overcome by sealing calcium-hydroxide paste or zinc-iodide-iodine solution as a dressing for 24–48 hours. Either medicament may diminish periapical secretion. The difficulty in obturating the canal may be overcome by filling the canal with: (1) gutta-percha cone in reverse, that is, the butt end in contact with the apical foramen, as the primary cone in a condensation technique; (2) a thermoplasticized or similar type of gutta-percha filling that can flow against the walls near the apical foramen and form an adequate apical seal; or (3) a retrograde filling placed into the root apex during a periapical surgical procedure.

Pulpectomy. Total vital pulp extirpation, pulpectomy, is performed on a fully developed tooth whose clinical crown has been extensively fractured, resulting in pulp exposure. To restore such a tooth, a post-core crown is needed. This restoration requires the completion of endodontic treatment prior to the preparation of the post-core crown. Pulpectomy should be delayed, and a pulpotomy performed in the tooth with an incompletely developed root apex or one with a fractured root until apexogenesis and healing occur and endodontic treatment can be safely completed.

Fracture of Root

When a horizontal or diagonal fracture of the root occurs, one should immobilize the tooth by splinting it to adjacent teeth to keep it at rest. If the fracture is in the apical third of the root, the prognosis is favorable, provided the tooth is immobilized and it is not placed under undue pressure during mastication. The apposing tooth or teeth should be ground down, to minimize incisal-occlusal stress.

One should not remove the pulp unless it is known to be completely necrotic (Fig. 16–2). Tests for pulp vitality, such as cold application and electric pulp testing, are not reliable indicators of the status of the pulp because a "stunned pulp" may not be capable of a positive response to such tests for at

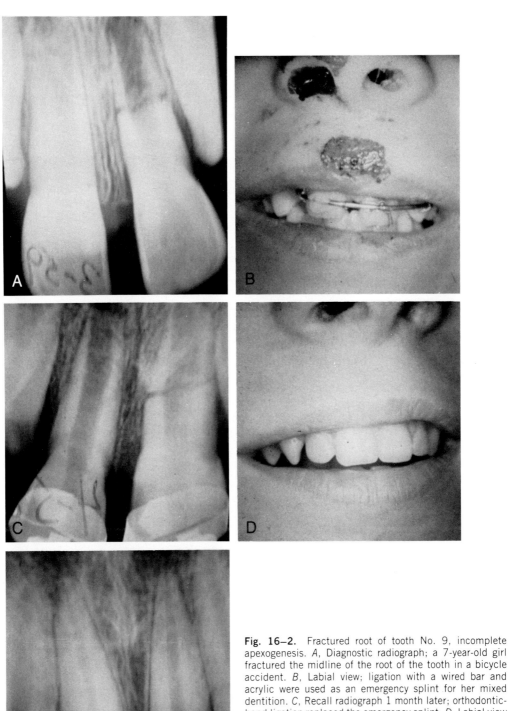

Fig. 16–2. Fractured root of tooth No. 9, incomplete apexogenesis. *A*, Diagnostic radiograph; a 7-year-old girl fractured the midline of the root of the tooth in a bicycle accident. *B*, Labial view; ligation with a wired bar and acrylic were used as an emergency splint for her mixed dentition. *C*, Recall radiograph 1 month later; orthodontic-band ligation replaced the emergency splint. *D*, Labial view 4 years later. *E*, Recall radiograph 4 years later.

least 6 to 8 weeks after the injury. According to Bender and Freedland,[8] pulps may retain their vitality following an intra-alveolar root fracture in as many as 75 to 80% of cases. The presence of vital pulp in the canal of a tooth with a fractured root enhances the possibility of hard tissue repair of the fragments.

Splinting may be done by ligating the fractured tooth to several adjacent teeth by extracoronal ligation. Several different methods can be used: (1) acid-etch technique cementation of plastic orthodontic brackets in composite, wired together with .01 dead-soft stainless steel wire and reinforced with resin; (2) acid-etch technique cementation of bonded resin with ligation using 20-lb monofilament plastic fishline and; (3) solid facial bonding of crowns of teeth adjacent to each other. Other splints can also be used, such as intracoronal acid-etch bonded resin, orthodontic-band wire ligation, or acrylic or cast splint cementation. The splint should be removed in 3 to 6 weeks, depending on the status of the alveolar bone surrounding the tooth, tooth mobility, and the overall root length of the tooth. The pulps of such teeth should be checked periodically for vitality, and radiographs should be taken. In most cases, the pulp remains vital. Successful cases followed over a period of years have been reported by Easlick,[16] MacLennan,[31] Michanowicz,[34] Spring,[42] Thoma,[46] and Wilbur.[48]

When a fracture occurs in the middle or coronal third of the root, the prognosis is less favorable because of the difficulty of immobilizing the tooth. Repair does not occur because of the constant movement of the tooth, as well as exposure of the pulp to the oral environment. In time, the tooth becomes loose and must be removed, or it may even be completely exfoliated as resorption occurs. On occasion, however, the apical fragment may be sufficiently long and may be supported by the surrounding periodontium to be satisfactorily retained. Intentional orthodontic extrusion (eruption) of the apical root is done to conserve existing alveolar bone and to expose sufficient root surface above the alveolar crest to enable one to construct post-core crown with tapered margins around the erupted root surface.[23,25,39]

A tooth whose root is fractured in its apical third has an excellent prognosis because the pulp in the apical fragment usually remains vital, and the tooth may remain firm in its socket. A mobile tooth should be ligated. If the pulp in the coronal fragment remains vital and the tooth is stable, with or without ligation, then no additional treatment will be indicated. In the event that the pulp in the coronal fragment dies, then endodontic treatment can be done, preferably limited to the coronal fragment. If the tooth fails to recover, the apical root fragment can be removed surgically (Fig. 16–3).

Andreasen and Hjorting-Hansen described three types of root repair following treatment of root fracture: (1) calcified tissue; (2) connective tissue; and (3) granulomatous tissue.[6] When the fragments are united by hard tissue, a form of dentin is found adjacent to the pulp, and a cementum-like tissue is found laterally. Repair may also occur by the deposition of cementum over the fractured surfaces of the fragments, with connective tissue growing between them. At times, bone may grow into the area between the separated fragments. When the treatment fails, granulomatous (inflamed granulation) tissue forms between the fractured segments of the root. At times, root resorption around the fracture site can be observed.

Following fracture, complete union of the parts does not usually occur. Healing of the fractured parts depends on the periodontal ligament. When the pulp remains vital, the

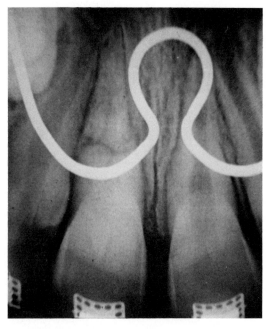

Fig. 16–3. Recall radiograph 2 years after fracture of the apical third of the root of tooth No. 8; a retainer is present. Note the calcification of the root canal in the coronal segment of the tooth.

blood clot organizes, and macrophages dispose of damaged tissue. A meshwork of granulation tissue develops; then fibroblasts appear on the scene and lay down fibrous tissue. This tissue is replaced by calcified tissue through the action of cementoblasts that cover the fractured root surfaces with cementum and, if the pulp is vital, odontoblasts that cover the medial fractured root surfaces with a dentin-like tissue. At times, the cementum extends into the canal and covers the irregular dentinal surface for a short distance. Connective tissue fills the space between the cementum-covered fragments. If however, a wide gap exists between the fragments, the fibrous tissue will either remain or be replaced by bone or bone-like substance.

At times, a layer of calcified repair tissue deposited across the pulp tissue at the line of fracture seals the upper and lower portions of the pulp. This repair tissue consists of both tubular dentin and uncalcified organic matrix, as reported by Manley and Marsland.[32] The histopathology of root fractures has been discussed by Blackwood,[11] Claus and Orban,[13] and others. Essentially, repair of the fractured root segments depends on the close, or at least near, apposition of the fragments, as well as on reasonable immobilization and the absence of infection.

Zachrisson and Jacobsen reported on 66 root-fractured teeth; the follow-up period ranged from 1 to 19 years, with a mean observation period of 5.2 years.[50] Repair of fractured sections occurred in 51 (77%) of the teeth. Necrotic pulps were present in 13 (20%). These investigators concluded the prognosis depends on the location of the fracture; the more apical the fracture, the better the prognosis.

Vertical Fracture

Vertical fracture of posterior teeth is not as amenable to conservative endodontic treatment as horizontal fracture (Fig. 16–4). The diagnosis is often difficult to establish by radiograph, percussion, or other means. In most cases, the patient complains of sensitivity and may or may not be able to locate the affected tooth. The tooth may react normally to the electric pulp test, or it may become hypersensitive. In the early stage, when a hair-line fracture is present and before separation of the fragments is evident, no radiographic changes are visible either in the tooth or in the adjacent bone. At times,

having the patient chew on a cotton applicator or rubber polishing wheel helps in identifying the tooth. Meister and colleagues have reported 32 cases of vertical root fracture and believe that most were due to condensation of gutta-percha.[33] In the other cases, the fractures were due to tapping inlays in place. Lommel and associates have reported 6 cases of vertical root fracture due to excessive pressure during condensation of gutta-percha, to cementation of an inlay in an endodontally treated tooth, and to cementation of a post.[29] Bender and Freedland are of the opinion that many root fractures are caused by excessive enlargement of the root canal with engine-driven instruments to receive a post-crown; occasionally, they may be due to traumatic occlusion.[9] Polson has described four cases of vertical root fracture that contributed to periodontal lesions.[38] Fracture lines were not always seen radiographically.

The prognosis of a tooth with a longitudinal (vertical) fracture depends on the location of the fracture. If the fracture passes through the clinical crown of a multirooted tooth and through its furcation, the prognosis may be favorable, provided the tooth can be hemisected. For example, a buccolingual fracture through the crown of a mandibular molar, extending into the bifurcation, can be treated. Endodontic therapy, followed by hemisection and full-coverage restoration of the mesial and distal segments, usually suffices.

If a vertical fracture occurs through the crown furcation of a maxillary molar in a mesiodistal plane, one should complete the endodontic treatment, and consider the following instead of extraction, whenever possible.

1. Section the crown through the trifurcation along the plane of fracture into two segments, the palatal segment and the buccal segment. Restore each segment with a coping that fits into a full-coverage temporary crown that can be made into a permanent restoration after recovery of the tooth. Failure can occur because of periodontal breakdown, the result of poor maintenance and improper home care in the trifurcation. Improper debridement results in pocket formation, root decay, and loss of supportive bone.

2. Section the crown into two segments, palatal and buccal, in the mesiodistal

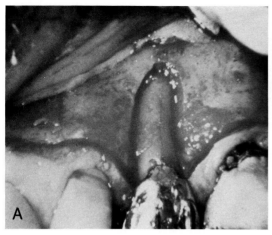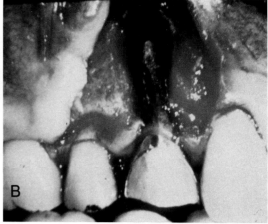

Fig. 16–4. *A* and *B*, Vertical root fracture. Buccal bone destruction results in an elliptic area of rarefaction in a radiograph. (Courtesy of Dr. I. Stephen Brown, Philadelphia, PA.)

plane of fracture, as before. Then remove either the distobuccal or mesio-buccal root, so that the trifurcation is accessible for home care after restoration of the remaining segments.

3. Section the crown into the two segments, palatal and buccal, and extract the less strategic of the two. Restore the remaining segment with a full-coverage restoration that has a narrower, contoured occlusal table, to limit the occlusal forces to the long axis of the roots of the retained segment.

4. Section the crown into two segments, and move the segments with orthodontic appliances into separate and adjacent units, splinted by full-coverage restorations.

When a longitudinal fracture of a root occurs, the prognosis for that root is usually hopeless. Oliet reported a series of cases in which the fractured segments were extracted, the segments were recemented with cyanoacrylate into a complete tooth, endodontic treatment was completed extraorally within 30 min, and the tooth was replanted into its original socket.[36] Although each of the teeth appeared to recover initially, treatment in all of them failed within 24 months because of failure of the cement bond, pocket formation, root resorption, or recurrent decay.

The successful termination of root fracture depends on the location of the fracture, on the proximity of the fractured surfaces, on whether the fracture is simple or comminuted, and on the ability to immobilize the fragments. In multirooted teeth, hemisection or radisectomy may be indicated.

LUXATED TEETH

Luxation is the displacement or dislocation of a tooth from its socket. Luxation may be partial, in which the tooth is partly displaced from its socket, or total, in which the tooth is completely avulsed from its socket. Luxated teeth may be intruded, that is, forced into the alveolar bone, but in most cases they are extruded, that is, forced out of the socket (Figs. 16–5 and 16–6).

WHO has classified tooth luxation (WHO Classification 873.66) into: concussion, in which a tooth is sensitive to percussion, but is not displaced; subluxation, in which a tooth has abnormal mobility, but is not displaced; and luxation, in which a tooth is loose and displaced. The WHO classification for intrusion (873.67) indicates displacement of the tooth into its socket accompanied by fracture of the alveolar socket, and extrusion (873.67) is partial displacement of a tooth out of its socket.[47]

When a tooth is partially luxated from a blow, the soft tissues become swollen and covered with blood, and the tooth may appear loose, especially if it is extruded. The periodontal ligament in such cases is usually torn in several places, if not entirely, depending on the amount of displacement. Grossman reported that luxated teeth are seldom fractured simultaneously.[21] He suggested that a blow that luxates teeth is usually received almost parallel with the long axis

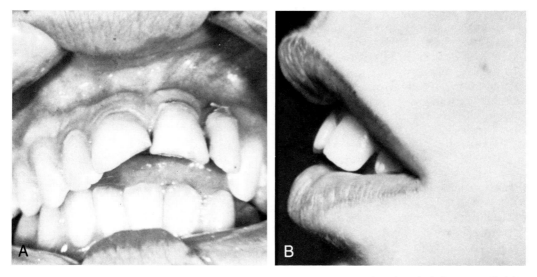

Fig. 16–5. *A*, Open bite. *B*, Overjet. Both conditions predispose persons to avulsion of teeth during traumatic injury.

of the tooth, rather than at right angles, and that a fracture is less likely to occur. Andreasen wrote that "most frequently, two or more teeth are luxated simultaneously, and that a number of luxations show concomitant crown or root fractures."[2]

With the exception of a diffuse ache in the area, effected by the blow, the patient complains of surprisingly little discomfort considering the appearance of the tissues. The tooth may feel numb shortly after the blow. Dumsha and Hovland found evidence of pulp necrosis in 51 of 52 partially displaced teeth, as determined by the development of periapical lesions, the absence of response to the electric pulp test, the painless entrance into root canals of unanesthetized teeth with an instrument, and the lack of bleeding.[15] One should be careful while testing the

degree of mobility of the tooth not to displace it further.

When the tooth is intruded, only a small portion of the crown may be visible because of swelling of the tissues and the amount of tooth intrusion. Intrusion occurs with greater frequency in primary teeth than in the permanent dentition. An intruded tooth is usually stable, in contrast to the mobility of extruded teeth. Diagnosis is readily established from the patient's history and by means of radiographic examination.

Treatment

An intruded tooth usually requires no immediate treatment, unless it is a primary tooth that can adversely affect the permanent tooth bud, because the tooth will slowly re-erupt. Emergency treatment is usually

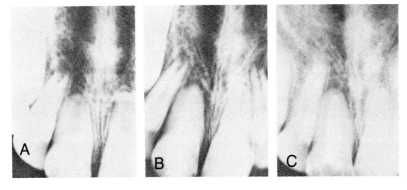

Fig. 16–6. *A*, Upper central incisor was accidentally avulsed; the tooth was washed in water and was replaced in its socket within 5 minutes by the child's mother. *B*, After endodontic treatment and obturation of the root canal. *C*, Eight years later; no evidence of root absorption or ankylosis is present.

accomplished by applying cold, to alleviate the swelling and pain and by stopping any bleeding. When return of the tooth to its original position in the socket is slow, the tooth may be actively erupted and properly positioned using an orthodontic appliance. Endodontic treatment may not be necessary unless the pulp of the intruded tooth dies; then, endodontic treatment must be done, for the tooth to recover. Frequent tests for vitality of the pulp should be made accordingly. When needed, root canal treatment should be done as soon as possible to forestall inflammatory root resorption.[35] The long-term prognosis for intruded teeth is poor.

Extruded teeth should be forced back into the socket as soon after the accident as possible. This procedure is preferably done with an anesthetic and by means of gentle finger pressure, or pressure may be exerted on a wooden tongue blade placed against the incisal surfaces of the adjacent teeth to force them back into their sockets. The affected tooth should be splinted using the extracorronal acid-etch resin technique. The tooth should be ground out of occlusion to prevent additional trauma. Depending on the degree of displacement, the pulp may survive and remain vital because the vascular supply to the pulp is not always severed or even impaired. The tooth should be tested for vitality once a month. Grossman reported a case of luxation of 5 teeth, with gradual recovery of vitality of the pulps in 3 teeth.[21] Return to a normal vitality index may be slow, but it should be complete or nearly complete within 6 months. When progressively more current is required to elicit a response to the electric pulp test, and when response to the cold test becomes weaker with time, a dying pulp should be suspected. If the pulp is found to be dead, endodontic treatment should be instituted at once, to prevent periapical involvement. If calcific metamorphosis becomes evident, endodontic intervention becomes a proper prophylactic measure.

BIBLIOGRAPHY

1. Anehill, S.: Svensk Tandlack. Tidskr., 62:367, 1969.
2. Andreasen, J.O.: Traumatic Injuries of the Teeth, 2nd Ed. Philadelphia, W.B. Saunders, 1981, p. 153.
3. Andreason, J.O.: Traumatic Injuries of the Teeth, 2nd Ed. Philadelphia, W.B. Saunders, 1981, p. 19.
4. Andreasen, J.O.: Traumatic Injuries of the Teeth, 2nd Ed. Philadelphia, W.B. Saunders, 1981, p. 40.
5. Andreasen, J.O.: Scand. J. Dent. Res., 78:273, 1970.
6. Andreasen, J.O., and Hjorting-Hansen, E.: Oral Surg., 25:414, 1967.
7. Bakland, L.K.: In Endodontics, 3rd Ed. (Edited by J.I. Ingle and J.F. Taintor). Philadelphia, Lea & Febiger, 1985, p. 708.
8. Bender, I.B., and Freedland, J.B.: J. Am. Dent.Assoc., 107:595, 1983.
9. Bender, I.B., and Freedland, J.B.: J. Am. Dent. Assoc., 107:413, 1983.
10. Bergenholtz, G.: Odontol. Revy., 25:347, 1974.
11. Blackwood, H.J.: Oral Surg., 12:360, 1959.
12. Brown, L.R., and Rudolph, C.B.: Oral Surg., 10:1094, 1957.
13. Claus, E.C., and Orban, B.: Oral Surg., 6:605, 1953.
14. Cvek, M., et al.: J. Endod., 8:391, 1982.
15. Dumsha, T., and Hovland, E.J.: J. Endod., 8:410, 1982.
16. Easlick, K.: Tex. Dent. J., 70:284, 1952.
17. Ellis, R.G.: The Classification and Treatment of Injuries to the Teeth of Children, 4th Ed., Chicago, Yearbook, 1961, p. 19.
18. Engstrom, B., and Frostell, G.: Acta Odontol. Scand., 19:23, 1961.
19. Grossman, L.I.: Endodontic Practice, 10th Ed. Philadelphia, Lea & Febiger, 1981, p. 345.
20. Grossman, L.I.: J. Dent. Res., 46:551, 1967.
21. Grossman, L.I.: Ann. Dent., 1:121, 1942.
22. Grundy, J.R.: Br. Dent. J., 106:312, 1959.
23. Heithersay, G.S.: J. Br. Endod. Soc., 8:74, 1975.
24. Heithersay, G.S., and Morile, A.J.: Aust. Dent. J., 27:368, 1982.
25. Ingber, J.S.: J. Period., 47:203, 1976.
26. Jacobsen, I., and Kerekes, K.: Scand. J. Dent. Res., 85:589, 1977.
27. Kantz, W.E., and Henry, C.A.: Arch. Oral Biol., 19:91, 1974.
28. Keudell, K., et al.: J. Endod., 2:146, 1976.
29. Lommel, T.J., et al.: Oral Surg., 45:909, 1978.
30. MacDonald, J.B., et al.: Oral Surg., 10:318, 1957.
31. MacLennan, W.D.: Dent. Pract., 32:492, 1957.
32. Manley, E.B., and Marsland, E.A.: Br. Dent. J., 93:199, 1952.
33. Meister, F., et al.: Oral Surg., 49:243, 1980.
34. Michanowicz, A.: Oral Surg., 16:1242, 1963.
35. Nicholls, E.: Endodontics, 3rd Ed. Bristol, England, J. Wright and Sons, 1984, p. 350.
36. Oliet, S.: J. Endod., 10:391, 1984.
37. Oliet, S.: Bull. Phila. Dent. Soc., 31:8, 1966.
38. Polson, A.M.: J. Period., 48:27, 1977.
39. Potashink, S.R., and Rosenberg, E.S.: J. Prosthet. Dent., 48:141, 1982.
40. Ritchie, G.M.: Br. Dent. J., 113:459, 1962.
41. Sinai, I.: J. Endod., 10:327, 1984.
42. Spring, P.N.: Ann. Dent., 18:44, 1959.
43. Sundqvist, G.: Bacteriological studies of necrotic dental pulps. In Umea University Odontological Dissertations. Umea, Sweden, Umea University Press, 1976.
44. Sweet, C.A.: J. Am. Dent. Assoc., 29:97, 1942.
45. Taklan, S.: J. Br. Endod. Soc., 7:75, 1974.
46. Thomas, G.E.: Fortnightly Rev., 24:7, 1952.
47. World Health Organization: Application of the International Classification of Diseases to Dentistry and Stomatology. IDC-DA, 2nd Ed. Geneva, World Health Organization, 1978.
48. Wilbur, H.M.: J. Am. Dent. Assoc., 44:1, 1952.
49. Wittgow, W.C., and Sabistan, C.S.: J. Endod., 1:168, 1975.
50. Zachrisson, B.V., and Jacobsen, I.: Scand. J. Dent. Res., 8:345, 1975.
51. Zadek, D., et al.: Oral Surg., 47:173, 1979.

17 Endodontic Surgery

The scope of endodontic surgery has expanded beyond apicoectomy (root resection, root amputation) to include periapical curettage, radisectomy, replantation, transplantation, implantation, trephination, incision for drainage, and root submergence. Root resection is still the most common form of periapical surgery (Fig. 17–1). Nevertheless, it is indicated in fewer than 5% of all endodontic patients. The success rate of surgical endodontics, however, is high, from 73 to 99%, depending on the criteria used for evaluating success.[32]

Persson reported a successful result following root resection in 73% of 26 teeth; 15% were doubtful, and 12% were failures.[33] Sommer reported a 95% success rate in more than 100 cases of root resection.[39] Phillips and Maxmen claimed a 99% success rate in more than 600 cases.[34] Oliet and Grossman reported that periapical surgery, when combined with endodontic treatment, was considered successful 90 to 99% of the time, depending on the criteria used for postsurgical evaluation.[32] Harty and associates have reported a success rate of 90% postoperatively.[18]

OBJECTIVE

As in all endodontic procedures, the objective of periapical surgery is to ensure the placement of a proper seal between the periodontium and the root canal foramina. When this seal cannot be achieved satisfactorily by working through the canal system (orthograde filling), a surgical procedure permits visual and manipulative control of the area and placement of the seal (retrograde filling) through the surgical site. The better the seal, the better the endodontic prognosis of the tooth; this feature accounts for the high percentage of healing in surgically treated teeth.

Periapical surgery can be classified as follows: (1) root resection or apical curettage following an orthograde filling, either in one stage, that is, immediate root resection, or in two stages, in which multiple appointments separate nonsurgical and surgical procedures; (2) orthograde filling during root resection or periapical curettage; (3) root resection and retrograde filling; and (4) root resection and retrograde filling following an orthograde filling (one- or two-stage procedures).

INDICATIONS

The primary indication for periradicular surgery is any circumstance in which direct vision and access to the periradicular region are needed for proper placement of a seal between the canal system and the periodontium. Therefore, whenever a root canal cannot be filled properly with an orthograde filling, endodontic surgery should be considered. Other possible indications are as follows:

1. Any condition or obstruction that prevents direct access to the apical third of the canal, such as:
   a. Anatomic: calcifications, curvatures, bifurcations, dens in dente, and pulp stones (Fig. 17–2).
   b. Iatrongenic: ledging, blockage from debris, broken instruments, old root canal fillings, and cemented posts (Fig. 17–3).
2. Periradicular disease associated with a foreign body: overfilled canals, excessive cement in the periodontium, broken instruments protruding into the apical tissue, and loose retrograde fillings.
3. Apical perforations: any perforation that cannot be sealed properly by a filling within the canal, or one that prevents the proper filling of the anatomic canal and perforation (Fig. 17–4).
4. Incomplete apexogenesis, with "blunderbuss" or other apices that do not respond to apical closure procedures (apexification) and are inadequately sealed with an orthograde filling.
5. Horizontally fractured root tip with periradicular disease.

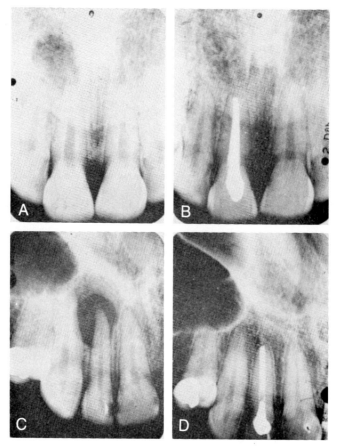

Fig. 17–1. A to D, Cysts of upper anterior teeth. A and C, Diagnostic radiographs. B and D, Check-up radiographs; note the complete repair of periapical bone.

6. Failure to heal following skilled nonsurgical endodontic treatment.
7. Persistent and recurring exacerbations during nonsurgical treatment or persistent, unexplainable pain after completion of nonsurgical treatment.
8. Treatment of any tooth with a suspicious lesion that requires a diagnostic biopsy.
9. Excessively large and intruding periapical lesion: marsupialization and decompression may be the preferred treatment (17–5).
10. Destruction of apical constricture of root canal due to uncontrolled instrumentation that results in an apical foramen that cannot be adequately sealed with an orthograde filling.

CONTRAINDICATIONS

The contraindications to periapical surgery are listed in the following sections.

General Considerations

1. Medically compromised or "brittle" patient: a patient with an active systemic disease such as uncontrolled diabetes, tuberculosis, syphilis, nephritis, blood dyscrasia, osteoradionecrosis, or any other medical condition in which the health of the patient restricts surgical treatment.
2. Emotionally distressed patient: a patient unable psychologically to withstand or cope with any surgical procedure.
3. Limitations in the surgical skill and experience of the operator.

Local Considerations

1. Localized acute inflammation: whereas emergency procedures such as incision and drainage or trephination may be indicated, elective periapical surgery should be avoided.
2. Anatomic considerations: procedures

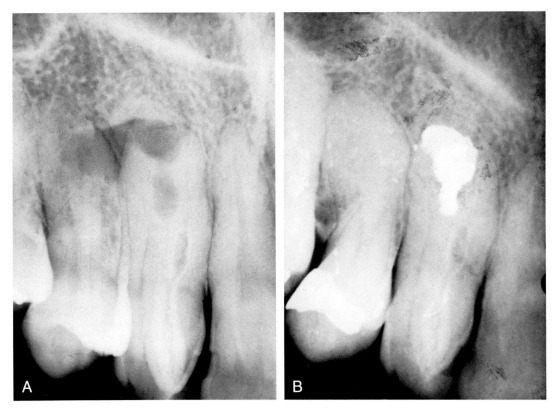

Fig. 17–2. *A,* Dens invaginatus of an upper premolar with an area of rarefaction. *B,* An amalgam resection was done to seal off the root canal, and the radiograph shows complete repair of periapical bone.

that penetrate the mandibular canal, maxillary sinus, mental foramen, floor of the nares, or that sever the greater palatine blood vessels should be avoided whenever possible.

3. Inaccessible surgical sites: inaccessible position and location of root apices, especially in posterior teeth, and the need to gain access to the surgical site through dense layers of bone, such as the lingual surface of molars or the external oblique ridge of the mandible, may preclude a successful result.

4. Teeth with a poor prognosis: short-rooted teeth, teeth with advanced periodontal disease, vertically fractured teeth, nonstrategic, and unrestorable teeth should not be considered for periapical surgery.

5. Finally, periapical surgery should not

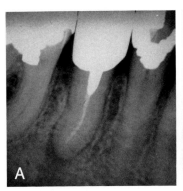
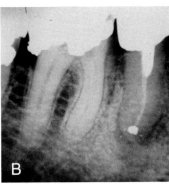
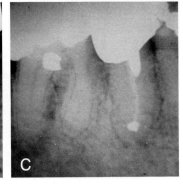

Fig. 17–3. *A,* Diagnostic radiograph; post-core restored premolar, previously filled with laterally condensed gutta-percha; recurrent sinus tract. *B,* Immediate postsurgical radiograph; amalgam retrofilling in the root apex. *C,* Recall radiograph at 6 months; bone regeneration is evident.

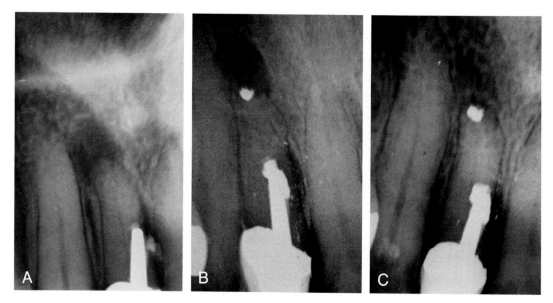

Fig. 17—4. *A,* Diagnostic radiograph; iatrogenic perforation with protruding post near the root's midline; untreated and unfilled root canal; periapical area of rarefaction. *B,* Postsurgical radiograph; lateral perforation has been sealed with amalgam, and retrofilled amalgam has been inserted in the root apex. *C,* Recall radiograph at 6 months; apical bone regeneration is evident; radiolucency persists at perforation site.

be considered as a cure-all to compensate for inadequate technique that resulted in failure to heal. Surgical treatment of teeth should not be done for expedience alone.

PREOPERATIVE CONSULTATION

A proper preoperative consultation is an essential part of the total surgical experience for both the patient and the clinician (Fig.

17—6). In addition to the necessary informed consent that the patient gives the clinician after a complete explanation of the contemplated procedures, the patient receives needed assurance that he will be treated expertly. The establishment of this rapport, the alleviation of the patient's anxieties, and the patient's reconfirmation of confidence in the dentist result in a coordinated team effort that should not be replaced or attempted by

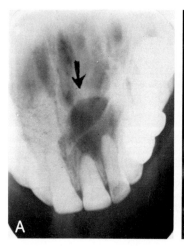
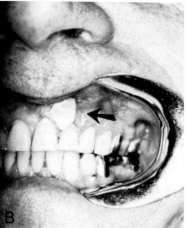
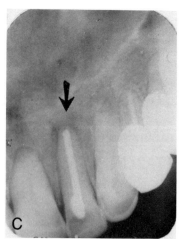

Fig. 17—5. *A,* Radiograph showing a large area of rarefaction over a left lateral incisor. Curettage at this time could disrupt and destroy the blood and nerve supply to adjacent teeth; the incision was made down to destroyed bone, and a rubber-dam drain was inserted (marsupialization). *B,* Rubber-dam drain in place. The drain was changed every 2 weeks until the area became smaller, when resection and curettage were done. *C,* Radiograph taken 1 year later.

SURGICAL ENDODONTICS (APICOECTOMY/CURETTAGE)
Information Sheet for Patients Requiring Endodontic Surgery

Informed Consent: Prior to any treatment you must be informed and understand:

    (a) What will be done.

    (b) How it will be done.

    (c) Why it will be done.

    (d) What constitutes a successful result (healing).

    (e) How likely are your chances of attaining success (healing).

    (f) What alternative treatments are available to you.

    (g) What risks you may encounter.

You may also be asked to sign a form granting the doctor permission to treat you with your full knowledge and understanding of the above.

Generally:

1. Surgical endodontics is a **PAINLESS PROCEDURE.**

2. Treatment is usually accomplished in the dental chair, using the same kind of anesthesia as for fillings.

3. Reactions can occur after treatment, such as:

    (a) Sore tooth and gum (pain).

    (b) Swelling, varying from slight to large.

    (c) Black-and-blue marks.

    (d) Paresthesia: a numbness or tingling sensation that persists in the treatment area, mainly the lower jaw, but usually disappears in time.

    Although these reactions do not occur routinely and are *not* usually dangerous, if any cause you concern, please call the office and notify the doctor so that he can continue to care for you properly.

4. Routine instructions will be given to you immediately following surgical treatment, regarding home care, diet, and medication.

5. No tooth will be treated unless there is a reasonable chance for success. If the chances for success are below average, you will be so informed.

6. Following completion of surgical endodontics, you will be referred back to your own dentist, who will restore the tooth with a filling or crown, if needed.

Fig. 17–6. Information and consultation sheet on root resection.

premedication alone. Frequently, a preoperative consultation obviates the need for premedication with barbiturates, antisialalogues, and other drugs, with their adverse side effects such as nausea, vomiting, and syncope.

PREMEDICATION

Premedication becomes necessary when a patient remains overly anxious and unaffected by the preoperative consultation. The premedication drugs selected should reduce anxiety, enhance the anesthetic to be administered, and favorably reduce salivation (antisialalogues), bleeding (epinephrine), or secondary infection (antibiotics).

Short-acting barbiturates, such as pentobarbital (Nembutal) and secobarbital (Seconal) are frequently used for sedation. Although they can be administered orally,

intramuscularly, intravenously, or by suppository, oral administration is most common, 50 to 150 mg, 30 min prior to the surgical treatment.

Tranquilizers are effective drugs for surgical premedication because they reduce apprehension, are sedatives, and act as muscle relaxants. They can potentiate the barbiturates and should be used cautiously in such combinations. Either meprobromate (Equanil), 400 mg 4 times daily for several days prior to treatment, or diazepam (Valium), 5 mg taken orally 30 min prior to treatment, is an effective tranquilizer and relaxant.

Narcotics can be effective premedication, but they are given infrequently to the ambulatory patient because of their lasting effect. The patient must be carefully monitored following the administration of these drugs, to prevent injury and accident after leaving the office. When sedatives or narcotics are given, the patient should be accompanied by a responsible adult.[8] Meperidine (Demerol), 50 mg, combined with premethazine (Phenergan), 25 mg, given intravenously, will provide excellent sedation. Unfortunately, these drugs may have unwanted side effects, such as nausea and vomiting, which can interfere with the surgical procedure.

SURGICAL INSTRUMENTS AND MATERIALS

A surgical setup should consist of all sterile instruments and materials needed to complete the contemplated procedure (Fig. 17–7). Too few instruments cause consternation for the surgeon who cannot efficiently and effectively complete the task. Too many

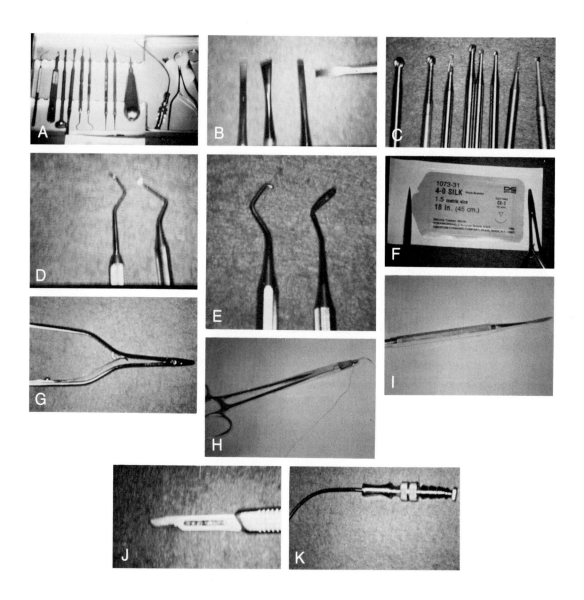

Fig. 17–7. *A*, Root resection kit. The sterilizable tray contains a periodontal probe, a Bard-Parker scalpel with a No. 15 blade, a Buckley chisel, a periosteal elevator and chisel, a periodontal curette (Goldman-Fox No. 3), a double-ended explorer, a plastic instrument, a retroamalgam plugger, a trephine, an aspirating tip, a needle holder, assorted burs, scissors, sutures with a needle, and cotton pellets. *B* to *K*, Surgical instruments. *B*, Chisels; *C*, SH burs, assorted round and tapered fissure burs; *D*, Goldman-Fox No. 3 double-ended curette, excavator; *E*, Retroamalgam plugger and plastic instrument; *F*, Atraumatic needle and silk suture, needle holder, scissors; *G*, Needle holder; *H*, Needle holder with scissors (Union Broach Co.); *I*, Periosteal elevator; *J*, Bard-Parker—blade No. 15—scalpel; and *K*, Aspirator tip.

instruments lead to confusion and hesitation during the surgical process. Because many instruments can be used for similar tasks, the operator can supplement or replace any instrument listed, to accommodate personal preference. A suggested surgical setup for periapical procedures follows:

1. Anesthesia. Aspirating syringe, disposable needle, and several Carpules of desired local anesthesia such as lidocaine HCl, 2%, epinephrine 1:50,000.
2. Isolation of the operative site. Sterile 2×2 cotton gauze squares, and cotton pellets or Racellets (alcohol sponges or topical antiseptic solution should be available to swab the operative site).
3. Incision. Bard-Parker handle, No. 15 blade, and periodontal probe (to help determine flap design).
4. Flap elevation and retraction. Periosteal elevator (Union Broach No. 9*).
5. Penetration and removal of cortical bone plate, root resection, and preparation for retrograde filling in the root apex. Assorted S.H. (straight-handpiece) burs Nos. 2, 4, 6, 8, 33½, 34, 558, 701, and 702, hand chisel (Hu-Friedy No. 1),† sterile saline or anesthetic solutions for use as a coolant and for debridement, handpiece (straight or contra-angle), and microhead contra-angle (Union Broach).
6. Curettage. Goldman-Fox No. 3 curette,‡ surgical excavator (Hu-Friedy No. 9 or No. 11).
7. Retrograde filling. Apical amalgam carrier, plastic instrument, apical amalgam plugger, and amalgam.
8. Suturing. Needle holder or hemostat, 3-0 or 4-0 silk suture on an atraumatic needle (Atraloc X-8 needle§ and 3-0 silk suture, FS-2 needle§ and 4-0 silk suture) and scissors.
9. Surgical tray. Cotton pliers, explorer, mirror, and cotton or Racellets.

TECHNIQUES

Anesthesia

Infiltration anesthesia, using an aspirating syringe, is adequate for most maxillary per-

*Union Broach Co., Long Island City, New York.
†Hu-Friedy, Chicago, Illinois.
‡Star Dental Co., Valley Forge, Pennsylvania.
§Ethicon, Inc., Somerville, New Jersey.

iapical surgery. The anesthetic is injected subperiosteally over the operative site, which extends laterally for an additional tooth on either side. A palatal injection of anesthetic solution completes the procedure and ensures a pain-free operation. If additional anesthetic is needed during the surgical procedure, the anesthetic can be injected directly into the bony medullary spaces inside the open wound.

Conduction anesthesia, in which the anesthetic solution is deposited near the mandibular foramen, is used for mandibular periapical surgery. Use an aspirating syringe to avoid injecting any local anesthetic into a blood vessel. If any blood appears in the Carpule, withdraw the needle and inject anew. When the patient reports midline lip symptoms indicating the effectiveness of the mandibular block, anesthetize the long buccal nerve, and infiltrate the mucosa around the operative site with additional anesthetic solution.

The choice of anesthetic is a matter of personal preference; usually, lidocaine HCl containing epinephrine 1:100,000 is used for a block, and lidocaine HCl containing epinephrine 1:50,000 is used for infiltration. The kind of anesthetic used, however, can be affected by the patient's medical status, such as by cardiovascular disease or allergies. A joint conference of the American Dental Association and the American Heart Association concluded that "the concentrations of vasoconstrictors normally used in dental local anesthetic solutions are not contraindicated in patients with cardiovascular disease when administered carefully *and* with *preliminary aspiration*."[3] A presurgical conference with the patient's physician is essential for all patients who are medically compromised or whose medical status is uncertain.

At times, two other anesthetic blocks can be used for periapical surgery. The first is the mandibular mental block, for lower anterior teeth mesial to the injection site. The needle is inserted into the mental foramen from a distal to a mesial direction, usually apical to and between the roots of both premolars, and a few drops of anesthetic are deposited. The other, a palatal injection, is used to block off the nasopalatine nerves by inserting the anesthetic solution into the incisive foramen. The nasopalatine block is readily achieved if the needle is inserted alongside the incisive papilla (not through it) and if the barrel of the syringe is aligned parallel to the long axis of the central incisor as the needle is advanced into the incisive foramen. A few drops of anesthetic are deposited for an effective block extending palatally from right to left cuspid.

The infraorbital injection is rarely needed for elective periapical surgery, nor is the posterior superior alveolar block. These injections are used in endodontics only in emergency situations, such as incision and drainage or trephination, to avoid insinuating needles and depositing anesthetic solutions into acutely inflamed and swollen tissue.

Flap Design and Preparation

A flap is designed to allow maximum manual and visual access to the operative site during periradicular surgical procedures (Fig. 17–8). In addition to access, other factors affect the design of a flap, such as underlying bone topography, status of the surrounding periodontium, tooth-root alignment, anatomic danger zones within the surgical site, and factors that affect healing of the flap. A well-designed flap permits clear access for successful surgical care and reduces the risk of objectionable postoperative sequelae.

The major components of flap design are the horizontal incision, which determines the lateral extension of the exposed surgical site, and the vertical or releasing incisions, which determine the limits of apical retraction. Incisions are made using a Bard-Parker scalpel with a No. 15 blade. The horizontal incision should extend for at least a tooth on each side of the tooth to be treated. The releasing incisions should permit sufficient flap retraction for access without tugging or tearing of the flap. The most frequently used flaps are semilunar, trapezoidal, triangular, and horizontally scalloped (Leubke-Ochsenbein).

Certain cardinal principles apply to all flap design, namely: (1) the base of the flap should be wider than the free end, to ensure adequate circulation into the flap; (2) the sutured flap margins should rest on solid cortical bone plate, whenever possible; (3) incisions should be made with a firm, continuous stroke, perpendicular to the cortical bone plate; short, intermittent incisions result in tissue tags and ragged margins that tear, retard healing, and scar; except for periodontal considerations related to underlying bony defect, the incision should be made to the cortical plate and the periosteum retracted with the flap, that is, a full-thickness flap of mucoperiosteum; (4) the flap should be designed with continuous curvatures between the horizontal and vertical incisions, to avoid sharp angles that tear; (5) a sinus tract, when present, should be included in the flap; (6) releasing incisions should be made between bony eminences because tissue over such structures is thin and stretches and tears when sutured; and (7) properly designed, a retracted flap can be held in position with passive pressure by means of a periosteal elevator pressed against underlying solid bone (Fig. 17–9).

The semilunar incision is used when no underlying periodontal problems are present. The horizontal component of this flap rests on alveolar bone structure at least 3 mm apical to the gingival crest and ends in the attached or "stippled" gingiva. Sutures passing through this fibrous tissue are less likely

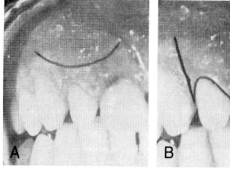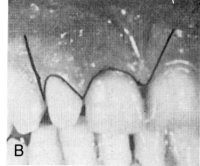

Fig. 17–8. Two types of incisions. *A*, Conventional semilunar incision extending toward the mesial and distal portions of adjacent teeth. *B*, Trapezoidal incision, used when extensive destruction of labial bone leaves one without a table of bone against which to suture.

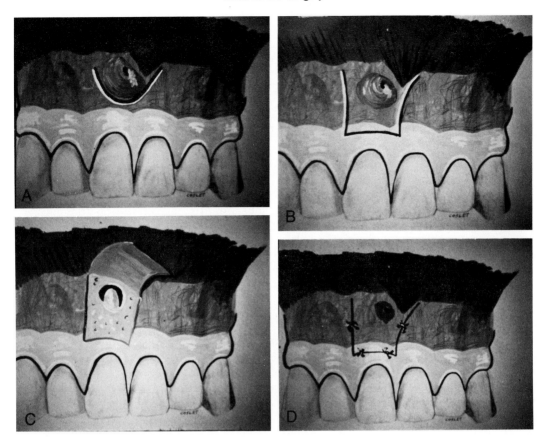

Fig. 17–9. Principles of flap design. *A,* Incorrect semilunar incision: Although the flap is wide enough and encompasses the sinus tract, it should extend into the attached (stippled) gingiva to increase access to the field of operation and to ensure retention of the sutures postoperatively. *B,* Trapezoidal incision: The base of the incision is wider than the incisal edge of the flap, to ensure an adequate blood supply and to aid in healing; the sinus tract is incorporated into the flap, and the horizontal incision lies in the attached gingiva and promotes suture retention; sharp margins permit correct flap replacement, but should be avoided, to prevent tissue tearing; round margins should be used instead. *C,* Elevated flap: Complete exposure of the operative field is possible, with access through the "window" in the cortical plate exposing the root apex and granulomatous tissue; the flap is retracted easily and has no tissue tension; flap margins end on the intact cortical plate. *D,* Coapted and sutured flap: Sutures are placed to hold the flap firmly in place without tension; intact sutures ensure healing by primary intention and are removed within a week. (From Oliet, S., and Grossman, L.I.: Compend. Contin. Ed., *4:*13, 1983; artist: Dr. George Coslet.)

to tear, and the gingival margins, especially around crowns, do not recede while healing.

The reverse or internal bevel incision is used when underlying periodontal problems exist around the teeth in the surgical site. The incision, made almost parallel to the long axis of the tooth into the crest of the gingival tissue to the crest of the existing alveolar bone beneath, connected by two vertical releasing incisions, exposes the entire tooth and supporting structures, to enable one to administer periodontal treatment, that is, curettage and root planing, during the surgical procedure. This incision protects the existing band of attached tissue, which can be sutured into a desired position alongside the tooth, and results in minimal loss or recession of

the tissue margins postoperatively. Because some recession does occur, the gingival margins around existing crowns are usually affected.

Flap Retraction

A full-thickness flap is retracted by inserting a periosteal elevator (Union Broach No. 9), into the vertical incision to the cortical plate and pushing the mucoperiosteum away from the bone with firm, continuous pressure. The opposite side of the flap can be released in a similar manner. The attached gingiva in the horizontal incision is separated and is firmly retracted apically. If the flap cannot be held with passive pressure after retraction, extend the vertical incision until the tension on the flap disappears. The flap can be held in a retracted position with the periosteal elevator or a Senn* retractor.

Removal of the Cortical Bone for Periapical Access

Once the flap is retracted, the exposed cortical bone over the periapical surgical site is removed (Fig. 17–10). This "window" is created by preparing 3 openings in the bone with a large, round bur, that is, an S.H. No.

*H. Schein, Inc., Port Washington, New York.

4 or No. 6, and sterile coolant, that is, sterile saline or anesthetic solution. Two of the openings penetrate the cortical plate adjacent to the mesial and distal sides of the root near its apical third. The third opening is made slightly beyond the root apex. The 3 openings are connected with a superficial cut by means of fissure burs, that is S.H. No. 701 or No. 702, and sterile coolant. A hand chisel, Hu-Friedy No. 1, is used to elevate and to remove the cut bone for preparation of "the window" and exposure of the periapical tissue.

Frequently, especially in the maxillary

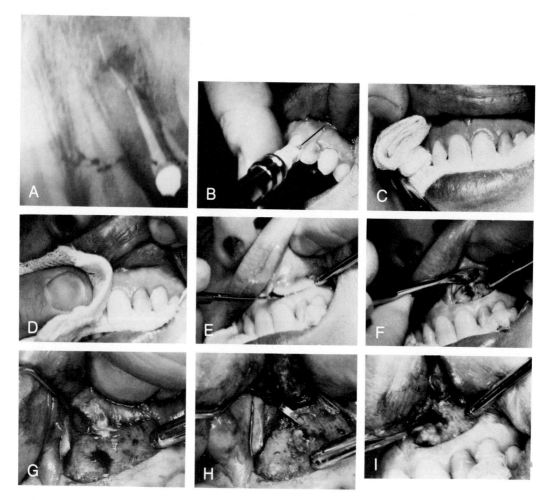

Fig. 17–10. Technique of root resection. *A,* Diagnostic radiograph of the upper left lateral incisor shows an area of rarefaction, with a gutta-percha filling through a perforated root. *B,* Anesthesia: Local infiltration of lidocaine HCl, 1:50,000 epinephrine, followed by anterior palatine block. *C,* Isolation of operative site: The patient bites gently on folded 2 × 2 sterile cotton gauze pads, additional pads are folded in the mucobuccal fold on both sides. *D,* Scrubbing of the surgical site: Scrub the surgical site with alcohol-wet sponges, including the upper and lower jaw, as well as the lips, chin, and adjacent facial tissue. *E,* Incision: Using a Bard-Parker scalpel, No. 15 blade, incise a semilunar, full mucoperiosteal flap in the attached gingiva. *F,* Retraction: Retract the released flap with a periosteal elevator. *G,* Curettage: Remove the extruded gutta-percha from the root perforation lying in the soft tissue and seal the perforation with the extruded gutta-percha. *H,* Exposure of the root tip: Remove the outer cortical bone plate and explore the periapical area with a curette to locate the root apex. *I,* Enlargement of the operative site: The "window" may be enlarged by hand chisel.

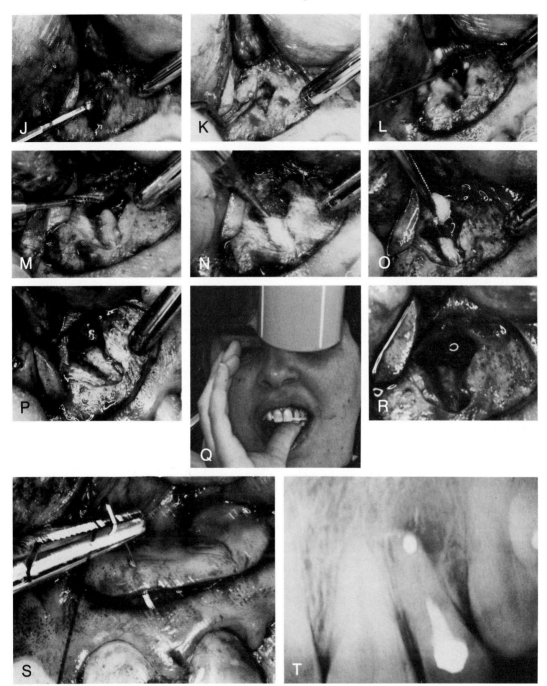

Fig. 17–10 continued. *J* Engine-driven SH burs can be used to enlarge the "window." *K*, Periapical curettage: Remove all granulomatous tissue with curettes or excavators. *L*, Debridement: Wash the periapex with sterile saline or anesthetic solution; aspirate. *M*, Root-tip resection: Bevel the root apex with a tapered fissure bur. *N*, Root-end preparation: Prepare a cavity at the apical foramen using round and inverted cone burs; keep the circumference as small as possible and extend the preparation about 2 mm into the canal; avoid root-end perforation. *O*, Isolation of exposed root-end preparation: Using sterile cotton pellets or cotton sponges isolate the cleaned root end to collect any amalgam "scatter" during condensation. *P*, Retroamalgam seal: Pack and condense amalgam into the prepared cavity, wipe margins clean, remove cotton sponges, irrigate, and aspirate to remove any unseen amalgam particles ("scatter"). *Q*, Radiograph: Verify proper position of the amalgam seal, locate any amalgam "scatter," check for any unexpected problems, such as additional roots. *R*, Blood clot: Allow blood clot to cover the entire surgical site; if necessary, create blood clot by curetting cancellous bone. *S*, Suture: Coapt and suture the flap using atraumatic needles with 3-0 or 4-0 silk suture. *T*, Postsurgical radiograph: Root-end is sealed with amalgam, and the midroot perforation is sealed with gutta-percha.

anterior region, the cortical plate can be penetrated with hand chisels or hand trephines alone. Penetrating the periapical tissue with hand instruments is more efficient than with burs, is less likely to gouge the root, and is less frightening for the patient. Once the initial access is completed and the root apex is located, the "window" can be extended by hand chisels. If the cortical bone is too thick, however, round or fissure burs and coolant should be used.

Hand instrumentation can be done in most cases when a sinus tract has penetrated the cortical plate or when an extensive area of "bone breakdown" exists around the root apex. Conversely, gaining access to the apex of a root with normal bone surrounding it is difficult, both to penetrate the solid bone and to distinguish between the root apex and bone in which it is embedded.

To determine the locale of the "window" and to locate the root apex when it is surrounded by normal bone, use the radiograph as a "road map." The radiographic tooth length and root anatomy can be measured and transferred to the mouth for orientation. The osseous topographic features overlying the root, that is, troughs in the mesial and distal aspects of the root and the eminence overlying the root itself, are useful, as well as the exposed tooth crown, for additional orientation. If the radiograph is accurate, then the measured length will be accurate, and the root apex may be localized under the bone plate. This area becomes the site for access preparation through the bone.

A radiopaque marker, such as a small piece of gutta-percha, can be placed on the cortical bone over the projected site of the root apex, and a radiograph can be exposed in the usual manner. This method is accurate for determining which structure is immediately beneath the marker, and it is especially useful in periapical surgery on posterior teeth, when accessibility is limited and orientation is uncertain.

Periapical Curettage and Root Resection

On removal of the cortical "window" bone, the tissues in the periradicular area become visible and accessible. Explore the exposed tissue, and locate the root apex while probing with an explorer or curette. Overfilling of the root canal, with gutta-percha protruding through the root apex, acts as an excellent marker for locating and identifying the root apex. Curette and remove all the pathologic

soft tissue surrounding the root down to the hard surrounding bone with a Goldman-Fox No. 3 curette or a surgical excavator. If complete curettage is hindered or obstructed by the presence of the root, the tip should be reduced carefully by shaving off about 1 to 3 mm with a tapered fissure bur, No. 702, until all the granulomatous tissue can be removed for biopsy.

Occasionally, the root and apex are difficult to localize even after removing the cortical bone plate, especially when the root is completely surrounded by intact bone and periodontal membrane. Using a Hu-Friedy No. 1 hand chisel, remove the overlying bone carefully without gouging the root until the root is exposed to sight. The root can be distinguished from its surrouding bone by its color, morphologic features, and hardness. Root structure is harder than the soft cancellous bone, with a defined anatomic outline and a different color when viewed in a washed and debrided operative field. Cambruzzi and associates described the use of methylene blue during endodontic surgery, to identify and isolate different structures around the root apex.[12]

On removal of all the soft pathologic tissue, the root is visually and tactilely inspected. The decision to resect the apical tip depends on the quality of the seal between the root canal and the surrounding periodontium. If the seal is satisfactory, such as usually follows an orthograde filling that is well condensed and preferably overfilled, periapical curettage and removal of the pathologic tissue and the extruded filling material will suffice.

The old concept of always resecting a root tip is no longer valid. A root is resected when its canals cannot be properly obturated, such as when an obstruction inside the canal precludes the placement of an adequate seal. Other indications for root resection are: (1) root perforation; (2) apical root fracture; (3) pathologic root defects; or (4) any anatomic factors that prevent the proper preparation and sealing of the canal such as calcified, bifurcated, or lateral and accessory canals.

On occasion, root resection alone converts an inadequately sealed canal to one that is well sealed and requires no retrograde filling, such as when shaving the root tip and removing the unfilled delta up to the gutta-percha filling, removing a horizontally fractured root tip and contouring the remainder of the retained root containing a properly sealed canal, removing a pathologic or iatrogenic defect in the apical root tip up to the level where the canal is properly sealed.

Retrograde Filling

A retrograde filling is placed in the apically resected root when the canal is poorly sealed from the surrounding tissue (Fig. 17–11). The technique used for resection and retrograde filling depends on the accessibility of the root tip in the operative site, the presence of hazardous anatomic structures surrounding the surgical site, the configuration, location, and accessibility of the apical foramina in the resected root, and the filling material to be used. The root is beveled, to achieve the access needed to expose, prepare, and fill all the foramina present on the resected root surface.

Therefore, a maxillary anterior tooth whose root apex is adjacent to the nasal fossa or is inaccessible because of root elongation or lingual inclination requires the removal of more root structure and a more obliquely beveled preparation. In addition to accessibility, the following factors can affect the root-end preparation: (1) the location of the apical foramen on a curved root; (2) the number, position, and shape of the foramina on the resected root apex; and (3) the location of a foramen on the root surface, such as occurs with root perforation or a lateral canal. Unlike with an anterior tooth, a retrograde filling in the root of a mandibular molar requires that more apical tooth structure be sacrificed to bevel the root tip, so the apical foramina can be exposed and sealed. For all molars, this procedure is complicated by the presence of the maxillary sinus, mental foramen, mandibular canal, and external oblique ridge. It is better to sacrifice more root structure than to lose the entire tooth eventually because of failure to seal the root apex properly. On the other hand, sufficient root must remain embedded in supporting bone to allow the tooth to be retained in a functional, healthy state after healing.

The cavity in the beveled surface of the root is prepared for a retrograde filling with small, round burs, No. $\frac{1}{2}$, 1, or 2, followed by inverted-cone burs, No. $33\frac{1}{2}$, 34, or 35. The microhead contra-angle (Union Broach) is a miniature handpiece that can be used effectively in the limited space of the operative site. The dimensional outline of the beveled root tip and the location of the apical

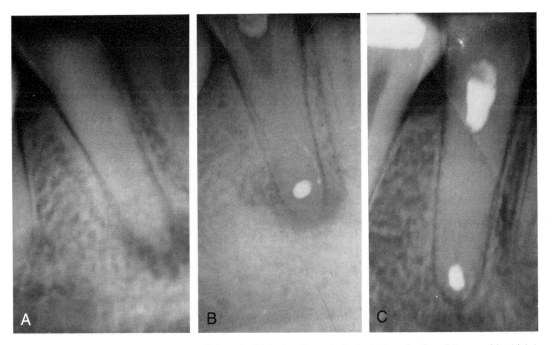

Fig. 17–11. Root resection with retrograde filling. A, Original radiograph: Periapical rarefaction of the cuspid, which has a calcified root canal; the patient has a history of pain and swelling around this tooth; the diagnosis is chronic alveolar abscess. B, Postsurgical radiograph: An attempt to find the root canal has been unsuccessful; the root has been resected and sealed with retrograde amalgam. C, Recall radiograph 1 year postoperatively: Bone regeneration is evident, and the patient has no symptoms. (From Oliet, S., and Grossman, L.I.: Compend. Contin. Ed., 4:14, 1983.)

foramen determine the size and shape of the surface preparation. The ideal preparation has the smallest exposed surface at the apex while encompassing all foramina and extends about 2 mm inside the root canal.

The rationale for keeping the exposed surface of the filling small and extending the filling deep into the root is to ensure an adequate, continual seal. Because root resorption can occur around the cut apex, a small, deep restoration is less likely to result in marginal leakage or to become a loose foreign body in the periapical tissues.

Apical Seal

The filling at the interface of the canal and periapical tissue should seal the root canal from the surrounding tissue. The most successful seal reported consists of the orthograde filling of condensed gutta-percha and cement, completing the obturation of the canal to the root apex.[24,37] Because an orthograde gutta-percha filling is easier to condense inside a prepared root canal preoperatively and results in a better seal than any retrograde filling placed intraoperatively, it is preferable to fill the root canal prior to the surgical procedure and to avoid placing a retrograde filling, whenever possible. In addition, gutta-percha is better tolerated and causes less periapical tissue toxicity than most retrograde filling materials.

Rud and colleagues have shown that the conventional orthograde filling of a root canal followed by resection resulted in a higher percentage of successful cases than retrograde sealing of the apex with amalgam.[38] Arwill and co-workers,[5] Barry and associates,[8] Holland and colleagues,[21] and Lehtinen and Aitasalo[26] also found retrograde amalgam fillings less successful than conventional canal obturation.

On occasion, however, a retrograde filling must be placed, usually when an orthograde gutta-percha and cement filling cannot be used to seal the canal to its apex. Some of the materials used for a retrograde filling are zinc and zinc-free amalgam, zinc-oxide-eugenol cements, Cavit, polycarboxylate cements, glass-ionomer cements, composite fillings, zinc-phosphate cement, silver cones, and gold foil. None of these materials are completely suitable for use as a retrograde filling, including amalgam, which is used most often.[35]

The technique of packing amalgam into a prepared cavity in the apical root tip follows:

1. Debride the operative site, wipe and dry the root tip, and isolate the root tip with sterile cotton pellets, to prevent any seepage into the cavity and to collect any excess amalgam particles that fall into the wound during packing and condensation. Place a varnish over the prepared cavity.
2. Pack the amalgam into the cavity using a KG retrofilling amalgam carrier (Union Broach), or a plastic instrument, PFI W3,* acting as an amalgam carrier, and condense the amalgam with a retrofill amalgam plugger, E-3*.
3. Wipe and adopt the margins of amalgam to dentin with a moist cotton pellet.
4. Remove all the cotton pellets surrounding the root apex cautiously, to prevent amalgam particles trapped in the cotton from falling into the surrounding tissues.
5. Irrigate the wound with sterile saline or anesthetic solution, and aspirate the solution thoroughly to debride the wound site.
6. Examine the root tip, filling, and surrounding tissue, both visually and radiographically, to ensure that the canals have been properly sealed, that the margins of amalgam to dentin are well adapted, and that no foreign-body amalgam particles or pathologic tissue debris remain in the wound site.

Some clinicians prefer to pack bone wax around the root apex and into the surgical site to control hemorrhage and collect amalgam ''scatter.'' Aurelio and colleagues reported a local chronic inflammatory reaction when bone wax was used,[6] and Robisek and associates reported the presence of bone wax in the lungs of animals shortly after it was placed in the cut sternum.[37] Bone wax is unnecessary and need not be used during root resection.

Amalgam, used as a retrograde filling, is not an ideal apical sealant (Fig. 17–12). Friend and Browne found that amalgam was well tolerated by periodontal tissues after 3 months,[15] and Feldmann and Nyborg reported that amalgam was tolerated better than gutta-percha in the periapical tissues.[14] Nevertheless, we have observed that amalgam can fail as a filling after several years of

---

*Premier Dental Products, Norristown, Pennsylvania.

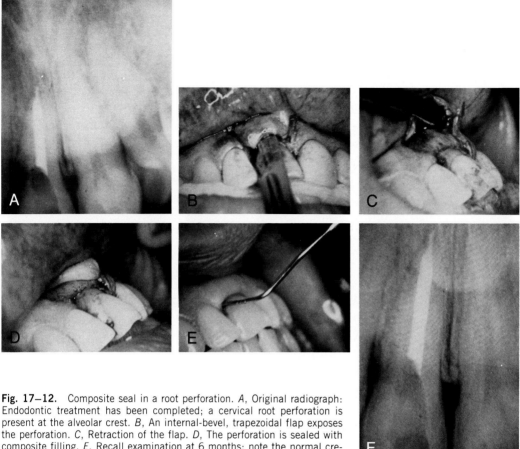

Fig. 17–12. Composite seal in a root perforation. *A,* Original radiograph: Endodontic treatment has been completed; a cervical root perforation is present at the alveolar crest. *B,* An internal-bevel, trapezoidal flap exposes the perforation. *C,* Retraction of the flap. *D,* The perforation is sealed with composite filling. *E,* Recall examination at 6 months; note the normal crevicular depth. *F,* Recall radiographs at 6 months.

apparent success. When bone trabeculation reappears around the root apex, as indicated by recall radiographs, subsequent recall radiographs taken 3 to 5 years later often show the presence of recurrent or persistent periapical rarefaction around the root apex (Fig. 17–13). Whether marginal adaptation is lost or resorption of the root occurs because of noxious stimuli from the surgical procedure, or from the chemophysical effect of the amalgam in situ, is unknown.

Other clinicians have recognized the need for a better retrograde filling, and other retrograde filling mateials have been used and evaluated. Mitchell reported poor results after using copper amalgam.[28] Gold foil has limited application and is too difficult to manage.[24] Polycarboxylate cement fillings seal poorly,[7,13] and root apices filled with Cavit, a zinc-oxide-polyvinyl cement fared poorly when compared with amalgam retrograde fillings.[16] Nicholls evaluated zinc-oxide-eugenol-type cements.[30] Although these cements are easy to manipulate, Niel-

sen reported that they resorb when exposed to periapical tissue fluids.[31] Stabholz and colleagues tested the marginal adaptation and sealability of five fillings: Restordent* sealed best, followed by, in descending order, zinc-phosphate cement, Cavit-W,† Duralon (Premier), and amalgam.[40]

Abdal and co-workers found glass-ionomer cements (ASPA)‡ Dentsply and Adaptic§ superior to amalgam when tested with a fluorescent dye for leakage.[1] Kos and associates reported that poly-HEMA is a better retrograde filling than zinc-free amalgam or gutta-percha,[25] whereas Kimura found little difference in periapical tissue reaction when zinc and nonzinc alloys were used for retrograde amalgam fillings, a reaction slightly in favor of the nonzinc alloys.[23]

Tronstad and colleagues have shown that

---

*Lee Pharmaceuticals, South El Monte, California.
†Premier Dental Products, Norristown, Pennsylvania.
‡Dentsply, Milford, Delaware.
§Johnson & Johnson, New Brunswick, New Jersey.

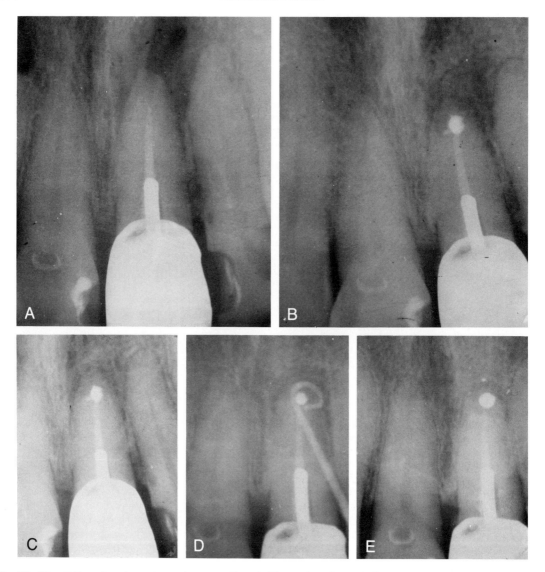

Fig. 17–13. Failure of a retrograde amalgam resection. *A,* Diagnostic radiograph of an upper left central incisor: Present are a periapical area of rarefaction, a poorly obturated root canal, and a post-crown restoration. *B,* Postsurgical radiograph: Retrograde amalgam is present in the root apex. *C,* Recall radiograph at 12 months: The area of rarefaction appears smaller. *D,* Diagnostic radiograph 4 years after the surgical procedure: A gutta-percha pointer inside the sinus tract extends to the resected root apex. *E,* Recall radiograph: 6 months after the original retrograde amalgam was replaced, the area appears smaller.

placing a varnish over the prepared cavity, followed by a retrograde amalgam filling, ensures a better seal.[41] Lin and associates are of the opinion that retrograde amalgam fillings should be done on all root apices, even though the canal has been obturated with gutta-percha.[27] Kaplan and associates found cold-burnished gutta-percha superior to heat-sealed gutta-percha or amalgam when these materials were tested for leakage with methylene blue.[22] If the apical seal is inadequate, or if cutting off the root tip adversely

affects the apical seal, as when root canals are filled with silver cones,[17] then a retrograde filling should be placed in the prepared root apex.

Completion of the Surgical Procedures

When the root apex has been sealed, the operative site is debrided thoroughly. A strong irrigating stream of sterile saline or anesthetic solution is flushed through and is aspirated from the surgical area. This procedure rids the wound of small bone splinters, soft tissue, and debris. It also helps to clear the wound of blood, to make it more visible for inspection, and to ensure that all pathologic tissue has been removed.

A radiograph is taken to verify that the retrograde seal is properly placed, that all roots have been properly prepared, that no root "spurs" or fragments remain, and that all foreign bodies, such as amalgam particles, cement, and gutta-percha, have been removed. This radiograph often shows a root canal filling apparently short of the resected root tip, owing to the beveling of root surface and to parallax. The filling appears at the radiographic apex only when the root end is cut at a right angle to the long axis of the tooth. This procedure cannot always be done, nor is it necessary.

Following irrigation, the wound is curetted to promote bleeding because "a normal blood clot is the best physiologic dressing for a wound." At times, various medicaments and materials have been placed into the wound to aid in clotting (Gelfoam), to combat infection (various topical antibiotic powders), and to enhance healing (hydroxyapatite). The practice of inserting foreign bodies into the wound site should be discontinued. Zillick[42] reported that the use of tricalcium phosphate (Synthos) or hydroxyapatite to fill the wound is questionable.

Suturing is done using an Atraloc X-8 needle and 3-0 silk suture or an FS-2 needle and 4-0 silk suture. Because sutures are easily torn from their sites, given the nature of the mucosal tissue, they should be inserted into fibrous tissue, that is, "stippled" or attached tissue, whenever possible. In addition, sutures should pass through the interproximal tissue between the teeth rather than the tissue surrounding the labial or buccal crown surface. For resection of a single tooth, 3 or 4 sutures are generally sufficient, except when suturing the tissue around the lower anterior teeth, where more sutures are necessary to offset the muscular pull from the lower lip during speech and mastication.

Following the surgical procedure, a brief discussion of the procedure and what it accomplished is followed by instructions to the patient on postsurgical care. Always assure the patient that you are available in case of need. Written instructions, to reinforce the oral instructions, should be given to every patient routinely, to avoid misunderstanding or confusion regarding postoperative care.

POSTOPERATIVE SEQUELAE

The following postoperative sequelae can occur after endodontic surgery:

1. Swelling. Although swelling does not occur in all cases following resection, it is sufficiently common to warrant every effort to prevent it, such as by keeping trauma to a minimum during the operation, by preventing undue development of heat during grinding of bone, by retracting the flap gently, albeit firmly, and by avoiding tugging of the tissue. Swelling will still occur in some cases, however. The most effective method for reducing swelling is the application of a cold compress on the face over the surgical area for approximately 20 min every hour postoperatively. Enzyme preparations and corticosteroids have been used, but are not recommended for routine use. Corticosteroids are contraindicated in patients with peptic ulcers, nephritis, diabetes, hypertension, congestive heart failure, and tuberculosis. When corticosteroids are used, the patient should be given an antibiotic because corticosteroids may interfere with repair of tissues and may predispose the patient to infection.

2. Pain. A modicum of pain is to be expected after an operation such as root resection, but some patients have no pain and others have considerable. Although the amount of pain is unpredictable, pain is usually a minor complaint and can generally be controlled with mild analgesics such as buffered aspirin.

3. Ecchymosis. Ths discoloration of the skin from extravasation and breakdown of blood in that area generally occurs adjacent to the surgical area, but it can travel along fascial tissue planes and may appear near the angle of the jaw, under the eye, and even in the neck and chest. These "black-and-blue" marks usually disappear within 2 weeks.

4. Paresthesia. A transient paresthesia sometimes lasts from a few days to a few weeks after root resection in any part of the jaw. Although paresthesia of the maxilla is rare, its occurrence has been observed following resection of the upper anterior teeth, and it lasts a few weeks. Paresthesia is more likely

to occur following resection of teeth in the mandible, especially the molars and premolars. It may last for several months to years, and, in rare instances, it may become permanent. Patients should be advised of this possibility before the operation.

5. Stitch abscess. Occasionally, a stitch abscess develops. Possible causes are local laceration of tissue during suturing, accumulation of food debris at the site of suturing, tying the knot in the line of incision, or irritation by the suture material itself.

6. Hemorrhage. Secondary hemorrhage is seldom observed following root resection. Slight oozing of the wound for several hours is usual. When hemorrhage occurs some time after the operation, a breakdown of the blood clot should be suspected. If cold compresses pressed over the site do not stop the bleeding, an injection should be made into the area, and the wound should be recurretted, irrigated with local anesthetic solution, and sutured.

7. Perforation. Perforation of the antrum may occur postoperatively in any of the maxillary teeth from cuspid to molar. Perforation into the antrum is not serious, provided no foreign bodies are introduced, a blood clot forms, and a suitable flap has been coapted and sutured properly. A prophylactic antibiotic should be considered, such as penicillin or erythromycin.

8. Iatrogenic damage to adjacent teeth. When the area of rarefaction is extensive and intrusive, it is always possible to disrupt the blood and nerve supply to adjacent teeth during curettage. To prevent this complication, routine root canal treatment and filling of the canal may be done first, followed by curettage limited to the affected root tip. The wound is packed with a rubber-dam drain, which is changed weekly for several weeks. When the area of rarefaction becomes smaller, a result similar to that achieved with the marsupialization technique, resection may be done without risk of damaging the blood supply to the adjacent teeth.

9. Incision failure. Failure of the incision to heal occurs infrequently. In most cases, it is due to extensive pathologic destruction of the labial alveolar bone to the degree that no table of bone exists under the sutured flap. It may also be due to persistence of infection, to fibrous adhesions that prevent the flap from being properly coapted, to irritation from a sharp edge of bone or resected root tip, or to accidental trauma to the flap. When flap failure occurs, the line of incision should be freshened with a Bard-Parker blade, granulation tissue under the flap should be curetted to stimulate the formation of a new clot, and the flap should be closely sutured. When a flap fails because of a missing table of bone, a laterally repositioned flap may be considered in selected patients.

Postsurgical Instructions

The patient should be instructed to apply an ice pack for 20 to 30 min each hour the first day, to reduce pain and swelling. The patient should not raise the lip to peek at the sutures or engage in extended conversation because such activity can tear out the sutures. The patient should avoid brushing the teeth near the surgical site; the sutures can be ripped out inadvertently by the toothbrush. In addition, a softer or semisolid diet, excluding gritty or chewy foods such as toast or steak, should be prescribed for the first few days. After eating, the patient should debride the wound by flushing it with a saline or bicarbonate-soda mouthwash. Most postoperative pain can be controlled with mild analgesics, such as aspirin, 5 to 10 mg, or acetaminophen (Tylenol), 300 mg taken every 4 hours as needed. If pain is severe, prescribe Tylenol No. 3 (acetaminophen containing half a grain of codeine), or Percodan, (oxycodone and aspirin), every 4 to 6 hours.

If warranted, antibiotics should be prescribed. The antibiotic of choice is penicillin V, orally administered, 1000 mg to start, followed by 500 mg 4 times daily for 3 to 4 days. The alternate antibiotic of choice in penicillin-allergic patients is erythromycin, 500 mg initially, then 250 mg every 6 hours for 3 to 4 days. Other antibiotics with similar spectra can be substituted. No antibiotic should be given routinely or indiscriminately to all patients, however. Use judicious care when prescribing narcotics or antibiotics for patients.

Additional instructions include the following: (1) in case of bleeding, apply constant, steady pressure, using an ice pack on the face over the surgical site for 20 to 30 min; (2) in the event of an emergency, call the dentist immediately; and (3) return to the office approximately 7 days later for suture removal (Fig. 17–14).

REPAIR

The initial repair that follows a periapical surgical procedure occurs across the margins of the line of incision. This healing by first intention usually occurs within 5 days, provided the sutures remain intact. Because healing takes place across the incisional margin, the length of the incision is not a factor in how quickly initial healing occurs. If the sutures tear or fail, however, then healing will occur through the formation of granulation tissue (second intention), a process lasting 4 to 6 weeks. At times, complete closure of such a wound can take over a year.

Repair of the periapical tissue is usually complete within a year, and progressive repair should be noticeable on a radiograph 6 months after the operation (Figs. 17–15 to 17–17). In many cases, the root canal appears to be incompletely filled because the cut root end is at an obtuse angle to the direction of the x-rays. When the periosteum has been destroyed during the operation and when the lingual or palatal plate of bone has been either pathologically destroyed or accidentally perforated, a radiolucent area ("surgical defect") will persist even though repair around the root apex, including the lamina dura, is complete. In such cases, repair occurs by means of noninflamed fibrous tissue, rather than bone. Such an area persists even if the tooth is extracted.

During the resection, necrotic bone, necrotic cementum, and granulomatous or cystic tissue, for example, are removed and are replaced by a blood clot. The formation and organization of the blood clot initiates the process of repair. This is followed by calcification. With a decreased need for vascularity and an increase in collagen, the capillaries disappear, and ossification begins, leading to healing eventually.

According to Andreasen and Rud, three main types of repair occur following root resection: (1) complete repair with restoration of the damaged periodontal ligament, with either mild or no inflammation; (2) repair with scar tissue adjacent to the periodontal ligament, with some degree of inflammation; and (3) scar tissue, with moderate inflammation.[4] Bhaskar reported minimal scar tissue in approximately 2400 teeth with periapical areas that had undergone resection and biopsy.[9] Successful repair following root resection, as determined by histologic examination, has been reported by Aisenberg,[2] Herbert,[19] Hill,[20] Moen,[29] Andreasen and Rud,[4] and others.[10,11]

Repair with new bone may occur 6 months to a year after root resection. This compares favorably with repair following extraction of a tooth, which may take much longer. In some cases, repair is slower, but repair following

---

INSTRUCTIONS FOLLOWING ROOT CANAL SURGERY

1. Apply ice (in plastic bag or ice pack) to face, at least 20 min in every hour. Repeat all day today and tomorrow if necessary to control swelling.

2. To prevent tearing of sutures and slowing of the healing process:
   (a) Do *not* raise the lip to look at operated area.
   (b) Keep talking to a minimum the first few days.
   (c) Do *not* brush area. Brush other parts of the mouth. Use mouth wash if desired, gently.

3. Do not eat gritty (i.e. toast) or chewy (i.e. steak) food for 3 to 5 days. Eat a soft diet; e.g., eggs, mashed potatoes, hamburgers, fruit juices, soups, malted milk, ice cream. Use a diet or vitamin supplement, if desired.

4. After the first day, use a warm salt-water mouth wash, gently, after meals (½ tsp salt to a glass of water).

5. If you are in pain, take prescription as directed; similarly, if antibiotics are needed, they will be prescribed with specific directions. **If any question or concern occurs, please call the office to notify the doctor.**

6. If bleeding occurs, place ice pack over area and hold with continuous gentle pressure until bleeding stops (approx. 20 min).

7. Return in approximately one week at scheduled appointment to have sutures removed.

Fig. 17–14. Information sheet for postsurgical home care.

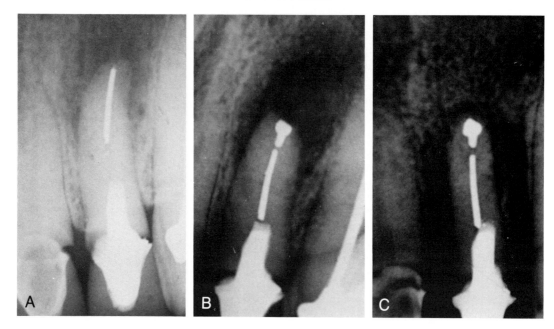

Fig. 17–15. Repair. *A*, Diagnostic radiograph: The periapical area is evident in a previously treated tooth whose root canal is obstructed by a post-core restoration. *B*, Postsurgical radiograph: Retrograde amalgam seal. *C*, Recall radiograph at 1 year; bone regeneration is evident.

root resection usually occurs more rapidly than that following simple root canal treatment for an equivalent periapical area.

Boyne and associates found, on reopening areas that had been resected, that the labial bone cortex was completely reformed after 5 months when the lesion was small, whereas larger areas had become smaller in that length of time, but had not completely healed.[11]

OUTLINE OF TECHNIQUE FOR IMMEDIATE ROOT RESECTION

The technique of immediate root resection may be summarized as follows:

1. On completion of the examination and diagnosis, consult with the patient to explain the reason for treatment, the method of treatment, and the possible postoperative sequelae. The consultation should establish a confident rapport between patient and dentist and should reduce the patient's anxiety concerning the proposed treatment.

2. Anesthetize the maxillary teeth by infiltration with approximately 1.8 ml of 2% lidocaine solution containing 1:50,000 epinephrine both buccally and palatally. The maxillary anterior teeth can be infiltrated labially, followed by conduction anesthesia of the nasopalatine

nerves with an injection into the incisive foramen. The mandibular teeth are anesthetized by conduction anesthesia, to block the mandibular nerve as it enters the mandibular foramen; use 2% lidocaine with 1:100,000 epinephrine, then a long buccal injection, followed by infiltration anesthesia in the tissue around the tooth. If pain occurs during the surgical procedure, an intraosseous injection into the medullary spaces of the bone surrounding the operative site will suffice.

3. Apply the rubber dam, and disinfect the operative field.

4. Establish the access opening into the pulp chamber aseptically.

5. Irrigate and debride the pulp chamber with a 5.2% sodium-hypochlorite solution, and aspirate.

6. Locate and instrument all the canals to the root apex with reamers or files in the presence of sodium-hypochlorite solution, and progressively increase the instrument sizes used until white shavings appear between the flutes, or up to three instrument sizes beyond the first instrument to bind near the root apex.

7. Irrigate the canal again, aspirate, and dry with sterile absorbent points.

8. Fit a gutta-percha cone into the root

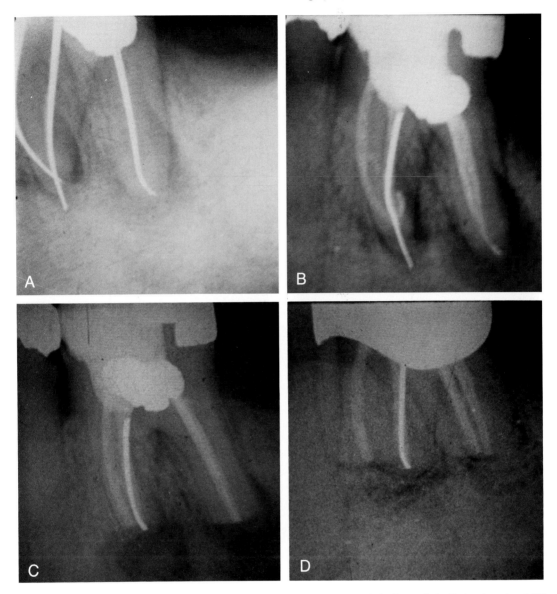

Fig. 17–16. Root resection. *A*, Diagnostic radiograph: A molar failed to heal following endodontic treatment and filling with silver cones. *B*, Retreatment radiograph: Several months after retreatment and filling of 3 of the 4 root canals with condensed gutta-percha, a sinus tract developed; the fourth root canal could not be retreated because of obstruction by an irretrievable silver cone. *C*, Postsurgical radiograph: The roots have been resected. *D*, Recall radiograph at 1 year: Bone regeneration is evident.

canal, by cutting a gutta-percha cone to the known working length of the tooth and inserting it into the root canal; when seated, the gutta-percha cone should bind at the root apex. No objection exists to overfilling the root canal. When the cone has been selected, the canal is dried and is coated with root canal cement, and the cone is inserted into the apex with pressure. Additional gutta-percha cones are compressed inside the canal, to form a tight seal.

Check the accuracy and quality of the filling with a radiograph. Overfilling is desirable because it helps the operator to locate the root end during root resection. The excess cement in the pulp chamber is removed, and the access cavity is sealed.

9. Remove the rubber dam. Replace the instruments and filling materials with a surgical tray and sterile set-up. Drape the patient with a sterile napkin, and don sterile rubber gloves to protect the

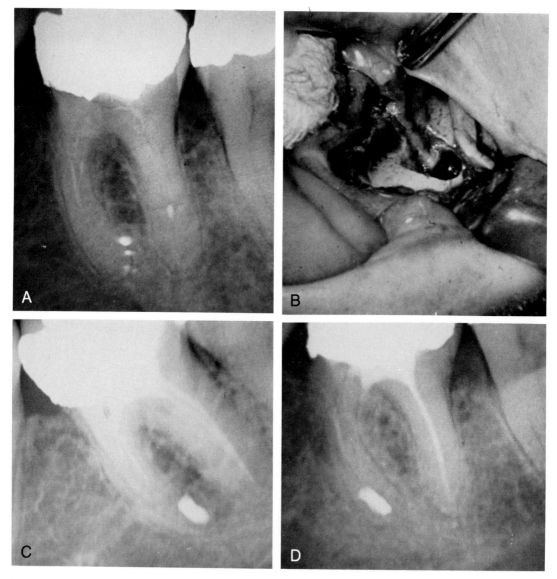

Fig. 17–17. Molar retrograde filling. *A*, Diagnostic radiograph: Recurrent acute symptoms from a mandibular first molar; a prior attempt to fill calcified root canals was apparently unsuccessful; the tooth was retreated, and the distal root canal was filled with gutta-percha; the mesial root canal was untreated because of root canal blockage. *B*, Surgical site: The mesial root is exposed in preparation for a retrograde amalgam seal. *C*, Postsurgical radiograph: The mesial root is sealed with retrograde amalgam. *D*, Recall radiograph at 6 months.

patient as well as yourself from secondary or coincidental infection.

10. Isolate the field of operation with sterile gauze, and scrub the patient's teeth and mucosa with an antiseptic solution.

11. Make a semilunar incision to the bone using a Bard-Parker scalpel with a No. 15 blade, and extend the incision beyond the distal surface of each adjacent tooth, to crest in the "stippled" or attached fibrous tissue surrounding the tooth.

12. Lift the flap away from the bone and retract it with a No. 9 periosteal elevator (Union Broach). An arched opening is made through the bone with engine-driven burs and a No. 1 Hu-Friedy hand chisel, to expose the root tip and adjacent soft tissue.

13. Curette the osseous bed thoroughly (Goldman-Fox No. 3 or Union Broach No. 10 curette).

14. If necessary, shave off 1 to 2 mm of the root tip, with a No. 702 or No. 558 bur,

under a sterile coolant spray of anesthetic or saline solution.

15. Irrigate, aspirate, and debride the wound with a sterile saline or anesthetic solution to remove bone chips, dentin chips, clotted blood, and debris. Inspect the surgical site visually and radiographically.

16. Induce the formation of a blood clot to fill the wound. If necessary, additional curettage will promote hemorrhage.

17. Return the flap to its original position and suture, using Atraloc X-8 needle and 3-0 silk suture or FS-2 needle with 4-0 silk sutures, held with a No. 8 Hu-Friedy needle-holder or Union Broach needle-holder-scissor.

18. Issue written postoperative instructions, and discuss postoperative care with the patient.

19. Remove the sutures in approximately a week.

ADDITIONAL SURGICAL PROCEDURES

At times, the endodontist is called on to perform other related surgical procedures. Using the surgical skills and knowledge needed for periapical surgery, the operator can achieve these surgical objectives by modifying and applying the previously described techniques.

Incision and Drainage

When the buildup of exudate (pus) is confined to the hard tissues, a dull, boring, excrutiating pressure pain develops. As the exudate penetrates the cortical plate, swelling occurs, and pain diminishes. When the swelling "points," that is, it localizes into a soft, fluctuant, palpable mass, it should be incised and drained, a procedure that dramatically reduces the swelling and pain.

Some clinicians prefer to anesthetize the area with conduction anesthesia (mandibular or infraorbital block) or peripheral infiltration, around but not in the swollen tissues, prior to incising, More often, a topical anesthetic, such as ethyl-chloride solution, is sprayed over the swollen area immediately preceding the incision. Although a topical anesthetic is minimally effective, it usually suffices for the quick, sharp thrust of the scalpel through the center of the soft, fluctuant mass down to the solid cortical bone plate. If, however, additional blunt dissection of the tissue is needed, or if trephination is con-

templated, the area must be adequately anesthetized for such procedures. A rubberdam "T" drain may be inserted for several days to prevent closure of the incision, but it is frequently unneeded and omitted.

If the swelling remains hard or indurated, then the swollen tissue should be bathed in saline rinses for 5 min every hour until it becomes soft and fluctuant, ready for incision. Some clinicians advocate incising even hard tissue whenever pain is present; they suggest that the tissues will drain eventually, and the pain will disappear sooner.

Trephination (Trepanation)

In trephination, a procedure used to relieve pain, the cortical bone is perforated by engine-driven burs or a hand-operated trephine, to release the buildup of pressure and exudate around the root apex of a tooth. If done correctly, trephination will afford emergency relief because, in effect, an artificial sinus tract is prepared through which trapped exudate in the bone is released.

The site must be anesthetized, an incision made to expose and penetrate the bone through the cortical plate with a large, round bur, No. 4 to No. 8, and with sterile coolant. Because the path of penetration must be a direct line to the periapical tissue surrounding the root apex, any deviation can cause irreparable damage to the root itself, such as from gouging and perforation, or to the surrounding tissue, such as from penetration into the mandibular canal or mental foramen. Trephination is therefore used infrequently as a means of pain control.

BIBLIOGRAPHY

1. Abdal, K., et al.: Oral Surg., 53:614, 1982.
2. Aisenberg, M.S.: J. Am. Dent. Assoc., 18:136, 1931.
3. American Dental Association: J. Am. Dent. Assoc., 68:333, 1964.
4. Andreasen, J.O., and Rud, J.: Int. J. Oral Surg., 1:148, 1972.
5. Arwill, T., et al.: Odontol. Revy., 25:27, 1974.
6. Aurelio, J., et al.: Oral Surg., 58:98, 1984.
7. Barry, G.N., and Fried, I.L.: J. Endod., 1:107, 1975.
8. Barry, G.N., et al.: Oral Surg., 39:806, 1975.
9. Bhaskar, S.N.: Oral Surg., 21:657, 1966.
10. Bhaskar, S.N., et al.: JAMA, 201:113, 1967.
11. Boyne, P.J., et al.: Oral Surg., 14:369, 1961.
12. Cambruzzi, J.V., et al.: J. Endod., 7:311, 1985.
13. Delivanis, P., and Tabibi, A.: Oral Surg., 45:273, 1978.
14. Feldmann, G., and Nyborg, H.: Odontol. Revy., 13:1, 1962.
15. Friend, L.A., and Browne, R.M.: Brit. Dent. J., 125:291, 1968.
16. Finne, K., et al.: Oral Surg., 43:621, 1977.

17. Harrison, J.W., and Todd, M.J.: Oral Surg., *50*:264, 1980.
18. Harty, F.J., et al.: Br. Dent. J., *129*:407, 1970.
19. Herbert, W.E.: Br. Dent. J., *70*:173, 1941.
20. Hill, T.J.: Dent. Cosmos, *73*:799, 1931.
21. Holland, R., et al.: Rev. Fac. Odontol. Araçatuba, *3*:23, 1974.
22. Kaplan, S.D., et al.: Oral Surg., *54*:583, 1982.
23. Kimura, J.T.: J. Endod., *8*:359, 1982.
24. Kopp, W.K., and Kresberg, H.: N.Y. State Dent. J., *39*:8, 1973.
25. Kos, W.L., et al.: J. Endod., *8*:355, 1982.
26. Lehtinen, R., and Aitasalo, K.: Proc. Finn. Dent. Soc., *68*:209, 1972.
27. Lin, L., et al.: J. Endod., *9*:496, 1983.
28. Mitchell, D.F.: J. Am. Dent. Assoc., *59*:954, 1959.
29. Moen, O.: J. Am. Dent. Assoc., *27*:1071, 1941.
30. Nicholls, E.: Oral Surg., *15*:463, 1962.
31. Nielsen, T.H.: Acta Odontol. Scand., *21*:159, 1963.
32. Oliet, S., and Grossman, L.I.: Compend. Contin. Ed., *4*:9, 1983.
33. Persson, G.: Int. J. Oral Surg., *11*:96, 1982.
34. Phillips, W.A., and Maxmen, H.A.: Dent. Dig., *47*:60, 1941.
35. Pitt Ford, T.R.: Int. Endod. J., *13*:89, 1980.
36. Reynolds, D.C.: Dent. Clin. North Am., *15*:319, 1971.
37. Robisek, F., et al.: Ann. Thorac. Surg., *31*:357, 1981.
38. Rud, J., et al.: Int. J. Oral Surg., *1*:258, 1972.
39. Sommer, R.F.: Am. J. Orthod. Oral Surg., *32*:76, 1946.
40. Stabholz, A., et al.: J. Endod., *11*:218, 1985.
41. Tronstad, L., et al.: J. Endod., *9*:351, 1983.
42. Zillick, R.M.: J. Endod., *10*:258, 1984.

18 Endodontic-Periodontic Interrelationship*

The tooth, its pulp, and its supporting structures must be viewed as a biologic unit. The interrelationships among these structures influence each other during health, function, and disease. Because the vitality of the tooth depends on its ability to function, and not on the viability of the pulp, the health of the structures is of prime importance.

Until recently, a tooth with a sinus tract draining through its gingival crevice was condemned to extraction.[8] Such a tooth was considered to have a hopeless periodontal prognosis; therefore, endodontic treatment was contraindicated. As a result, many teeth were sacrificed unnecessarily. Fortunately, the combined endodontic-periodontic lesion that affects a single tooth can now be diagnosed and treated successfully, with a predictable prognosis in many instances.[11,20,21]

CLASSIFICATION

Differential diagnosis can be a problem. Understanding the endodontic-periodontic relationship is essential because it frequently dictates the plan of treatment. Oliet and Pollock suggested a classification for the combined endodontic-periodontic lesion based on treatment procedures.[21] Although other valid classifications exist, based on etiologic factors, histopathology, or anatomic pathways,[30] the following classification is less complicated and directs the clinician to the appropriate treatment with an improved prognosis.

The endodontic-periodontic lesion can be classified into 3 different treatment categories:

I. Lesions that require endodontic treatment procedures only
 1. Any tooth with a necrotic pulp and apical granulomatous tissue replacing periodontium and bone, with or without a sinus tract (chronic periapical abscess).
 2. Chronic periapical abscess with a sinus tract draining through the gingival crevice, thus passing through a section of the attachment apparatus in its entire length alongside the root.
 3. Root fractures, longitudinal and horizontal.
 4. Root perforations, pathologic and iatrogenic.
 5. Teeth with incomplete apical root development and inflamed or necrotic pulps, with and without periapical pathosis.
 6. Endodontic implants.
 7. Replants, intentional or traumatic.
 8. Transplants, autotransplants or allotransplants.
 9. Teeth requiring hemisection or radisectomy.
 10. Root submergence.

II. Lesions that require periodontal treatment procedures only
 1. Occlusal trauma causing reversible pulpitis.
 2. Occlusal trauma plus gingival inflammation, resulting in pocket formation.
  a. Reversible but increased pulpal sensitivity caused by trauma or, possibly, by exposed dentinal tubules.
  b. Reversible but increased pulpal sensitivity caused by uncovering lateral or accessory canals exiting into the periodontium.
 3. Suprabony or infrabony pocket formation treated with overzealous root

*Portions of this chapter have been contributed jointly with George G. Stewart, Professor of Endodontics, School of Dental Medicine, University of Pennsylvania, Philadelphia. Portions of this chapter have been adapted, by permission, from: Oliet, S.: Treatment of the endodontic-periodontic lesion. *In* Current Therapy in Dentistry, Vol. 6. Edited by H. Goldman, et al. St. Louis, C.V. Mosby, 1977, p. 129.

planing and curettege, leading to pulpal sensitivity.

    4. Extensive infrabony pocket formation, extending beyond the root apex and sometimes coupled with lateral or apical resorption, yet with pulp that responds within normal limits to clinical testing.

III. Lesions that require combined endodontic-periodontic treatment procedures

    1. Any lesion in group I that results in irreversible reactions in the attachment apparatus and requires periodontic treatment.

    2. Any lesion in group II that results in irreversible reactions in pulp tissue and also requires endodontic treatment.

ETIOLOGIC FACTORS

Examination of the etiologic factors that cause group III lesions, which require combined treatment, indicates that these factors originate from one of the other two groups. For example, a progressing infrabony pocket exposes the pulp tissue to the oral environment by "uncovering" a lateral canal and resulting in irreversible pulpal inflammation. Both endodontic and periodontic therapy are required for healing to occur. Similarly, furcation bone loss can lead to pulp exposure by "uncovering" a subpulpal-floor accessory canal, with concomitant sequelae.[3,9,16,29,35]

Thus, it is possible for periodontal disease to cause secondary pulpal disease (Fig. 18–1).

Conversely, pulpal disease can cause periodontal disease. A pulpal infection can spread through lateral and accessory canals or apical foramina and may cause furcation breakdown, infrabony pocket formation, and periapical lesions. Conceivably, a persistent sinus tract draining through the gingival crevice could become an infrabony pocket and could require combined therapy, for healing to occur.

The length of time the etiologic factors persist in a susceptible environment is directly related to the probability that combined therapy (group III) will be needed. In other words, duration can be a key factor in evaluating etiologic effects.

The following are other possible predisposing factors leading to combined treatment:

I. Atypical anatomic factors

    1. Malalignment of a tooth, a predisposing factor to trauma; examples are food impaction and occlusal trauma.

    2. Presence of a multirooted tooth in a position usually occupied by a single-rooted tooth, or additional roots, separate or fused, in multirooted teeth.

    3. Presence of additional canals, with resultant changes in root morphology in single and multirooted teeth.

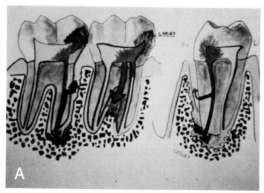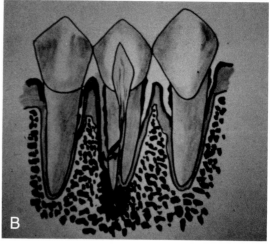

Fig. 18–1. *A*, Pulp disease progressing to periodontal disease through the apical foramina, lateral canal, or subpulpal-floor accessory canal and affecting the periradicular tissues. *B*, Periodontal disease progressing to pulp disease through the apical foramina in an infrabony pocket extending beyond the root apex, lateral canals, and accessory canals. (Artist: Dr. George Coslet.)

4. Cervical enamel projections into the furca of multirooted teeth.
5. Large lateral (accessory) canals in coronal and middle sections of roots.

II. Trauma

1. Combined with gingival inflammation, trauma can lead to deep periodontal pockets or, in multirooted teeth, furca exposure. If large lateral canals exit in the pocket area, the pulp will usually be exposed to the oral environment, and in addition to the periodontal problem, an irreversible pulpitis may occur.
2. Possible cause of crown fracture, root fracture, or root displacement, resulting in irreversible pulpitis, necrosis, or periapical disease.
3. Possible involvement of the pulp and disturbance of the periodontal membrane, with the resultant sinus tract draining through the periradicular tissue and exiting through the gingival crevice; a newly found "pathway of least resistance" that differs from the usual sinus tract, which drains through the labial or buccal mucosa.
4. Possible cellular changes in the pulp or periodontium leading to internal or external resorption associated with root perforation. Trauma to a tooth can originate from an accidental blow, cavity preparation and other restorative procedures, tooth separation, orthodontic treatment, malocclusion, and detrimental habits. Trauma appears to be a major etiologic factor in the formation of an endodontic-periodontic lesion.

III. Miscellaneous factors

1. Iatrogenic errors, such as perforation into the furcation of multirooted teeth during root canal therapy, root perforation during post preparation, or perforation in the apical part of a curved root during instrumentation.
2. Possibly, systemic factors, such as systemic disease as a cause of the combined lesion (for example, does diabetes increase the susceptibility of teeth and surrounding tissues causing combined lesions?).

Differentiation of a Sinus Tract from an Infrabony Pocket

It is clinically important to differentiate between a sinus tract draining into the gingival crevice and an infrabony pocket extending to the root apex of a tooth (Fig. 18–2). A sinus tract originates from the root canal and progresses occlusally from the apical foramina or from a lateral canal, whereas an infrabony pocket originates in the gingival crevice and progresses apically. Specifically, a sinus tract closes when routine endodontic procedures have been performed. Attacking the focus of infection within the root canal by instrumentation, by intracanal medication, or even by establishing drainage through an occlusal access opening usually results in tract closure in several days (group I). An infrabony pocket requires periodontal therapy, with or without endodontic treatment, to facilitate healing (group II or III). Fortunately, the clinical differentiation is simple because a sinus tract is narrow and can be traversed only with a thin diagnostic wire or gutta-percha cone, whereas an infrabony pocket, the result of extensive tissue destruction, can be probed with wider and large instruments.

CONTROVERSIAL ASPECTS CONCERNING THE COMBINED LESION

Pathways of Endodontic-Periodontic Disease

Pulpal disease can undoubtedly lead to periodontal disease; however, the concept that periodontal disease can cause pulpal disease remains controversial.[2,10,17,26] Chacker stated that periodontal disease would not usually cause pulpal disease because inflammation follows the venous drainage, and venous blood flows outward from the pulp into the periodontium.[4] Mazur and Massler reported no evidence of periodontal disease as a cause of pulpal disease, based on their studies of the pulp and periodontium.[19] One factor that was noticeably absent in their observations was the incidence of lateral or accessory canals and the possibility that such canals could be a pathway for progression of disease in either direction (Fig. 18–3). Czarnecki and Schilder also reported no causal relationship between periodontal disease and subsequent pulpal disease.[5]

Other investigators, such as Seltzer and Bender,[27] among others, showed that periodontal disease could cause pathologic pulpal changes, especially through the lateral or accessory canals. Stahl reported that experimentally induced gingival trauma in the

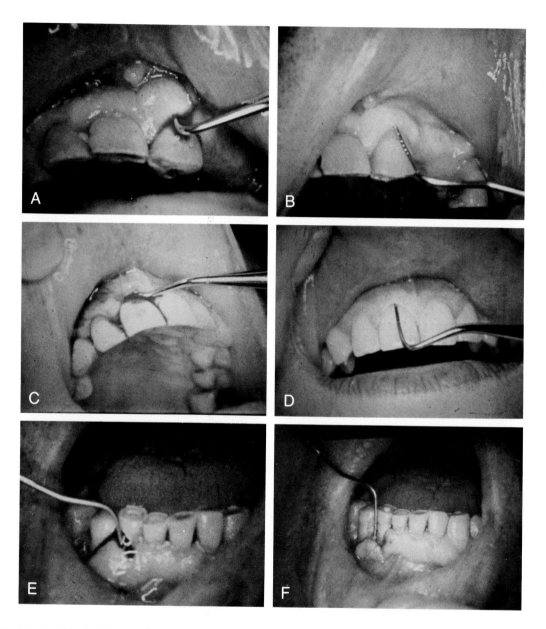

Fig. 18–2. *A* to *D*, Differentiation between sinus tracts and infrabony pockets. *A* and *C*, Sinus tracts draining through the sulcular crevice. *B* and *D*, Sinus tracts closed several days after the start of endodontic treatment. *E*, Infrabony pocket masked by swollen gingival tissue. *F*, Infrabony pocket evident several days later, after emergency periodontal care. An infrabony pocket is the result of extensive tissue destruction and may be differentiated from the fine, narrow sinus tract by the size and extent of the tract.

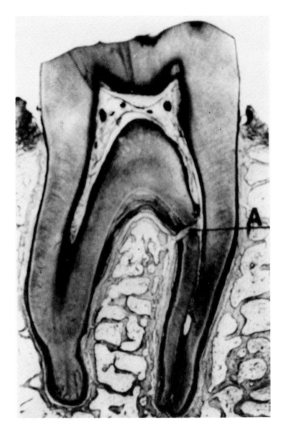

Fig. 18–3. Photomicrograph showing an accessory canal (A) at the midroot of a lower molar. (From Johnston, H.B., and Orban, B.: J. Endod., 3:21, 1948.)

molar regions of rats resulted in demonstrable deleterious effects on the pulp.[33] Apparently, the presence of patent lateral or accessory canals is an important factor in the development of pulpoperiodontal disease of the individual tooth.[20,21] Although other pathways exist,[31] such as open dentinal tubules, root perforations, or exposed apical foramina, the "uncovered" lateral canal may be a likely cause of periodontal disease progressing into pulpoperiodontal disease, the combined lesion.

Lateral or Accessory Canals

Yet the complete role of lateral or accessory canals in the endodontic-periodontic continuum is still uncertain. Does every exposed lateral or accessory canal result in irreversible pulpitis? Studies of the incidence and location of lateral and accessory canals describe these canals as common, with their foramina located anywhere on the root surface (Fig. 18–4). Perlich and associates found 5 teeth with accessory canals in the furcation area of 62 human molars examined under the

scanning electron microscope.[22] Kirkham examined 100 extracted teeth and found that only 2% had accessory canals in the periodontally involved furcation area.[15] Other investigators found significant numbers of molars, as many as 59%, with lateral canals exiting into the furcation area.[3,16,29,35] If one were to compare this frequency with the frequency of infrabony pocket formation or furcation breakdown, the numbers of combined lesions would be astounding. Obviously, the incidence of the combined lesion does not reflect such large numbers of cases. Although Seltzer and Bender and others have conclusively shown a localized pathologic reaction in the pulp tissue adjacent to an exposed lateral canal,[27] it would seem that not every exposed lateral canal results in an irreversible pulpitis; rather, the pulp, as a hardy tissue, has the capability of defense and repair of many exposed lateral (accessory) canals. The prognosis of the involved pulp depends on many localized factors such as tissue resistance, pathogenicity of the microbial flora, size and patency of the canal lumen, and possible systemic factors. Weine concluded that such canals can cause pain and may simulate periodontal disease.[36]

Sequence of Treatment

Another controversial aspect of the treatment of the combined lesion is the order of treatment procedures. Some clinicians suggest that initial treatment be either endodontic or periodontic, depending on the origin of the initiating disease. Others recommend that partial endodontic treatment be performed through canal preparation and medication, followed by periodontal therapy, before finally finishing the endodontic procedures once a successful periodontal result has been achieved.[24] We suggest that endodontic treatment should precede periodontal therapy, regardless of the cause of disease.

An example of a major clinical problem in treating the combined lesion is when the root of a molar is cut off, especially through the chamber, before endodontic treatment is completed. The destruction of the anatomic "guideposts," in addition to the loss of aseptic technique, complicates the treatment and reduces the endodontic prognosis unnecessarily. On exceptional occasions, the periodontal procedure should precede the endodontic treatment, such as when an unexpected need arises for radisectomy of a multirooted tooth exposed during a perio-

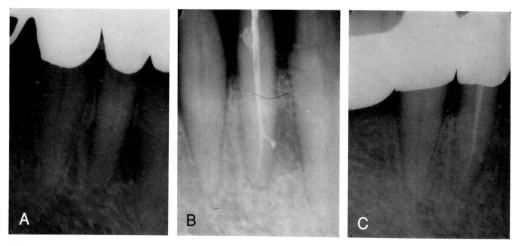

Fig. 18—4. Lateral canal in a lower premolar. *A,* Diagnostic radiograph: An area of rarefaction is visible near the apical third of the root. *B,* Obturation radiograph: Gutta-percha and cement are condensed into the lateral canal, whose foramen is near the area of rarefaction. *C,* Recall radiograph at 6 months: Bone regeneration is evident.

dontal surgical procedure; however, careful assessment of the anticipated treatment will keep such exceptions to a minimum.

Case Selection

Another problem requiring clinical judgment is the patient whose symptoms are borderline between group II (periodontal treatment only) and group III (combined therapy). For example, does one routinely use combined therapy whenever an infrabony pocket is extensive, sometimes reaching beyond the root apex? Actually, the problem is synonymous with the original controversy regarding the possibility of pulpal sequelae of periodontal disease. It is contraindicated to treat such a tooth with combined therapy routinely. The decision on treatment procedures depends on many factors. If the pulp tests normal to all clinical tests of vitality (electric pulp test, cold test), does not react abnormally (painfully) to heat application, and functions properly without causing pain, one might restrict treatment to the periodontal problem only, observe the results, and re-evaluate healing after a reasonable length of time. Endodontic treatment can be initiated at a later date, if necessary (Fig. 18–5).

On the other hand, the periodontist may request immediate endodontic treatment prophylactically to eliminate the possibility of imminent pulp disease that would interfere with periodontal healing. Justification for intentional extirpation of a "normal" pulp has clinical precedence, such as when a post-core is needed to retain a crown res-

toration on a tooth. At best, this treatment is based on the judgment of the clinician.

Other clinical problems that can be classified under group I (requiring endodontic treatment procedures only) are: horizontal root fractures, vertical root fractures, root perforations, root-end closures (apexification), hemisection and radisectomy, endodontic implants, replants, transplants, and root submergence (Fig. 18–6).

PERFORATIONS

Two causes of crown-root perforations are known: iatrogenic and pathologic. Iatrogenic and pathologic destruction of the clinical crown can be resolved, provided the root and supporting structures remain intact, by a full-coverage post-core restoration after endodontic preparation of the root. At times, crown perforation, coupled with extensive root destruction, such as occurs with internal or external resorption, can necessitate tooth extraction because endodontic treatment and proper restoration may not be possible (Fig. 18–7).

Iatrogenic Root Perforations

Iatrogenic root perforations are common. Root perforation by engine-driven burs and reamers occurs infrequently during post preparation, whereas the more frequent perforation of the curved root apex, caused by failure to negotiate the canal curvature during instrumentation, is often unrecognized. Another cause of root perforation is instru-

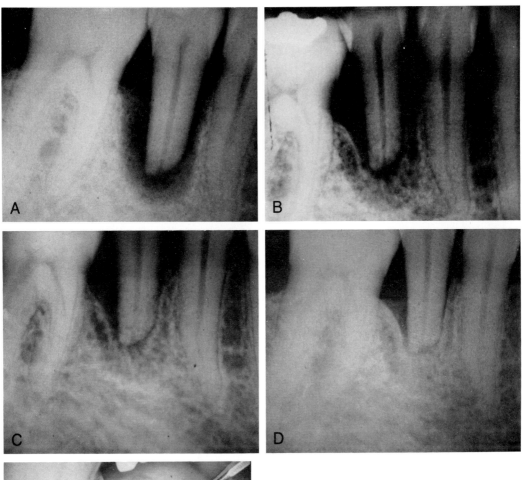

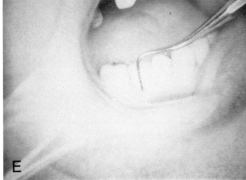

Fig. 18–5. *A*, Diagnostic radiograph: An infrabony pocket in a lower premolar extends beyond the resorbed root tip; the pulp tested vital within normal limits during electric and cold pulp testing. *B*, Recall radiograph 3 months after root planing and curettage. Recall radiographs at 6 months (*C*) and 2 years (*D*). *E*, Buccal view 2 years after treatment.

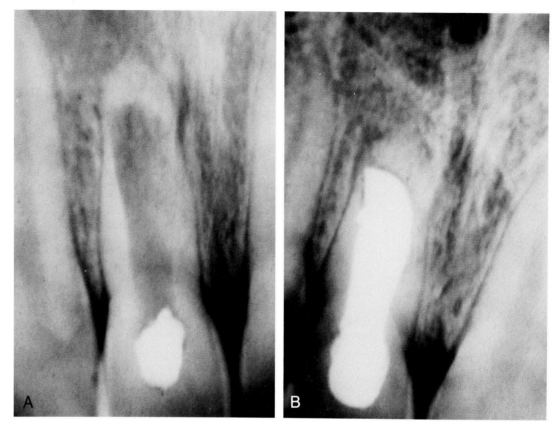

Fig. 18–6. *A*, Radiograph after apexification. *B*, Radiograph after obturation.

mentation of a root canal with instruments that are too large or too rigid, such as the use of a Gates-Glidden drill to enlarge the coronal orifice of a canal located in a narrow slender root. At times, with engine-driven instruments, combined with chelating agents to make the dentin friable, one can perforate the lateral wall or the apically curved root inadvertently. The apical perforation precludes access to the last 3 or 4 mm of the canal. Untreated or unfilled, this part of the apical canal remains a focus of infection, resulting in ongoing periapical disease. Skill and caution, with judicious use of instrument force and size, help to avoid this error.

Another problem with apical perforation occurs during endodontic implantation, sometimes intentionally. In placing an inflexible endodontic implant in a curved root, the root is perforated to seat this implant into the spongy alveolar bone. Some clinicians also perforate both sides of a previously treated

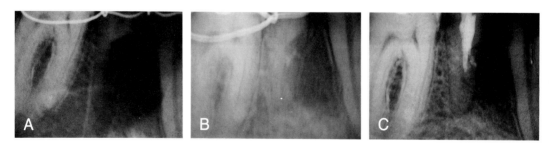

Fig. 18–7. Iatrogenic perforation of a lower premolar. *A*, Diagnostic radiograph: The root had been partially resected inadvertently during surgical removal of an adjacent impacted premolar; the tooth was ligated because of excessive mobility. *B*, Apexification radiograph: Calcium hydroxide paste is inserted for several months. *C*, Obturation radiograph: The root canal is filled with gutta-percha up to the perforation; the tooth is stable, and bone regeneration is evident.

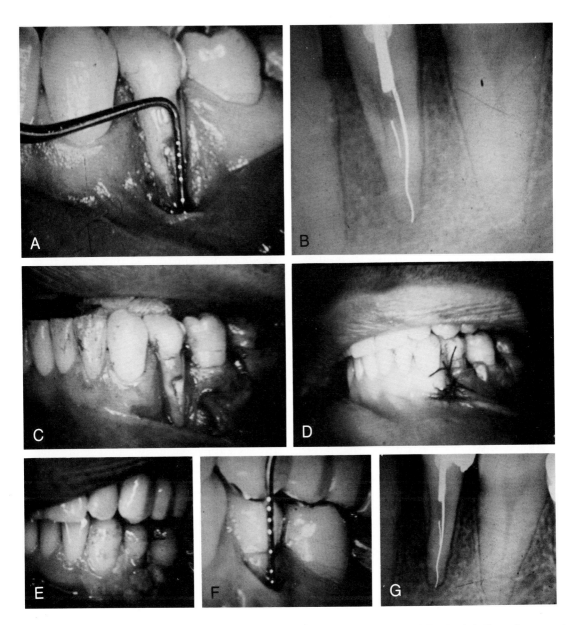

Fig. 18–8. Root decay of a lower premolar. *A*, Buccal view: A periodontal probe in the cleft extends to the root apex; root decay is evident on the buccal midroot surface. *B*, Obturation radiograph: The bifurcated root canals are filled with silver cones; the second root canal is filled through an access preparation created after removal of the decay. *C*, Releasing incisions free the full mucoperiosteal flap and also release the frenum and muscular pull. *D*, The laterally repositioned flap is sutured. *E*, Buccal view 3 weeks postoperatively. *F*, Buccal view at 2 years: Evident are recessed gingiva and normal crevicular depth. *G*, Recall radiograph at 2 years.

root to place an implant horizontally through the root of a malpositioned tooth because a conventional implant insertion would perforate the cortical bone plate and would fail. The prognosis for teeth treated in this way is guarded, and such treatment should be avoided whenever possible.

Pathologic Root Perforations

The causes of root perforation are root decay exposing the pulp cavity, internal resorption, and external resorption. Root decay implies the absence of attachment structures on a periodontally exposed root surface. If the root can be retained, the decay will be excavated and the root restored. The canal system must not be blocked with restorative material. Afterward, root canal therapy is completed, followed by the necessary periodontal procedures to correct the periodontal lesion. The periodontal procedure may consist of root planing, curettage, laterally repositioned flaps, or grafts, for example, depending on the circumstances (Fig. 18–8). Reattachment over any restoration is difficult, and the overall prognosis for this tooth (root) depends on the response to periodontal treatment. In selected cases of multirooted teeth, radisectomy following root canal therapy, that is, total removal of a root(s) and retention of the intact crown may be the treatment of choice.

The cause of internal resorption is still unknown. Frequently, the patient has a history of trauma, from placement of a gold foil or a deep restoration, for example. The subsequent pulp tissue change causes a cellular response resulting in resorption, rather than calcification with formation of reparative dentin. The process of internal resorption ceases when the pulp is removed; therefore, pulpectomy is the treatment of choice. When perforation into the periodontium occurs, the resorbed area, as well as the root canal, must be sealed from the adjacent periodontal tissues. In the past, this seal was created by filling the root canal with thermoplasticized or laterally condensed gutta-percha and root canal cement. If the resultant seal was inadequate, surgical intervention was considered, whenever possible, to save the tooth.

The current treatment is an attempt to induce a bone-like closure of the perforation by applying calcium-hydroxide paste (calcium hydroxide in a vehicle solution) in contact with the periodontium through the perforation. Over a period of several months, this calcium-hydroxide paste is reinserted to compensate for the continuing loss of previously inserted paste into the surrounding tissues. When closure occurs, the forceful placement of softened gutta-percha and cement seals the canals and the perforated area easily. Overfilling is usually negligible. This procedure can be done for any root perforation, iatrogenic or pathologic, as long as the perforated area is not exposed to the oral environment. Another advantage of this procedure is the elimination of endodontic surgery to achieve healing. Note that this method is also used in apexification techniques for the same end; that is, root-end closure of the "blunderbuss" opening to facilitate complete and proper canal obturation without overfilling and without a surgical procedure.

External resorption is another matter. After perforation, nonsurgical root canal therapy alone is unsuccessful because it does not permit a proper seal of the perforated area, nor does it necessarily stop external resorption. Many procedures have attempted to overcome this process of root destruction, such as surgical removal of the affected area or the affected root. Not all these empiric procedures are routinely successful in saving the root, however. Usually, they are desperate attempts to retain a hopelessly involved tooth.

Cvek reported that external resorption of the root appeared to stop and to heal before perforation when the pulp was removed and calcium-hydroxide paste was placed in the prepared canal.[6] Later, the root canals were filled in a conventional manner, and the tooth was retained in a healthy, repaired state.

Occasionally, external resorption appears on the root surface adjacent to the region of an improperly debrided and inadequately sealed portion of the root canal, even though the canal may be apically obturated, as in replantation. Whether external resorption can be induced by retained pulpal debris, the presence of a lateral canal in the area, or simply a coincidence must still be determined. Proper clinical treatment, however, requires proper canal preparation and complete obturation in every possible instance, including replantation. The use of amalgam apical seals for replanted teeth without treating obvious root canals reduces the potential for long-term healing.

The clinician must differentiate between

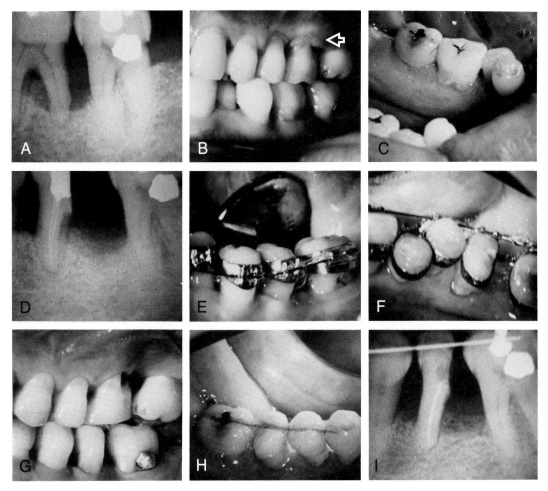

Fig. 18–9. Hemisection of a lower molar, with orthodontic treatment. *A,* Diagnostic radiograph: Extensive bone loss is visible around the distal root, involving bifurcation. *B,* Buccal view of tooth No. 21, in linguoversion (arrow); the arch is misaligned. *C,* Lingual view. *D,* Postoperative radiograph. *E,* Buccal view of the orthodontic appliance. *F,* Lingual view of the orthodontic appliance. *G,* Buccal view after completion of orthodontic treatment. *H,* Occlusal view of the intracoronal splint. *I,* Radiograph after completion of treatment. (Courtesy of Dr. I. Stephen Brown, Philadelphia, PA.)

internal and external resorption, including perforation, because treatment procedures and prognosis are specifically related to this diagnosis. Radiographic interpretation of internal and external resorption is generally accurate. When the resorptive process initiates on the mesial or distal surface of the pulp cavity wall (internal resorption) or the root surface (external resorption), radiographic differentiation is simple. Unfortunately, interpretation of rarefaction on the buccolingual surface (radiographic center) of any root is more difficult and is less precise. Interpretation is still possible by using a simple rule of thumb, however. Because internal resorption starts in the canal wall, the first anatomic change, as determined by the radiograph, is a loss of the canal's typical morphologic features. The amorphous rarefaction completely obliterates the outline of a root canal typically seen in a radiograph. Conversely, because external resorption starts on the root surface, the last anatomic area destroyed is the canal wall. Therefore, on a radiograph, if the morphologic features of a root canal are still evident in the rarefied area on the root, external resorption is the diagnosis.

HEMISECTION AND RADISECTOMY

Radisectomy denotes the removal of one or more roots of a molar. Hemisection refers to sectioning of the crown of a molar tooth, with either the removal of half the crown and its supporting root structure or the retention of both halves, to be used after reshaping and

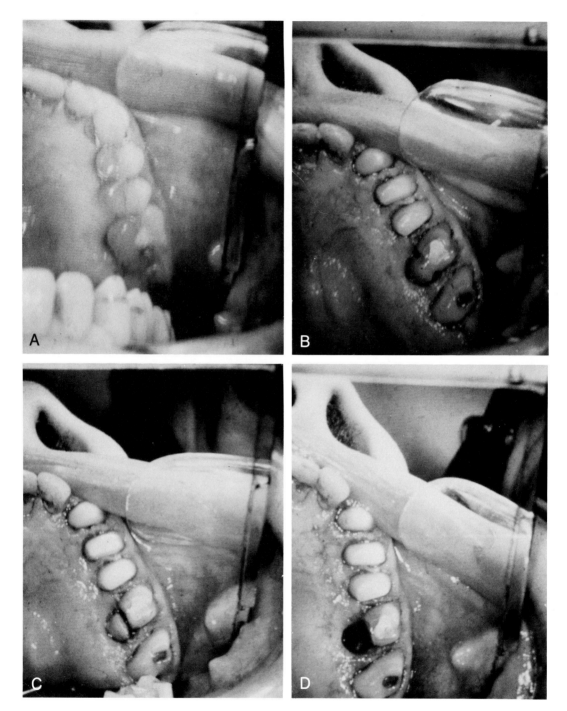

Fig. 18–10.   Hemisection of an upper molar. *A*, Occlusal view prior to treatment. *B*, Occlusal view: The tooth is prepared for full-coverage restoration prior to removal of the palatal root, to permit easy, accurate hemisection; this procedure is designed to conserve the structure of the tooth. *C*, Occlusal view: The palatal root is separated from the buccal segment. *D*, Occlusal view: The palatal root has been extracted. (Courtesy of Dr. Morton Amsterdam, Philadelphia, PA.)

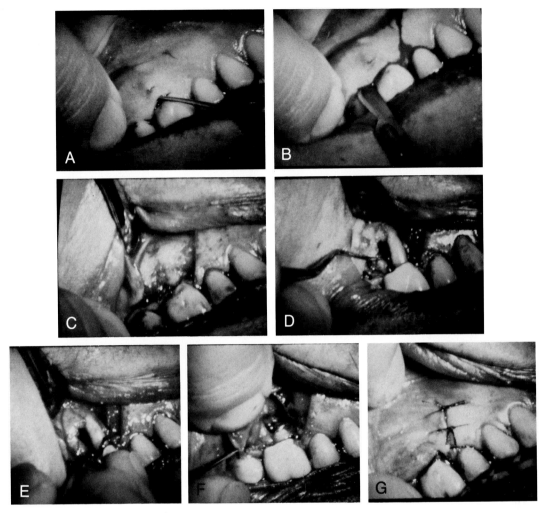

Fig. 18—11.   Radisectomy of an upper molar. *A,* Periodontal probe placed into the furcation infrabony pocket. *B,* Trapezoidal flap; internal bevel on the gingival root crest exposes the mesiobuccal root. *C,* Flap retracted to expose furcation and cortical bone. *D,* Mesiobuccal root exposed following curettage of granulomatous tissue. *E,* Radisectomy done with an SH No. 702 fissure bur. *F,* Contouring of segment remaining after root resection. *G,* Flap coapted and sutured.

splinting as two premolars. Radisectomy and hemisection are often desirable for periodontal reasons.

At times, a multirooted tooth has an untreatable periodontal lesion on one or more of its roots, but the remaining root or roots are well supported and treatable. For example, one root may have an extensive infrabony pocket with concomitant bone loss, and the other root may be surrounded by normal gingiva and supportive bone. To retain a portion of this strategic tooth and to avoid extraction of the entire tooth, hemisection or radisectomy can be performed (Fig. 18–9).

The indications for radisectomy are as follows: (1) when endodontic treatment of one root is technically impossible or when such treatment has failed; (2) when untreatable furcation involvement is present and removal of the root will facilitate oral hygiene in that area; (3) when extensive loss of bone has occurred around one root of an upper molar; (4) when a fractured root of an upper molar is present; (5) when a root has been perforated and cannot be treated endodontally; and (6) when a root has been destroyed by extensive decay.

The contraindications are as follows: (1) when loss of bone involves more than one root, and the remaining root would have inadequate support; (2) when the bridge span is long, and the abutment tooth would lend inadequate support; and (3) when the roots are fused.

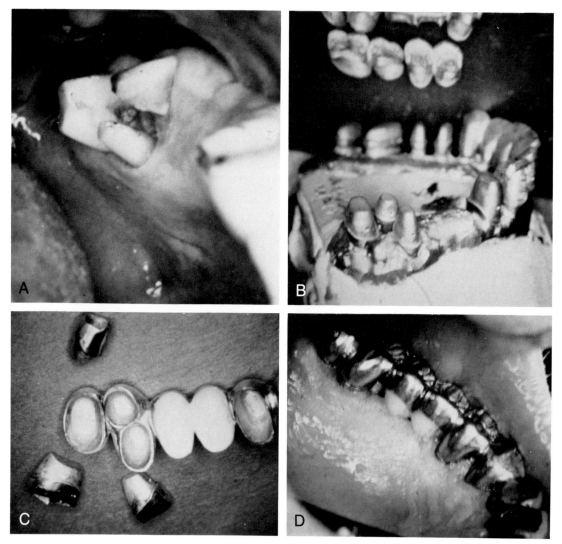

Fig. 18–12. Restoration of a hemisection. *A*, Occlusal view of hemisected upper molar. *B*, Model and dies. *C*, Copings and fixed prosthesis. *D*, Occlusal view (mirror image) of the restoration. (Courtesy of Dr. Morton Amsterdam, Philadelphia, PA.)

The indications for hemisection are as follows: (1) when periodontal involvement of one root is severe; (2) when loss of bone is extensive in the furcation area; (3) when caries involves much of the root. The contraindications are similar to those for radisectomy.

Whenever possible, endodontic treatment should precede root removal. It is difficult to treat a tooth properly when it has been sectioned through the pulp chamber because asepsis is impossible, anatomic guidelines used in treatment are removed or destroyed, and a medicated dressing cannot be adequately sealed between visits. In addition, the amalgam seal placed in the pulp chamber over the root to be removed should have set

before radisectomy, to avoid "amalgam scatter" in the adjacent tissues during radisectomy.

Another technique for radisectomy precludes the need for root canal therapy. When the root has been removed, calcium hydroxide is sealed over the exposed pulp. In essence, a vital pulpotomy (vital radisectomy) is performed in anticipation of pulp healing with dentin bridge formation. The conditions in which this procedure can be wisely done are limited, however, to when a vital, normal pulp is present, a tooth is not a strategic abutment, and a crown restoration is not needed, for example.

To remove a root or hemisect a tooth prop-

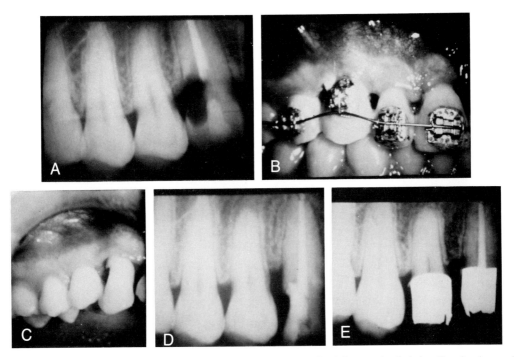

Fig. 18–13. Extrusion of an upper cuspid. *A*, Diagnostic radiograph: Distal decay extends below the alveolar crest. *B*, An orthodontic appliance is placed to erupt the cuspid actively. *C*, The tooth is extruded. *D*, Radiograph after treatment. *E*, Radiograph of temporary full-coverage restoration. (Courtesy of Dr. Robert Vanarsdall, Philadelphia, PA.)

erly, the clinician should visualize the end result before initiating treatment. When a full-coverage restoration is planned after hemisection or radisectomy, one would prepare this tooth for full coverage before removing the root (Fig. 18–10). Once the crown has been prepared, it is easier to see and to sever the root to be extracted from the remaining structures by hemisection and radisectomy; thus, maximum tooth structure is conserved, restorative problems are easier to solve, and periodontal healing is enhanced (Fig. 18–11 to 18–13).

Some clinicians prefer the use of diamond discs when performing hemisection; however, the use of carbide burs and diamond stones with water spray usually results in a controlled cut, with contoured sections having better margins and restorations. Frequently, a tissue flap is incised and is retracted to allow unrestricted observation of the planned sectioning and extraction. Reluctance to create a flap when necessary could result in an improper section, a section through an adjacent root, incomplete root removal, and "spur" formation, all of which jeopardize proper restoration and repair. Moreover, exposure of the operative site enables one to avoid the disastrous error of sep-

aration and removal of fused roots that were not readily evident in the radiographs.

BIBLIOGRAPHY

1. Bender, I.B., et al.: Oral Surg., *33*:458, 1972.
2. Bergenholtz, G., and Lindhe, J.: J. Clin. Period., *5*:59,1978.
3. Burch, J.S., and Hulen, S.: Oral Surg., *38*:451, 1974.
4. Chacker, F.M.: Dent. Clin. North Am., *18*:393, 1974.
5. Czarnecki, R.T., and Schilder, H.: J. Endod., *5*:242, 1979.
6. Cvek, M.: Transactions of the Fifth International Conference on Endodontics. Edited by L.I. Grossman. Philadelphia, University of Pennsylvania, 1973, p. 30.
7. Feldman, G., et al.: Dent. Radiog. and Photog., *54*:1, 1981.
8. Grossman, L.I.: Root Canal Therapy, 4th Ed. Philadelphia, Lea & Febiger, 1955, p. 167.
9. Gutmann, J.L.: J. Period., *49*:21, 1978.
10. Hattler, A.B., et al.: Oral Surg., *44*:939, 1977.
11. Hiatt, W.H: Oral Surg., *54*:436, 1982.
12. Hiatt, W.H.: J. Period., *48*:598, 1977.
13. Hildebrand, C.N., and Morse, D.N.: Dent. Clin. North Am., *24*:747, 1980.
14. Johnston, H.B., and Orban, B.: J. Endod., *3*:21, 1948.
15. Kirkham, D.B.: J. Am. Dent. Assoc., *91*:353, 1975.
16. Koenig, J.F., et al.: Oral Surg., *38*:773, 1974.
17. Langeland, K., et al.: Oral Surg., *37*:257, 1974.
18. Mandi, F.A.: J. Br. Endod. Soc., *6*:80, 1973.
19. Mazur, B., and Massler, M.: Oral Surg., *17*:592, 1964.
20. Oliet, S.: Bull. Phila. Dent. Soc., *31*:7, 1966.
21. Oliet, S., and Pollock, S.: Bull. Phila. Dent. Soc., *34*:12, 1968.

22. Perlich, M.A., et al.: J. Endod., *7*:402, 1981.
23. Rossman, L., et al.: Oral Surg., *53*:78, 1982.
24. Rossman, S.R., et al.: Oral Surg., *13*:361, 1960.
25. Ruback, W.C., and Mitchell, D.F.: J. Period., *36*:34, 1965.
26. Sauerwein, E.: Dtsch. Zahn. Mund. Kieferhelkd., *22*:289, 1955.
27. Seltzer, S., and Bender, I.B.: The Dental Pulp, 3rd Ed. Philadelphia, J.B. Lippincott, 1954, pp. 303, 306.
28. Seltzer, S., et al.: Oral Surg., *16*:1474, 1963.
29. Shoba, R., et al.: Oral Surg., *38*:294, 1974.
30. Simon, J., et al.: J. Period., *43*:202, 1972.
31. Simring, M., and Goldberg, M.: J. Period., *35*:22, 1964.
32. Sinai, I., and Soltonoff, W.: Oral Surg., *36*:558, 1973.
33. Stahl, S.S.: Oral Surg., *16*:9, 1116, 1963.
34. Torabinajed, M., and Kiger, R.D.: Oral Surg., *59*:198, 1985.
35. Vertucci, F.J., and Williams, R.G.: Oral Surg., *38*:308, 1974.
36. Weine, F.S.: Dent. Clin. North Am., *28*:4, 833, 1984.

19

Replantation, Transplantation, and Endodontic Implants

The terms "replantation," and "implantation" are often confused. Replantation, sometimes referred to as reimplantation, is the insertion of a tooth in its socket after its complete avulsion resulting from traumatic injury. Intentional replantation is the intentional removal of a tooth and its reinsertion into the socket after orthograde obturation and resection of the root tips, or resection of the root tips followed by retrograde obturation, an operation usually limited to posterior teeth. Transplantation is the removal of a tooth or tooth bud from one socket and transplanting it into another socket. Autotransplantation is the transplanting of a tooth or tooth bud from one socket to another socket in the same person. Allotransplantation is the transplanting of a tooth or tooth bud from a socket of one person and inserting it into the socket of another person (same species). Implantation is the insertion of an artificial "tooth" or stabilizer into a surgically prepared socket.

REPLANTATION

Total luxation or avulsion of teeth is treated by replantation. This term refers to replacement of a tooth in its socket, with the object of attaining reattachment when the tooth has been completely avulsed from its socket by an accident (Fig. 19–1). Replanted teeth have been reported by a number of clinicians, but except for Andreasen and Hjörting-Hansen,[5] Grossman and Ship,[30] and Kemp and colleagues,[41] few have evaluated long-term results in a large number of teeth.

Although the life span of replanted teeth is short, one sees occasional accounts of unusually long survival times (Fig. 19–2). Barry reported 2 upper central incisors that were avulsed, fell in the snow, were immediately replanted, and were vital 42 years later.[9] Henning reported that a 22-year old patient

washed an avulsed tooth in brandy, replanted it himself within 5 min of the accident, and had endodontic treatment 6 weeks later.[36] No evidence of root resorption was present 8 years afterward. Weill reported avulsion of a lower lateral incisor and cuspid, which the patient himself replanted and which remained vital and showed no evidence of resorption 20 years later.[78] White replanted 2 upper central incisors that had been in a swimming pool for 18 hours; these teeth were clinically normal in appearance, but showed some evidence of root resorption after 11 years.[81] Although these isolated case histories are not the norm, they do extend the potential of repair, longevity, and function beyond a few short months.

Guidelines for the Treatment of the Avulsed Tooth

A committee of the American Association of Endodontists has recommended a concensus of their respective approaches for the treatment of the accidentally avulsed tooth; these guidelines are a working document subject to revision on the basis of additional research.[1]

Extraoral Time

Because extraoral time is one of the most critical factors affecting prognosis, the avulsed tooth should be replanted immediately into its socket, whenever possible, to reduce this time to an absolute minimum. The dentist should instruct the patient or parent on replantation technique during the initial emergency telephone call and should stress the importance of coming to the office immediately for follow-up splinting and treatment.

Storage Media

By replanting the tooth into its socket as soon as possible, not only is the extraoral

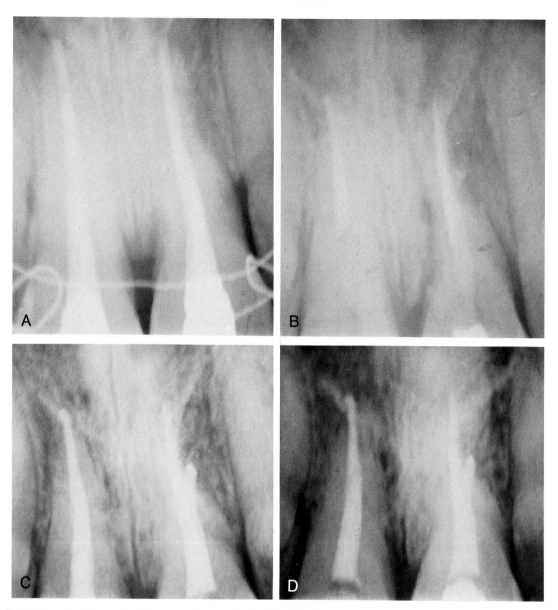

Fig. 19–1. Avulsion, replantation, resorption, and perforation of both upper central incisors. *A,* Replantation radiograph: The teeth were avulsed during an automobile accident; endodontic treatment was completed extraorally, the teeth were replanted in a hospital emergency room, and wire ligation was done. *B,* Treatment radiograph: Several weeks later, the upper left central incisor developed lateral resorption of the root with perforation; the gutta-percha filling was removed to the perforation, and calcium hydroxide was inserted. *C,* Treatment radiograph: Several months after calcium hydroxide treatment, the root canals were refilled with laterally condensed gutta-percha. *D,* Recall radiograph at 6 months: Bone regeneration is evident; however, resorption recurred, the tooth was extracted after 2 years.

time reduced, but also the tooth is restored to the best possible environment, conducive to maintaining vitality of the root surface cells and viability of the periodontal ligament. Alternate storage media for carrying the tooth to the dentist when replantation into the socket is not feasible are the patient's saliva, wherein the tooth can be held in the buccal vestibule or under the tongue, milk, or, last and least effective, water.

Management of the Socket

The less manipulation of the socket the better prognosis for the replanted tooth. Use light irrigation and gentle aspiration to remove any blood clot present in the socket, to permit replantation. Do not curette or vent the socket. Do not make a surgical flap unless bony fragments prevent replantation. After replantation, manually compress the facial and lingual bony plates.

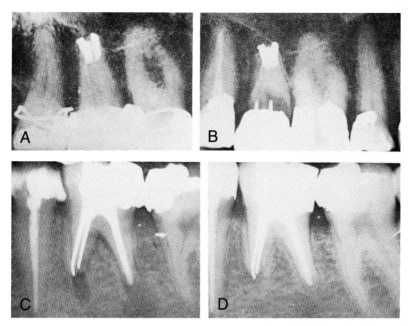

Fig. 19–2. *A*, Maxillary molar about a month after intentional replantation. *B*, Radiograph of the tooth in *A*, 16 years later. The tooth was removed because of caries. *C*, Mandibular molar immediately after the removal of a splint. *D*, Radiograph of the tooth in *C*, 11 years later.

Management of the Root Surface

To preserve the vitality of the root surface cells, do not handle, scrape, brush, or remove any of the root surface. If the root appears clean, replant as is. If the root surface is dirty, rinse it clean with tap water. If persistent debris remains on the root, use cotton pliers gently to pick away any debris, or, as a last resort, use a wet sponge to brush off debris gently. Do not apply any medicaments, disinfectants, or chemicals to the root surface.

When to Perform Endodontic Treatment

The guidelines suggest that endodontic treatment should be initiated within 7 to 14 days of replantation and when the tooth is in its socket. If the tooth apex is open, monitor the replanted tooth every 2 weeks for revitalization of the pulp. If pathologic signs are noted, then extirpate the pulp, and continue with an apexification procedure using calcium hydroxide until such time as endodontic treatment and root canal filling can be completed.

Filling Materials

Use calcium hydroxide for treatment fillings after a minimum delay of 7 days after replantation, and permanently obturate the root canal with gutta-percha later.

Splinting

The suggested splint is composed of acid-etch resin alone or with soft arch wire, orthodontic brackets with wire arch, or large monofilament fishing line. Leave the splint in place for 7 to 10 days if no bony fractures are present, or longer if necessary, and ask the patient not to bite on the splinted teeth; prescribe a soft diet.

Adjunctive Drug Therapy

Refer the patient for a tetanus consultation within the first 48 hours, and prescribe antibiotics only if indicated, such as in a medically compromised patient or a case of contaminated avulsion.

Prevention of Avulsed Teeth

The general dentist has an obligation to patients who engage in athletic activities to tell them how to prevent fracture and avulsion of teeth and what to do if a tooth is avulsed. Whenever possible, a mouthguard should be worn during rough play or strenuous athletics. In addition, an overjet of the teeth should be corrected because inadequate lip coverage predisposes patients to crown and root fractures and to avulsion of teeth.

Immediacy of Replanting Tooth

The length of time the avulsed tooth is out of the socket is critical and can affect the prognosis of the tooth. All investigators appear to agree that the shorter the extraoral time before replantation, the better the prognosis. This hypothesis has been proved by experimental study and clinical observation. Coccia evaluated 129 teeth during a 5-year period and found that the prognosis is more favorable if the time between avulsion and replantation is short.[15]

Once a tooth has been avulsed, an effort should be made to preserve the vitality of the periodontal ligament. In order of preference, the avulsed tooth should be rinsed in water and should be replanted immediately by the patient, parent, or friend because the best storage medium for maintaining the vitality of the root surface cells is the tooth's socket. As soon as possible, the patient should be taken to the dentist, to make certain that the tooth is in proper occlusion and is not extruded. The second order of preference is to rinse the tooth with water and submerge it in a container of milk. Both the patient and the avulsed tooth, which is immersed in milk, are taken to the dentist immediately, so the tooth can be replanted in the socket without delay. Blomlöf has shown that milk preserves the vitality of the periodontal ligament longer than saliva, 6 hours versus 2 hours, respectively, but milk has no restorative effect when the periodontal ligament has already become dehydrated.[12] The third order of preference is to rinse the tooth and to place it in the vestibule of the mouth, where it will have proper moisture and temperature, and immediately have the dentist replant it. The least preferable method is to rinse the tooth, place it in a cup of water, and have it replanted by the dentist without delay.

Almost all valid experimental work in lower animals, as well as observations in human subjects, emphasizes that the key to success in replantation rests in the vitality of the periodontal ligament cells. Two important factors are: (1) the degree of damage to the periodontal ligament from trauma during avulsion; and (2) the length of time the tooth is out of the mouth, with resulting dehydration and death of the cells. Most experimental studies indicate that if the extraoral time is less than 30 minutes, the periodontal ligament will survive.

Söder and associates found viable cells of the periodontal ligament of human teeth after a drying period of half an hour in 4 of 4 teeth, in 3 of 4 teeth after 1 hour, and no viable cells after 2 hours.[74] In a study by Löe and Waerhaug, it was found that when the periodontal ligament was removed prior to replantation, anklyosis invariably resulted; when the periodontal ligament was dried for short periods of time, localized areas of normal ligament persisted in an amount proportional to the drying time; and when the periodontal ligament was intact and the tooth was replanted immediately, normal reattachment of the tooth occurred, and ankylosis was not observed.[45] Hamner and colleagues removed the periodontal ligament and cementum on the distal surfaces of replanted teeth of baboons, but did not disturb these structures on the mesial surfaces of these teeth; massive root resorption occurred on the distal surfaces, whereas only limited focal resorption occurred mesially.[32] Additional studies by Oswald and co-workers,[62] as well as Van Hassel and associates,[77] confirmed the need for maintaining the periodontal ligament in a viable state in an avulsed and replanted tooth, to deter root resorption.

Other studies examined the treated roots of replanted teeth. Mahajan and Sedhu intentionally replanted teeth in 88 patients and reported their results after 6 and 12 months of observation.[48] The teeth were divided into 3 groups: (1) periodontal ligament scraped and soaked in a 2% solution of sodium fluoride for 4 min; (2) periodontal membrane left intact and soaked in 2% sodium fluoride for 4 min; and (3) periodontal ligament left intact without any soaking in sodium fluoride. Less resorption occurred in teeth that were untreated (group 3), and ankylosis rather than repair occurred in the fluoride-treated groups. Shulman immersed extracted teeth of monkeys in an acidulated sodium-fluoride solution at pH 5.5 for 20 min, with the object of prolonging the survival of these teeth,[70] but Barbakow and colleagues found that the application of an acidulated sodium-fluoride solution on roots of replanted teeth in monkeys did not prevent or retard root resorption or ankylosis, when compared to control subjects during an 8-week observation period.[8] Nolbandian and Hellden, on the basis of experimental work in dogs using small 4-mm Teflon implants in roots that were then examined histologically, are of the opinion that if the entire root is coated with Teflon, root resorption and ankylosis will not occur.[57]

In an evaluation of 81 completely and partially avulsed teeth, Hines concluded that avulsed teeth had a better prognosis if replanted immediately, without endodontic treatment.[37] Cvek and associates have recommended that an avulsed tooth that has been dry for more than 15 min should be placed in an isotonic salt solution for about half an hour before replantation, to revive the cells if they are still alive.[17] Later, the root canal should be filled with a calcium-hydroxide paste for at least 6 months before the root canal is obturated. Heithersay has also found the application of calcium hydroxide effective as a temporary root canal dressing in immature, incompletely developed, avulsed teeth,[35] although Andreasen and Kristerson have stated that calcium hydroxide placed in the root canal of replanted teeth may diffuse through the apical foramen and may injure the apical portion of the periodontal ligament.[6]

Endodontic Treatment—Before or After Replantation?

The question is often asked whether to carry out endodontic treatment before or after the tooth has been replanted. A good rule to follow is: if the periodontal ligament is still vital, replant the tooth without delay, and plan on endodontic treatment at a later time; if the periodontal ligament is dried out and dead, the endodontic treatment may just as well be done before replanting the tooth. According to Andreasen, root resorption is less likely if the root canal of the replanted tooth is not filled prior to replantation than if the pulp is left in the canal or is extirpated and the endodontic treatment is done.[2] Andreasen and Hjörting-Hansen found no evidence of vitality, but rather necrosis, when endodontic treatment has not been carried out on replanted teeth.[5] In experimental work in dogs, Knight and associates found less resorption in teeth that had undergone root canal treatment than in those not treated endodontally.[43] Woeherle replanted teeth in dogs.[82] Minimal pathosis was seen when root canal treatment was done; abscesses developed in teeth whose pulps were removed but no treatment was done; periapical pathosis developed when the pulps were not removed and the teeth were replanted. Nasjleti and colleagues compared obturation and lack of obturation of replanted teeth in monkeys and found that periapical complications developed in the unobturated teeth.[55]

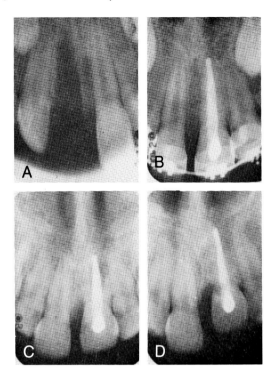

Fig. 19–3. *A,* Avulsed central incisor. *B,* The tooth has been replanted after obturation of the root canal; an orthodontic band splint was used. *C,* Recall radiograph at 2 years. *D,* Recall radiograph at 5 years: The tooth is mobile; one sees almost complete root resorption and some resorption of the gutta-percha cone.

Replantation Resorption

The major cause of failure in replantation of avulsed teeth appears to be resorption of the root, frequently followed by ankylosis (Fig. 19–3). Andreasen described three types of resorption: (1) surface resorption, which is a small, localized area of cemental resorption that may also superficially affect the dentin and can be related to tears occurring during tooth avulsion; such areas are repaired with secondary cementum; (2) inflammatory resorption, which is probably due to the presence of microorganisms in the dentinal tubules or to necrotic tissue in the root canal that causes inflammation of bone and destruction of both the root surface and bone, with replacement by granulomatous tissue; and (3) replacement resorption, characterized by gradual root resorption, including periodontal ligament, cementum, and dentin of the root, with replacement by bone.[4] The distinction between root and bone is lost, and the tooth is said to be ankylosed.

Two major deterrents to external resorption of the roots of avulsed and replanted teeth are: (1) the reduction of extraoral time of the avulsed tooth to less than 30 min before replantation; beyond 30 min, the root surface cells dehydrate and die, and the viability of the periodontal ligament is impaired; and (2) the initiation of endodontic treatment a week after replantation. Immediate replantation without endodontic treatment of the avulsed tooth reduces the extraoral time. In addition, intracanal medication of the replanted tooth with calcium hydroxide should be delayed until the first week after replantation, to prevent the calcium hydroxide from adversely affecting the viability of the root surface cells. Finally, endodontic treatment must include thorough debridement of the root canal and the elimination of necrotic pulpal debris and microorganisms, as well as obturation of the root canal. Endodontic treatment can be completed within 6 months of replantation.

Technique for Delayed Replantation

The technique and precautions for replantation of the avulsed tooth are discussed earlier in this chapter. On occasion, however, the recommended procedures are modified. When much time has elapsed and the periodontal ligament has completely dried out, the detached tooth is first washed thoroughly and is held in moist sterile gauze during the endodontic procedure. The pulp tissue is completely removed, and the root canal is instrumented, irrigated, and obturated in the usual manner with gutta-percha cones. Excess gutta-percha protruding through the apical foramen should be removed, and the root tip should be shortened 2 mm and trimmed smooth. With the patient under anesthesia, the blood clot should be removed, but the socket should not be curetted because such a procedure may remove periodontal ligament remnants. The socket should be aspirated. The prepared tooth is replaced in its socket and is ligated to adjacent teeth by stainless steel wire and acrylic, acid-etch resin and soft arch wire, or acid-etch resin and monofilament fish line.

Regardless of the type of splint, it should be removed in 7 to 10 days. Andreasen and Hjörting-Hansen advocate splinting a tooth for that length of time because prolonged splinting may induce replacement resorption.[5] Moreover, Andreasen found a higher incidence of replacement resorption in replanted teeth that had not been splinted than in those that were splinted.[3]

No case of tetanus has been reported following the replantation of a "dirty" tooth picked up off the ground, perhaps because freshly stimulated saliva inhibits the growth of tetanus bacillus, according to the findings of Bartels and Blechman.[10] The patient should be referred to a physician within the first 48 hours for tetanus consultation, however. Antibiotic therapy is not recommended, except in medically compromised patients or in cases of contaminated avulsion.

Although replanted teeth may become reattached satisfactorily, they have a short life span, especially when the extraoral time exceeds 30 min, because root resorption usually takes place, and the tooth is eventually exfoliated. Such teeth become ankylosed from loss of periodontal ligament viability and dehydration of the root surface cells. In most cases, one sees gradual root resorption, followed by progressive loosening of the tooth. Isolated areas of resorption may be recognized on the radiograph within 2 to 3 months of replacement of the tooth and may continue to such an extent that extraction of the tooth is often necessary in about 2 years. Despite an uncertain prognosis, replantation is still worthwhile in children and young people whose jaws have not yet attained maximum growth and development, when a replacement would be difficult, and when the psychologic impact of loss of the tooth may cause irreparable harm.

Intentional Replantation

Although Fauchard is often credited with a description of intentional replantation,[20] it is likely that the operation was practical before his time. Fauchard described four cases of intentional replantation, all of which were successful. In one report, he stated, "this tooth had remained on my table nearly a quarter of an hour after drawing it before I replaced it; however, it united so well and tightened in its own socket that it is still today as firm as it was in the beginning."[20]

The term intentional replantation means the removal of a tooth for the purpose of extra-oral endodontic treatment and the replacement of that tooth in its socket almost immediately (Fig. 19–4). During this time, every effort is made to keep the periodontal ligament viable by moistening the tooth frequently in sterile saline solution, anesthetic solution, or milk. The planned operation can usually be performed within 15 min (Fig. 19–5). Intentional replantation of teeth should be differentiated from autotransplan-

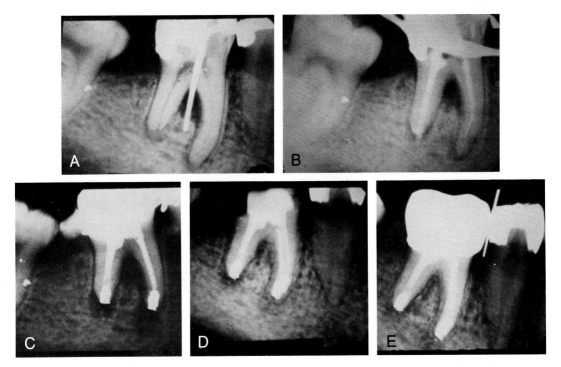

Fig. 19–4. Intentional replantation of a lower molar, with an endodontic-periodontic lesion. *A,* Diagnostic radiograph: Chronic alveolar abscess with bifurcation bone loss; a probe is present in the sulcular crevice. *B,* Treatment radiograph: Endodontic treatment has been attempted; the tooth has been overfilled in the distal root and filled in the mesial canals to the fractured instrument. *C,* Replantation radiograph: The tooth has been intentionally replanted, and the apices have been sealed with amalgam extraorally. *D,* Recall radiograph at 6 months. *E,* Recall radiograph at 1 year: The crevicular depth is normal when probed.

tation of immature teeth, in which the tooth is transplanted from one part of the mouth to another part of the same mouth. Andreasen and Hjörting-Hansen,[5] Deeb,[18] Emmertsen and Andreasen,[19] Grossman and Chacker,[29] and Kingsbury and Wiesenbaugh[42] have reported on a significant number of cases of intentional replantation. Flanagan and Myers have shown that teeth that were extracted and replaced in their sockets within 30 min showed no deleterious effect, whereas any further delay had an adverse effect.[22]

Emmertsen and Andreasen evaluated 100 intentionally replanted molar teeth, a few of which had been followed-up for as long as 13 years.[19] No evidence of resorption of the roots was noted in 67% of the replanted teeth (Fig. 19–6).

In a 2-year evaluation of 117 intentionally replanted teeth, Deeb reported a success rate of 67%.[18] Failures were ascribed to toxic products, trauma from excessive manipulation during extraction, and curettage of the periodontal ligament on the root and in the socket. In a histologic study of intentionally replanted teeth in monkeys, Grossman and Chacker observed all 3 groups of periodontal ligament fibers in 7 of 8 teeth.[29] The periodontal fibers were dense and well arranged, and the gingival fibers were re-established. Cemental tears and crestal bone damage, the result of extraction, had been repaired. The periodontal ligament was completely reattached on both sides of the cementum and alveolar bone, and it had a normal vascular pattern. In a 4-month specimen, the attachment apparatus was almost indistinguishable from that of the control teeth.

In a short-term study of intentionally replanted teeth, Hurst observed thick fibers running parallel to the teeth and "smaller fibers" oriented horizontally in the transseptal region.[39] Caffesse and associates noted cervical and apical root resorption following intentional replantation of teeth in monkeys, but aborted resorption areas were repaired by cementum.[14] The periodontal fibers became reattached to bone and cementum, but they did not have the original orientation. These investigators state, however, that "total clinical success seems possible in spite of the

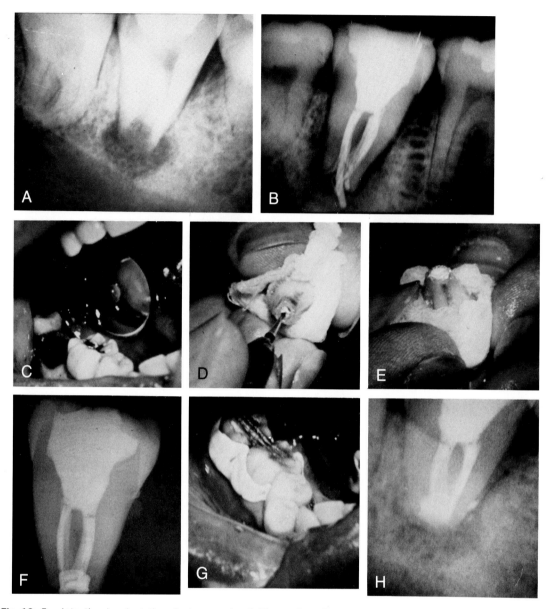

Fig. 19–5. Intentional replantation of a lower molar. *A*, Diagnostic radiograph: Chronic alveolar abscess with incomplete apexogenesis. *B*, Obturation radiograph: Overfilled root canal with failure of the tooth to heal. *C*, Buccal view: The tooth has been extracted. *D*, Extraoral treatment: The periapical cavity is prepared while the tooth is held in a sterile gauze pad moistened with anesthetic solution. *E*, Retrograde filling: Gutta-percha is packed into the apical cavity preparation. *F*, Extraoral radiograph: Retrograde gutta-percha filling. *G*, Buccal view: The tooth was replanted within 15 min, ligated, and the periodontal pack was placed. *H*, Recall radiograph at 6 months: Bone regeneration is incomplete.

common histopathologic evidence of abnormal periodontal relationship after tooth reimplantation."[14] Nasjleti intentionally replanted teeth in monkeys within half an hour and splinted with an acid-etch splint for either 7 or 30 days; those splinted for 7 days showed no evidence of resorption, whereas those splinted for 30 days had increased areas of root resorption and ankylosis.[54]

Andreasen and colleagues reported that teeth of monkeys that had been placed in tissue culture medium for 5 to 14 days showed less inflammatory resorption, with increased pulp survival than teeth that were extracted and immediately replanted.[7] Barbakow and co-workers did not find topical treatment of the roots of teeth with sodium fluoride and thyrocalcitonin to have any effect on the healing response.[8]

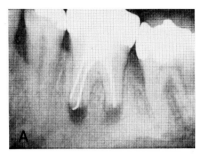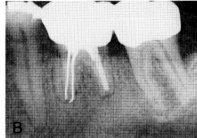

Fig. 19–6.   *A,* Intentional replantation of a mandibular molar immediately after clipping off the root apices and return of the tooth to its socket. *B,* Radiograph 18 years later.

Indications and Contraindications

Intentional replantation is indicated in few instances. It should not be done when resection is possible. The operation should be limited to posterior teeth in which resection is not feasible for anatomic reasons, risk of paresthesia, or inaccessibility to endodontic treatment (Fig. 19–7). The indications for the operation are as follows:

1. When an instrument has been broken in the root canal and projects through the apical foramen.
2. When mechanical obstruction of the root canal is present, such as from a pulp stone, fractured instrument, or glass bead that cannot be removed.
3. When a perforation of the root cannot easily be contained.
4. When the root canal is calcified or partly calcified, making it impossible to enter with a root canal instrument, and an area of rarefaction is present.
5. When a root canal has been grossly overfilled and the protruding filling is irritating the periapical tissues.
6. When the root canal is sharply curved and cannot be negotiated.
7. When the root canal is bifurcated as it approaches the root apex and cannot be negotiated.
8. When a foreign body is lying free in the periapical tissue and is acting as an irritant, such as an excess piece of gutta-percha that has broken off from the main stem, or a grossly overfilled canal, or root canal cement, or when an absorbent point has been pushed completely through the apical foramen.
9. When root canal treatment has already

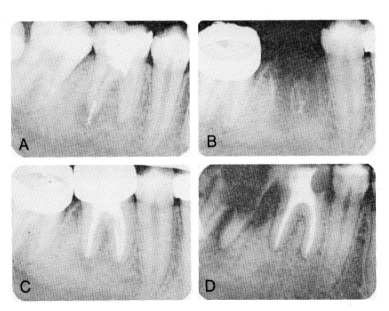

Fig. 19–7.   Intentional replantation. *A,* Molten metal is present in the root canal and through the apical foramen into bone. *B,* The tooth is extracted. *C,* The tooth is replaced and stabilized with an orthodontic splint. *D,* Radiograph 11 years later.

been done, a periapical lesion is present, and the canal filling cannot be removed.

The contraindications to intentional replantation are as follows:

1. Periodontal involvement with extensive mobility of the tooth.
2. Buccal or lingual plate that is destroyed or missing.
3. Septal bone at the bifurcation and trifurcation that is destroyed or missing.
4. Likelihood that extraction of the tooth will fracture the crown.

The tooth to be replanted intentionally should have a strong enough crown to resist the mechanical forces necessary to extract it. Whenever possible, the root canals should be filled the day before the operation. The crown should also be restored with an amalgam restoration. One should pack the amalgam into the pulp chamber as well as the access cavity, to strengthen the tooth and thereby to prevent its being crushed between the beaks of the forceps.

Technique

Intentional replantation is simpler if done by 2 persons. One person should be given the responsibility of extraction and care of the wound and socket, the other of carrying out the necessary endodontic treatment and replacing the tooth in its socket. The entire procedure should be done as aseptically as possible, following regular operating-room technique, including scrubbed hands and sterile gloves. The following should be on hand: a sterile beaker containing about 20 ml sterile saline solution or sterile anesthetic solution, sterile 2 × 2 gauze, and a pair of sterile rongeur forceps. In addition, when an amalgam resection "in the hand" will be done, sterile amalgam pluggers, squeeze cloths, Nos. 1 and 2 round sterile burs, and Nos. 34 and 35 inverted cones should be prepared in advance.

When suitable anesthesia has been induced, the tooth and tissues are painted with an antiseptic solution. The tooth is then cautiously extracted. The wound and periapical tissue are debrided, and any foreign body, such as excess gutta-percha, cement free in the tissue, or pathologic tissue, is carefully curetted if necessary. The wound is packed with sterile gauze, and the patient is asked to close his teeth together to immobilize the pack.

The endodontic procedure is started the moment the tooth is removed intact from its socket. The tooth is wrapped in sterile gauze and is saturated with the sterile solution such that only the root tips protrude from the gauze. The purpose is to keep the periodontal ligament viable. The operator then clips about 2 or 3 mm from the root apices with a pair of rongeur forceps. Alternately, the root tips can be resected using a high-speed drill, sterile burs, and sterile spray. The amount of root tip resected depends on the individual case and the discretion of the operator. In most cases, however, cutting off the root at the 2- or 3-mm level suffices for the procedure of blocking off the foramen with amalgam. If the root canals have been well filled and only the root tips need to be removed, the tooth can be returned to its socket within a minute or so of its removal from the jaw. Such teeth have a better prognosis than those in which an amalgam resection needs to be done.

When the root canal is blocked by calcification, when a perforation is present, or when the canal is blocked by a foreign object and the canals cannot be filled in advance to a reasonable level, an extraoral amalgam resection is indicated. When the root tips have been cut off, a cavity is prepared in each of the resected roots with a small No. 1 or 2 round bur to a depth of at least 2 mm. The cavities are then undercut with an inverted-cone No. 34 or 35 bur and varnished. Amalgam is packed into the cavities, with care to keep the cavities dry and the periodontal ligament moist, by means of the wet gauze. Excess amalgam is removed with sterile cotton, and the tooth is returned to its socket.

A splint is now prepared to stabilize the replanted tooth and to prevent it from being displaced or dislodged. Andreasen and Hjörting-Hansen found that in monkeys whose teeth were replanted, replacement resorption (ankylosis) occurred more often in teeth that were not splinted than in teeth that were splinted.[5] An acceptable splint that is easy to apply is the acid-etch resin splint for direct bonding. Splints can be constructed by direct bonding of orthodontic brackets on the buccal enamel surface of the replanted tooth, as well as the adjacent teeth, mesial and distal to the replanted tooth; they are ligated using arch wire around the brackets and are sealed with composite.

The technique of direct bonding consists of the following: (1) pumice and wash the buccal surfaces of the crowns of the involved teeth; (2) isolate the teeth with cotton rolls and air dry them; (3) apply etchant for 30 sec or as long as the manufacturer of the product recommends; (4) wash with water to remove all acid and breakdown products for approximately 30 sec; (5) air dry the crown surfaces for another 30 sec; (6) when the "frosty" appearance is present on the dry and isolated buccal crown surface, apply the adhesive resin to the tooth and bracket base, and press the bracket into position; the excess resin can be removed if necessary; (7) once the resin has set, usually within a few minutes, ligate the teeth by connecting the brackets with arch wire; this splint should be removed in 7 to 10 days.

The "A" splint or intracoronal splint, can also be quickly prepared to stabilize the replanted tooth. Prepare a groove between the occlusal surfaces of the replanted tooth and the adjacent teeth, insert a small arch wire inside the groove, extending the length of the three teeth, and seal the groove with composite or any other suitable filling that will set rapidly. This splint can be left in place for several weeks.

When the periodontal ligament has not been damaged to a great extent during extraction and replacement of the tooth, and if the tooth has been out of the mouth a minimal amount of time and the periodontal ligament has been kept moist, the prognosis is excellent. On the other hand, when damage to the periodontal ligament has been considerable, either because of trauma or dehydration, resorption of the root will occur. The resorptive process may be rapid or slow, depending on the individual case. Nasjleti and associates have shown that, regardless of the state of the root canal, reattachment of the periodontal ligament occurs, and teeth replanted without subsequent endodontic treatment develop periapical lesions, whereas endodontically treated teeth do not.[55]

Grossman has intentionally replanted a number of posterior teeth and has observed 2 cases for as long as 20 years without evidence of root resorption (Fig. 19–8). In some cases, resorption has occurred within 1 or 2 years, whereas in other cases, resorption is slow and may become static. Approximately 65 to 75% of cases may be considered successful.

TRANSPLANTATION

Transplantation of teeth is not as successful as intentional replantation because of the immunologic factor. Massler stated "tooth autotransplants are more successful than tooth allotransplants, in all species. Autotransplantation (i.e., transplantation of a tooth in the same individual) is the method of choice. Allotransplantation (i.e., from one person to another) is still to be considered an experimental procedure with a relatively high rejection rate (50%)"[49] (Fig. 19–9).

Homograft (from one person to another) rejection of teeth is similar to rejection of tissues elsewhere in the body and is mediated by cells derived from the reticuloendothelial system. In soft tissue, the cell that attacks and infiltrates the homograft is the lymphocyte; in hard tissue, the multinucleated osteoclast gradually removes the hard tooth substance. As early as a week after transplantation, degenerative changes begin to appear. Fong has compared these changes in autologous (same person) and homologous (different person) tooth transplants.[23] Although little difference between the two is seen in the monkey during the first week, the autologous transplant eventually undergoes repair, whereas the homologous transplant continues to degenerate. The pulp becomes completely acellular, the periodontal ligament and cementum gradually disappear, and the picture is that of resorption and ankylosis.

In experimental studies in rabbits and mice, Shulman concluded that replantation of allogenic teeth caused an immunologic reaction that resulted in failure due to resorption and ankylosis of these teeth.[70] Enamel and dentin, as well as pulp and periodontal ligament, carry transplantation antigens and are capable of producing an immunologic reaction. Shulman showed that a second-set reaction will occur if an embedded tooth is challenged by a skin graft.

Mincer and Jennings,[52] as well as Robinson and Rowlands,[68] have also shown that tooth substance has antigenic properties. Mincer and Jennings have shown that fragments of teeth produce a second-set reaction in different strains of mice when skin grafts are exchanged, and Robinson and Rowlands have stated that the periodontal ligament provokes an immunologic reaction and the tooth socket is not an immunologically privileged site. Although dental tissues are antigenic, they are of a low order of antigenicity according to Weinreb and Sharav.[79] Hasselgren and associates have shown that pulps do not survive a transplantation procedure

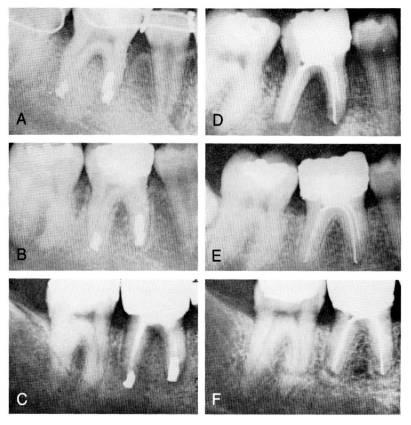

Fig. 19–8. Two molar teeth intentionally replanted in the mouth of the same patient using two different methods of obturating root canals. *A*, Radiograph immediately after replantation: A wire splint is visible; the root canals were obturated apically with amalgam. *B*, Radiograph 13 years later. *C*, A large amalgam filling in the crown had become loose, possibly exposing the root canal apices; endodontic treatment had therefore been done; this radiograph was taken 20 years post-operatively. *D*, The root canals were obturated prior to replantation in the opposite molar; the root apices were cut off with Rongeur forceps, the socket was carefully curetted, and the tooth was immediately replanted. *E*, Radiograph 13 years later. *F*, Radiograph 20 years later. (*C* and *F*, Courtesy of Dr. Jan Levy.)

and endodontic treatment should be done for the successful outcome of the transplant.[34]

Fong and Berger,[24] as well as Nordenram and Bergman,[58] stated that radiation, with the object of suppressing the antigenic factor, did not prevent ankylosis and root resorption of transplanted teeth in monkeys. Natiella and associates have reviewed the problems of replantation and transplantation of teeth in great detail.[56]

Even though mature tooth transplants are not permanent, transplantation of anterior teeth is indicated at times, to tide a child over a period of growth of the jaws or to help a teenager psychologically during a period of maturity. Clinical studies on tooth transplantation have been made by Cserepfalvi,[16] Mezrow,[51] and Hansen and Fibaek,[33] not only on anterior teeth, but on posterior teeth as well, some of which have been retained by

ankylosis for a number of years. Grossman has kept a transplanted tooth under observation for 12 years, from childhood to manhood, during an important psychologic period in the development of a person. Although tooth transplantation is an intriguing area of dental practice, its usefulness is circumscribed.

Current research in transplantation of teeth holds promise, following the experimental and clinical studies of Litwin, Söder and their colleagues.[44,47,74] The immunologic reaction to the protein in tooth substance can be eliminated by tissue culturing the tooth over an extended period of time. Söder and Lundquist have developed an operation in which the crown of the tooth is removed and endodontic treatment is carried out in the root, which is then tissue cultured.[73] After some time, an incision is made, a socket is

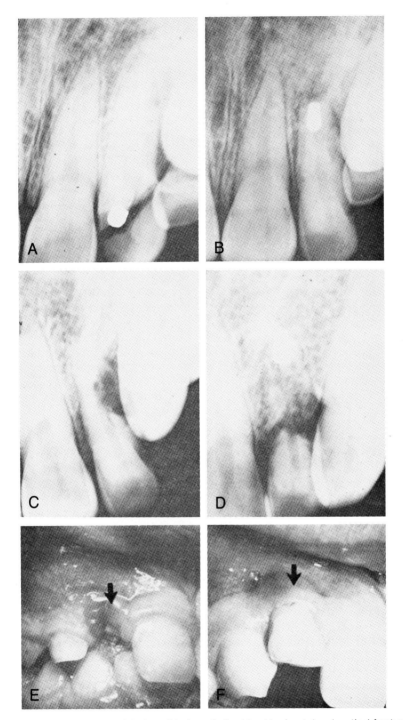

Fig. 19–9. Transplantation of an upper right lateral incisor. *A*, Combined horizontal and vertical fractures extending into the root. *B*, Tooth from a "tooth bank" 1 month after transplantation. *C*, Root resorption 3.5 years later. *D*, Radiograph 8 years later: Root resorption has progressed, but the tooth is immobile because of ankylosis. *E*, Appearance of the area before transplantation; the horizontal fragment was removed because of extreme mobility. *F*, Appearance of the tooth and gingiva 8 years later; the patient was advised to have the tooth removed if the tooth became mobile.

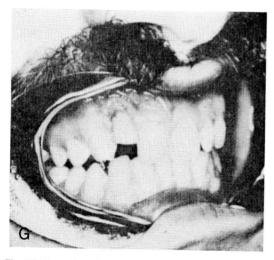

Fig. 19–9 continued. *G,* Photograph 12 years after transplantation, just prior to removal of the tooth.

prepared, and the root is submerged in the bone and is completely covered by the flap. When one sees radiographic evidence of a "take," the root is exposed, and an artificial crown is made. Such a tooth, together with others, can serve as a support for a splint or partial denture.

Youdelis and Filipchuk have described a method of transplanting and submerging a root from another part of the same mouth, later uncovering the root, preparing a post and coping, and using the root as an abutment, similar to the Söder and Lundquist technique.[83] Although failures have occurred, some roots have been functional for 7 years.

ENDODONTIC IMPLANTS

An endodontic implant is a metallic extension of the root with the object of increasing the root-to-crown ratio, to give the tooth better stability in the arch (Fig. 19–10). Souza described a metallic implant for stabilization of teeth,[75] but Orlay and Frank must be given credit for popularizing the method.[25,61]

Endodontic implants are useful for treatment of the following: (1) periodontally involved teeth requiring stabilization; (2) transverse root fracture involving loss of the apical fragment or the presence of two fragments that cannot be aligned; (3) pathologic resorption of the root apex incident to a chronic abscess; (4) a pulpless tooth with an unusually short root; (5) internal resorption affecting the integrity and strength of the root; (6) a tooth in which additional root

length is desired for improving its alveolar support.

Endodontic implants have a high failure rate (Fig. 19–11). The success of an endodontic implant depends on proper case selection and on close adherence to the following criteria: (1) routine endodontic treatment can be carried out without difficulty; that is, a normal-appearing root canal without curvature or deflection, so the implant can be inserted the desired distance and remain wholly between the labial and lingual plates of bone; and (2) alveolar bone is sufficient for retention and stability of both the tooth and the implant. In other words, a successful implant depends on careful selection of the tooth to be treated (Figs. 19–12 and 19–13). Teeth with multiple canals, curved canals with curved root apices, and calcified or obstructed canals should be avoided whenever possible. Caution must be exercised to avoid penetration by the implant of the mandibular canal, maxillary sinus, nasal fossa, or the bone plates on the labial or lingual sides of the maxilla or mandible. Teeth with insufficient bone support and a hopeless periodontal prognosis cannot be salvaged by an endodontic implant.

The Achilles heel of the endodontic implant is its apical seal. In preparing a wide apical foramen, with instrument sizes No. 60 to No. 90, the root apex is ground away by the large endodontic instruments, which can also fracture the root tip. This complication is followed by resorption of the root tip. The result is an imperfect apical seal and the formation of a periapical lesion. Holland and colleagues attributed the failure of implants in dogs' teeth to a defective seal between the implant and the root apex that resulted in small areas of periapical radiolucency, which became larger with time.[38] Zmener found Tubli-Seal* more effective in sealing endodontic implants than zinc phosphate or polycarboxylate cements, as determined by methylene-blue diffusion studies.[85] Silverbrand and associates claimed a 90% success rate for endodontic implants, despite the presence of periapical lesions in 18% of their cases.[71] Ohno and co-workers histologically examined periapical tissue around implants that were placed in dogs' teeth for up to 6 months.[59] The implant and sealer were found to be encapsulated by fibrous connective tis-

---

*Kerr Manufacturing Co., Romulus, Michigan.

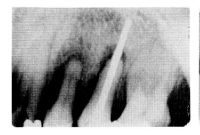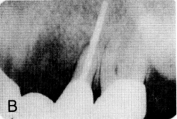

Fig. 19–10. Endodontic implant. *A*, After endodontic treatment and cementing of the implant. *B*, Recall radiograph at 6 months.

sue; apical resorption or deposition was present in 55 of 59 (93%) roots. Simon and Frank removed an endodontally implanted tooth after 3 years.[72] No corrosion of the implant material was seen under the scanning electron microscope; however, evidence of resorption of dentin and cementum was present at the root apex because of a faulty seal. Zmener has shown that Vitallium endodontic implants that have been in place, in contact with bone, for 5 or more years were corroded.[84] Goldberg reported a case in which a tooth with an endodontic implant had to be removed after 9 years for prosthetic reasons.[27] On histologic examination, a pseudo-periodontal ligament had developed and covered the cementum and the apical portion of the root.

The following are sound clinical criteria for a successful endodontic implant: (1) a

normal gingival crevice containing a normal epithelial attachment; (2) a radiographically normal attachment apparatus including the bone, cementum, and dentin; (3) a stabilized, functional, and symptomless tooth.

The disadvantages of endodontic implants, which can result in failure, are: (1) poor apical seal resulting in periapical rarefaction around the root apex; (2) extrusion of excessive sealer through the apical foramen into the periapical tissues, with resulting irritation; (3) limitation in the length of the osseous portion of implant by local anatomic factors in the maxilla or mandible, such as the maxillary sinus, nasal fossa, and mandibular canal, or labio- or linguoversion of the tooth in the jaw; (4) perforation of the lateral root surface or perforation of a curved root near the root apex; and (5) a structurally weakened tooth, instrumented to a much larger size than usual, to receive an inflexible implant, which may fracture during function.

Technique

The equipment needed for endodontic implantation is the same as for endodontic treatment, with the addition of a series of extra-long reamers, 40 mm, in sequential sizes and implants of corresponding size. The steps in technique are as follows (Fig. 19–14). First, anesthetize the tooth and involved area with a local anesthetic. Next, with the rubber dam in place, aseptically complete the usual treatment of access preparation, enlargement, and irrigation of the root canal. The access preparation should differ from the usual in that it must be larger and wider in the clinical crown, to accommodate the placement of a rigid implant that requires "straight-line" insertion into the canal. In addition, the root canal must be enlarged to at least the size of a No. 60 instrument. In a tooth with multiple canals or an apical root curvature, the canals should be

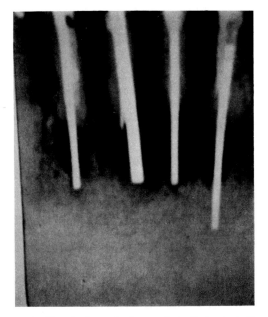

Fig. 19–11. Radiograph of an endodontic implant: Periapical areas of rarefaction developed 6 months after placement of implants.

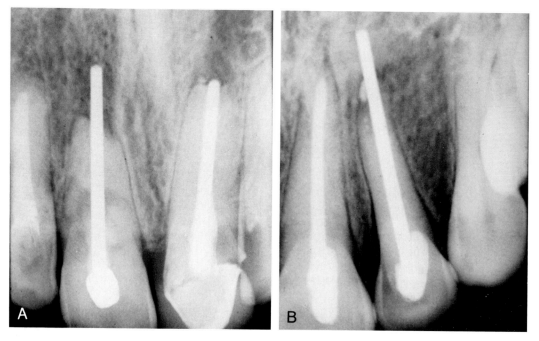

Fig. 19–12. *A,* Maxillary central incisor fracture in two places: An area of rarefaction is present, along with diagonal root resorption; a Vitallium endodontic implant was used to unite the fractured segments and to stabilize the tooth. *B,* The patient was in an automobile accident, and the lateral incisor was partially avulsed; note the thickened periodontal ligament space of that tooth as well as of the adjacent central incisor, near the cervix; the lateral incisor was stabilized with a Vitallium endodontic implant.

filled and sealed with gutta-percha and cement in the usual manner. Unfilled canals or a partially unfilled canal in a curved root tip, as occurs with penetration of the osseous layer from the root canal in a "straight-line" preparation, will result in failure and formation of subsequent periapical rarefaction. A marker is then set on the 40-mm reamers at a level equivalent to the length of the tooth plus the number of millimeters the implant will extend beyond the root apex. The first 40-mm reamer used to perforate the root apex should be several sizes smaller than the last-sized instrument used to complete the preparation of the root canal. The last 40-mm reamer used should be at least equivalent in size to the last endodontic instrument used in the root canal alone, and the bone is reamed to the desired length. Irrigate the root canal with anesthetic solution or sterile saline solution rather than sodium hypochlorite, which can irritate the periapical tissue. Irrigation of the canals debrides as well as controls hemorrhage within a few minutes. Dry the canal with sterile absorbent points.

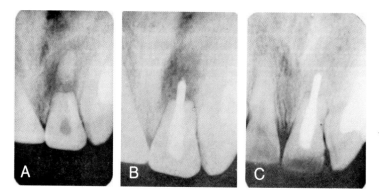

Fig. 19–13. Endodontic implant. *A,* Fracture of a root, with mobility of the crown. *B,* After removal of the root tip and cementing of the endodontic implant. *C,* Recall radiograph at 9 months: Bone repair is evident, and the tooth is stable.

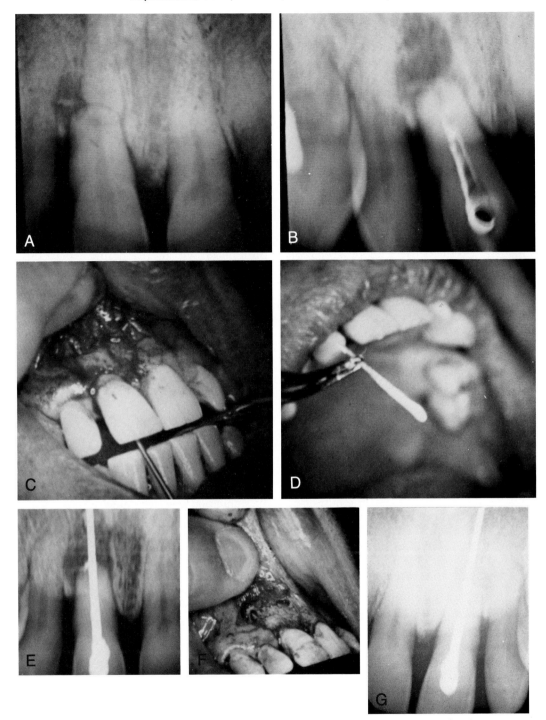

Fig. 19–14. Endodontic implant in an upper central incisor with an apical root fracture. *A*, Diagnostic radiograph: Apical root fracture; the tooth is stable despite minimal root structure and bony support. *B*, Treatment radiograph: The fractured root tip has been removed, and the root canal is instrumented; the opaque material lining the walls of the root canal is debris. *C*, Labial view of the surgical site: The implant extends into bone through the root canal. *D*, The measured, fitted, and prepared implant is coated with cement prior to placement through the root canal into the periapical bony cavity. *E*, Radiograph immediately after implantation. *F*, The implant has been cemented; it extends beyond the cavity into cancellous bone. *G*, Recall radiograph at 6 months.

Select an implant of equivalent size to the last instrument used, score it lightly to indicate the desired length, that is, from the occlusal tip through the root canal to the exact length cut into the cancellous bone, and insert it into the root and bone. The implant must fit tightly and must penetrate the bone to the prepared length. If necessary, enlarge the root canal a little more to accommodate the implant, but the implant must fit at the apical foramen, Dry the root canal again. Shorten the implant at its apical tip by 1 mm, to ensure that it will seat snuggly and will not bind in the cut osseous bed. Insert a plugger into the access opening until it binds, and measure the exact length it can be inserted unimpeded into the canal. This plugger will be used to seat the implant during cementation; because the butt end of a Vitallium or chrome-cobalt implant must be cut off prior to insertion into the tooth because of the hardness of the metal.

Using a diamond or carborundum disc, cut the butt end of the fitted implant and remove a length equivalent to that measurement obtained by inserting the plugger blade into the root canal. Insert cement into the dried canal (Grossman suggests a polycarboxylate cement; Frank suggests AH 26 cement), and try to avoid cement extrusion beyond the canal. Using a hemostat to hold the sterilized implant, insert the implant slowly into the canal and bone. Seat the implant by pressing the plugger blade firmly against the butt end of the implant until it binds completely in the canal. When a post-type crown is to be made, seat the implant to the level corresponding to the midroot and leave sufficient space to cement a post-core crown afterward.

ENDODONTIC TREATMENT AND OVERLAY DENTURES

The pervasiveness of endodontic treatment is felt in several branches of clinical dentistry. The orthodontist often requests that a first permanent molar be saved by endodontic treatment because it is the keystone of the dental arch. The pedodontist prefers that a tooth be treated endodontally rather than be extracted, to prevent a collapse of the bite. The periodontist requests that the pulp be removed because of hypersensitivity following periodontal treatment or that a tooth be treated conjointly because of a periodontal-endodontal lesion. The crown-and-bridge prosthodontist asks that certain teeth be treated endodontally to permit restoration to proper occlusion, and the full-denture prosthodontist often uses root-supported complete dentures (overlay dentures), which require that the remaining teeth be treated endodontally, so that the crowns can be reduced in height.

An overlay denture is a complete denture that derives support from the mucosal soft tissues and auxiliary support from endodontally treated teeth that have been reduced in length. These treated teeth may or may not have metal attachments. The supporting or contact area between the denture and the reduced teeth may be a gold coping, a chrome-cobalt bearing area, a stud attachment, or a thimble crown, or the denture may derive support by simply resting on an amalgam surface of a reduced tooth.

Basker and associates reported cephalometric measurements over a 5-year period that showed an average bone loss of 0.6 mm in the overdenture group, as against 5.2 mm in the conventional denture group.[11] Moreover, although not so well documented, sensory feedback from the periodontal ligament of the retained roots is a factor in masticatory function.

Roots may be endodontally treated and submerged under the mucosa to retain alveolar bone for support of full dentures, a procedure termed root submergence. Whitaker and Shankle studied the reaction of submerged root segments with vital pulps and root-filled root segments in monkeys.[80] In 2 to 25 weeks, vital segments had a higher success rate than those with obturated canals. When the procedure was successful, a cementum-like tissue was seen between the connective tissue and the dentin. Bowles and Daniel doubt the success over the long term of overdentures placed over submerged roots for preserving the alveolar ridge because of chronic inflammation of the pulp with abscess formation.[13]

Reames and associates treated 8 teeth of 2 monkeys endodontally, surgically reduced the roots to between 2 and 3 mm below the crest of alveolar bone, then studied the adjacent tissues histologically.[65] Bone formed over the amputation sites, and soft tissue covered the roots, except in 2 cases. Although some inflammation was present, it may have been due to the coronal sealant. Plata and Kallin reduced vital teeth about 2 mm below the alveolar bone in dogs and sutured the tissue to cover the submerged roots.[64] Histologic examination disclosed that the pulps remained vital, and the cut dentin was covered with cementum. Ground and colleagues treated root canals of dogs, extracted the teeth and reduced the roots so they would be 2 to 3 mm below the crest of alveolar bone, intentionally replanted the roots, and sutured the flaps.[31] Some coronal osseous regeneration occurred after 60 days. Inflammation from Tubli-Seal may have interfered with formation of more coronal bone. O'Neal and associates filled the root canals of lower premolar teeth of dogs and then reduced them to 2 mm below the bone level.[60] On histologic examination, no resorption of the submerged roots had occurred after 120 days, and some new bone was seen over the reduced root surfaces, but inflammation was present around the sealer.

One of the problems of submerging roots is dehiscence, that is, splitting open of soft tissue with exposure of the root. Masterson reduced vital teeth 2 mm below the crestal bone and observed dehiscence in 6 of 10 cases.[50] Garver and colleagues observed dehiscence in a number of their 28 cases and concluded that sectioning the teeth on a horizontal plane could be improved by contouring of the retained roots.[26]

Another problem with abutment teeth for overdentures is caries. Toolson found that the application of fluorides or silver nitrate to abutment teeth produced a significant decrease in caries, when compared to those that received no preventive treatment.[76] Fenton and Hahn also observed a reduction in caries after the application of a fluoride gel.[21] Reitz and associates,[66] however, have stated that periodontal disease is more of a problem than caries. Although they have recommended the application of fluorides, they have also urged better oral hygiene for prevention of periodontal disease.

Because the height of the ridge is maintained in the region of the supporting teeth or roots, less alveolar resorption occurs with an overlay denture than with a full denture. Moreover, because of the reduced height of the teeth, the root-to-crown ratio is improved, so the teeth are less susceptible to periodontal involvement. Furthermore, proprioceptive discrimination is more sensitive in wearers of overlay dentures than in those with complete dentures, according to Loiselle and colleagues,[46] Pacer and Bowman,[63] Richard and associates,[67] Nagasawa and colleagues,[53] and Kapur and Collister.[40]

Schweitzer and co-workers have stated: "the retention of a few natural teeth over which a complete denture may be telescoped provides better retention and stabilization than is possible with the usual complete denture."[69]

On the other hand, an overlay denture may be bulky if the labial surface of the tooth cannot be reduced or if a coping or stud is used for additional retention. Moreover, teeth under overlay dentures are more susceptible to caries and the development of gingival pockets.

Endodontic treatment is carried out in the usual manner for teeth that are to serve as supporting abutments for an overlay denture. Gutta-percha should be the filling material of choice and it should preferably not extend beyond the apical foramen. In some cases, when the teeth are short, an endodontic implant rather than the usual gutta-percha cone should be considered.

BIBLIOGRAPHY

1. American Association of Endodontists: J. Am. Dent. Assoc., 107:706, 1983.
2. Andreasen, J.O.: J. Endod., 7:245, 1981.
3. Andreasen, J.O.: Swed. Dent. J., 5:115, 1981.
4. Andreasen, J.O.: Traumatic Injuries of the Teeth, 2nd Ed. Philadelphia, W.B. Saunders, 1981, p. 184.
5. Andreasen, J.O., and Hjörting-Hansen, F.: Acta Odontol. Scand., 24:263, 287, 1966.
6. Andreasen, J.O., and Kristerson, L.J.: J. Endod., 7:349, 1981.
7. Andreasen, J.O., et al.: Int. J. Oral Surg., 7:104, 1978.
8. Barbakow, F.H., et al.: J. Endod., 4:265, 1978, and 7:302, 1981.
9. Barry, G.N.: J. Am. Dent. Assoc., 92:412, 1976.
10. Bartels, H.A., and Blechman, H.: Oral Surg., 12:1141, 1959.
11. Basker, K.M., et al.: Br. Dent. J., 154:285, 1983.
12. Blomlöf, L.: J. Dent. Res., 62:912, 1983.
13. Bowles, W.H., and Daniel, R.E.: J. Am. Dent. Assoc., 307:429, 1983.
14. Caffesse, R.G., et al.: Oral Surg., 44:666, 1977.
15. Coccia, C.T.: J. Endod., 6:413, 1980.
16. Cserepfalvi, M.P.: J. Am. Dent. Assoc., 67:35, 1963.
17. Cvek, M., et al.: Odontol. Revy., 25:43, 1974.
18. Deeb, E.: In Transactions of the Fourth International Conference on Endodontics. Edited by L.I. Grossman. Philadelphia, University of Pennsylvania, 1968, p. 147.
19. Emmertsen, E., and Andreasen, J.O.: Acta Odontol. Scand., 24:327, 1966.
20. Fauchard, P.: The Surgeon Dentist. Vol. 1. Translated by L. Lindsay. London, Butterworth, 1946, p. 40.
21. Fenton, A.H., and Hahn, H.: J. Prosthet. Dent., 40:492, 1978.
22. Flanagan, V.D., and Myers, H.I.: Oral Surg., 11:1179, 1958.
23. Fong, C.: Seminars in Dental Tissue Transplantation. University of California, 1965, p. 2.

24. Fong, C., and Berger, J.E.: Oral Surg., *29*:275, 1970.
25. Frank, A.L.: J. Am. Dent. Assoc., *74*:451, 1967.
26. Garver, D.G., et al.: J. Prosthet. Dent., *40*:23, 1978.
27. Goldberg, F.: Int. Endod. J., *15*:77, 1982.
28. Grossman, L.I.: J. Am. Dent. Assoc., *92*:1111, 1966.
29. Grossman, L.I., Chacker, F.M.: *In* Transactions of the Fourth International Conference on Endodontics. Edited by L.I. Grossman. Philadelphia, University of Pennsylvania, 1968, p. 197.
30. Grossman, L.I., and Ship, I.: Oral Surg., *29*:899, 1970.
31. Ground, T., et al.: Oral Surg., *46*:114, 1978.
32. Hamner, J.E., et al.: J. Am. Dent. Assoc., *81*:662, 1970.
33. Hansen, J., and Fibaek, B.: Int. Dent. J., *22*:270, 1972.
34. Hasselgren, G., et al.: Oral Surg., *44*:106, 1977.
35. Heithersay, G.S.: Aust. Dent. J., *20*:63, 1975.
36. Henning, F.R.: Aust. Dent. J., *10*:306, 1965.
37. Hines, F.B.: J. Orthod., *75*:1, 1979.
38. Holland, R., et al.: Rev. Asoc. Odontal. Argent., *65*:67, 1977.
39. Hurst, R.V.: J. Dent. Res., *51*:1183, 1972.
40. Kapur, K.K., and Collister, P.: *In* Second Symposium on Oral Sensation and Perception. Edited by J.F. Bosnia. Springfield, IL, Charles C Thomas, 1970, p. 332.
41. Kemp, W., et al.: J. Endod., *3*:30, 1977.
42. Kingsbury, B.C., and Wiesenbaugh, J.M.: J. Am. Dent. Assoc., *83*:1053, 1971.
43. Knight, M.K., et al.: Oral Surg., *18*:227, 1964.
44. Litwin, J., et al.: Scand. J. Dent. Res., *79*:536, 1971.
45. Löe, H., and Waerhaug, J.: J. Arch. Oral Biol., *3*:176, 1961.
46. Loiselle, R.J., et al.: J. Prosthet. Dent., *28*:4, 1972.
47. Lundquist, G., and Söder, P.O.: Transactions of the Fourth International Conference on Oral Surgery. Amsterdam, 1971.
48. Mahajan, S.K., and Sedhu, S.S.: Aust. Dent. J., *26*:42, 1981.
49. Massler, M.: Dent. Clin. North Am., *18*:455, 1974.
50. Masterson, M.P.: J. Prosthet. Dent., *41*:12, 1979.
51. Mezrow, R.R.: Oral Surg., *17*:375, 1964.
52. Mincer, H.H., and Jennings, B.R.: J. Dent. Res., *49*:381, 1970.
53. Nagasawa, T., et al.: J. Prosthet. Dent., *42*:12, 1979.
54. Nasjleti, C.E.: Oral Surg., *53*:557, 1982.
55. Nasjleti, C.E., et al.: J. Dent. Res., *57*:650, 1978.
56. Natiella, J., et al.: Oral Surg., *29*:397, 1970.
57. Nolbandian, J., and Hellden, L.: Oral Surg., *54*:452, 1982.
58. Nordenram, A., and Bergman, G.: Oral Surg., *29*:944, 1970.
59. Ohno, Y., et al.: Jpn. J. Cons. Dent., *20*:117, 1977.
60. O'Neal, R.A., et al.: Oral Surg., *45*:803, 1978.
61. Orlay, H.J.: Br. Dent. J., *108*:118, 1960.
62. Oswald, R.J., et al.: J. Endod., *6*:546, 1980.
63. Pacer, F.J., and Bowman, D.C.: J. Prosthet. Dent., *33*:602, 1975.
64. Plata, R.L., and Kallin, F.F.: Oral Surg., *42*:100, 1976.
65. Reames, R.L., et al.: J. Endod., *1*:367, 1975.
66. Reitz, P., et al.: J. Prosthet. Dent., *43*:457, 1980.
67. Richard, G.F., et al.: J. Prosthet. Dent., *38*:16, 1977.
68. Robinson, P.J., and Rowlands, D.T.: Transplantation, *14*:787, 1972, and *16*:261, 1973.
69. Schweitzer, J.M., et al.: J. Prosthet. Dent., *26*:357, 1971.
70. Shulman, L.B.: Oral Surg., *17*:389, 1964.
71. Silverbrand, H., et al.: Oral Surg., *45*:920, 1979.
72. Simon, J.H., and Frank, A.L.: J. Endod., *6*:450, 1980.
73. Söder, P.O., and Lundquist, G.: Transactions of the Fourth International Conference on Oral Surgery. Amsterdam, 1971.
74. Söder, P.O., et al.: J. Dent. Res., *85*:164, 1977.
75. Souza, M.: Odontol. Uraguay, *7*:13, 1953.
76. Toolson, L.B.: J. Prosthet Dent., *40*:486, 1978.
77. Van Hassel, H.J., et al.: J. Endod., *6*:506, 1980.
78. Weill, D.: J. Am. Dent. Assoc., *30*:782, 1943.
79. Weinreb, M.M., and Sharav, Y.: Int. Dent. J., *21*:488, 1971.
80. Whitaker, D.D., and Shankle, R.J.: Oral Surg., *37*:919, 1974.
81. White, E.: J. Endod., *1*:247, 1975.
82. Woehrle, R.R.: J. Dent. Res., *55*:235, 1976.
83. Youdelis, R.A., and Filipchuk, C.E.: J. Prosthet. Dent., *35*:307, 1976.
84. Zmener, O.: J. Endod., *9*:486, 1983.
85. Zmener, O.: Oral Surg., *52*:635, 1981.

Appendix A

Single-Visit Endodontics

Total endodontic care of a tooth in a single visit is an old concept in clinical practice. It was displaced by multivisit procedures as endodontic treatments became more exacting and sophisticated and thereby required more time to complete properly. Dentists were taught that endodontic care required multiple visits, and as a result, single-visit care fell by the wayside. Nevertheless, it never quite disappeared, and clinicians continued to practice single-visit endodontics, usually surreptitiously, because such treatment was considered radical and substandard in quality.

Historically, the single-visit procedure can be traced through the literature for at least 100 years.[3,7,8,11] Although the concept remained constant, the techniques varied. In the early years, pressure anesthesia was followed by root canal sterilization using hydrogen dioxide and sodium dioxide.[16,21] Root canals were filled with chloropercha, guttapercha, and formapercha. In 1901, Trallero used a bichloride wash, hot platinum-wire sterilization, and zinc oxide-eugenol and xeroform paste fill.[20] Inglis, in 1904, anesthetized with cocaine, applied the rubber dam, "sterilized" with potassium permanganate, and filled with chloropercha, sectional guttapercha, or formapercha; he excluded all "acute cases" and expected "absolute success when directions are followed."[9] In the same year, Philips reported that teeth he treated were "in perfect condition after three years," "color as when alive," and "no abscess in a thousand."[16] In 1908, Barnes irrigated root canals with sulfuric acid and filled them with chloropercha, but he excluded "abscessed roots" from treatment.[1] Claims of unparalleled success were largely testimonial and unsubstantiated.

In the middle of the twentieth century came a resurgence of single-visit endodontics. Initially, it started with the immediate root resection,[2,10,14] that is, endodontic treatment including apicoectomy in a single visit, but some clinicians began to practice single-visit endodontics without periapical surgical procedures (except in exacerbations when "artificial fistulation" was employed to reduce pain and swelling.[18])

In 1955, Lorinczy-Landgraf and Polocz reported that 10% of 1200 gangrenous teeth, treated in single visits, caused moderate to severe postoperative pain, with 3% requiring trephination.[12] Two years later, these investigators reported 82% healing. In 1959 Ferranti compared postoperative sequelae following single visit and 2-visit procedures and found little difference.[5] In the same year, Sargenti and Richter advocated either single-visit or multivisit endodontics and claimed that the root canal filling material, containing paraformaldehyde and other ingredients, prevented flare-ups and failure.[18] Fox and associates, in 1970, treated 291 teeth in single visits and reported severe pain within 24 hours in 7% of those patients.[6] These investigators indicated that more pain occurred postoperatively in teeth that had no radiographic areas, in female patients, and in teeth that had been overinstrumented or overfilled.

In 1978, Ether and colleagues compared single-visit and 2-visit endodontic procedures in 564 vital teeth and found moderate

349

to severe pain in 9% of the single-visit group and in 5% of the 2-visit group.[4] Soltanoff, in the same year, treated 80 teeth in single visits and reported slightly more pain in those patients than in those whose teeth were treated with multivisit procedures; he found similar healing in both groups.[19]

Oliet, in a long-term study, compared single-visit and two-visit endodontics for postoperative pain and swelling as well as healing.[15] Excluded from this study were patients with acute symptoms that were relieved by establishing drainage, such as patients with acute alveolar abscess, those whose teeth had a persistent, continuous flow of exudate and, those whose teeth had anatomic difficulties and so could not be treated fully within the prescribed appointment time. Examination of data showed that only 4 teeth in both groups had slight swelling that disappeared within 48 hours; 3% of the 264 teeth treated in 2 visits, caused severe pain within 24 hours, and approximately 7% of the single-visit group had moderate pain, as compared to 4% of the 2-visit group. The difference was not statistically significant. Similarly, no significant difference existed between both groups when they were compared according to the following categories: (1) tooth morphology: anterior teeth, premolars, and molars; (2) sex; (3) diagnosis: teeth with vital pulps versus teeth with necrotic pulps and areas of rarefaction evident on a radiograph; and (4) filling terminus: teeth filled short or within 0.5 mm of the radiographic apex of the root canal. Overfilling of the root canals of teeth treated in a single visit resulted in moderate to severe pain in 25% of cases, a statistically significant difference. Younger patients, aged 10 to 39 years, had significantly more pain than older patients.

In the foregoing study, 153 teeth treated in a single visit were compared for healing, after a minimum of 18 months, with 185 teeth treated in 2 visits. Approximately 89% of teeth in both groups healed. No significant differences were found in healing when other factors, such as age, sex, tooth morphology, and pulp status (vital versus nonvital with periapical area) were compared. A significant increase of failure to heal (18%) was noted in teeth treated in a single visit when the final filling of laterally condensed gutta-percha extruded beyond the root apex.

Rudner and Oliet described a concept and clinical technique for treating teeth in a single visit.[17] They reported that postoperative pain and swelling, as well as healing, remained equivalent to that of multivisit endodontics, provided one had an accurate diagnosis, proper case selection, and skill in technique.

BIBLIOGRAPHY

1. Barnes, H.: Summary (Dent.), 28:758, 1908.
2. Camara, J.A.: Dent. Surv., 30:1005, 1954.
3. Dodge, J.S.: Dent. Cosmos, 29:234, 1887.
4. Ether, S., et al.: J. Farm. Odontol., 8:215, 1978.
5. Ferranti, P.: Dent. Dig., 65:490, 1959.
6. Fox, J., et al.: Oral Surg., 30:123, 1970.
7. Gutmann, J.L.: J. Endod., 4:165, 1978.
8. Hofheinz, R.H.: Dent. Cosmos, 34:182, 1892.
9. Inglis, O.: Br. J. Dent. Sci., 47:122, 1904.
10. Kaplan, H., et al.: N.Y. J. Dent., 30:253, 1960.
11. Kells, C.E.: Dent. Cosmos., 29:366, 1887.
12. Lorinczy-Landgraf, V.E., and Polocz, G.: Dtsch, Zahnarztl. Z., 10:742, 1955, and 12:438, 1957.
13. Mainguy, H.: Dent. Cosmos, Jan.: 126, 1912.
14. Okun, J.: N.Y. J. Dent., 23:403, 1953.
15. Oliet, S.: J. Endod., 9:147, 1983.
16. Philips, T.S.: Br. J. Dent. Sci., 36:16, 1904.
17. Rudner, W.L., and Oliet, S.: Compend. Contin. Ed., 2:63, 1981.
18. Sargenti, A., and Richter, S.L.: Rationalized Root Canal Treatment. New York, AGSA Scientific Publications, 1959.
19. Soltanoff, W.: J. Endod., 4:278, 1978.
20. Trallero, T.: Dent. Cosmos., 43:1405, 1901.
21. Zsigmondy, L.: Dent. Cosmos, 34:126, 1912.

Appendix B

A Radiographic Technique for Endodontics*

Radiographs are the only visual method of gaining clinical knowledge of teeth and periapical tissues; therefore, they are essential to the practice of endodontics. Radiographs are indispensable for the diagnosis and prognosis of endodontic cases and are the most reliable method of monitoring endodontic treatment.

Proper positioning and stabilization of the radiographic film during endodontic procedures become difficult because of the interference from the protruding rubber-dam clamp or root canal instruments or obturating material protruding from the access cavity. That visualization of the tooth for proper film positioning and cone angulation is impeded by the presence of the rubber dam makes this process a guessing proposition.

RADIOGRAPHIC TECHNICAL REQUIREMENTS

1. The image of the tooth being evaluated or undergoing endodontic therapy should be in the center of the radiograph.
2. Radiographs should show at least 5 mm of bone surrounding the apex of the tooth being evaluated or undergoing endodontic therapy.
3. If a periapical lesion is too large to fit in one periapical film, supplemental diagnostic radiographs must be made.
4. A single radiograph taken from one direction only may not provide sufficient diagnostic information when multirooted teeth or teeth with curved roots are involved endodontally; under these circumstances, consideration should be given to taking at least 2 periapical radiographs to help gain a 3-dimensional perspective. One radiograph should be taken at normal vertical and horizontal angulation, the other at a 20° change in horizontal angle from either mesial or distal direction (Fig. Appendix B–1).
5. If a sinus tract is present, a tracing radiograph should be taken. This procedure is accomplished by carefully threading a No. 40 gutta-percha cone into the tract and taking a radiograph to identify the origin of the tract (Fig. Appendix B–2). This technique is also useful for localization and depth marking of certain periodontal defects.
6. Correct processing of the radiographic film is essential to evaluate success or failure of the case at a later date.

For endodontic pre- and postoperative radiographs, the long-cone paralleling technique is preferred over the short-cone

*Text and figures slightly modified from Del Rio, C., Canales, M.L., and Preece, J.W.: A Radiographic Technique for Endodontics. San Antonio, University of Texas Health Science Center, 1986. Reproduced by permission.

351

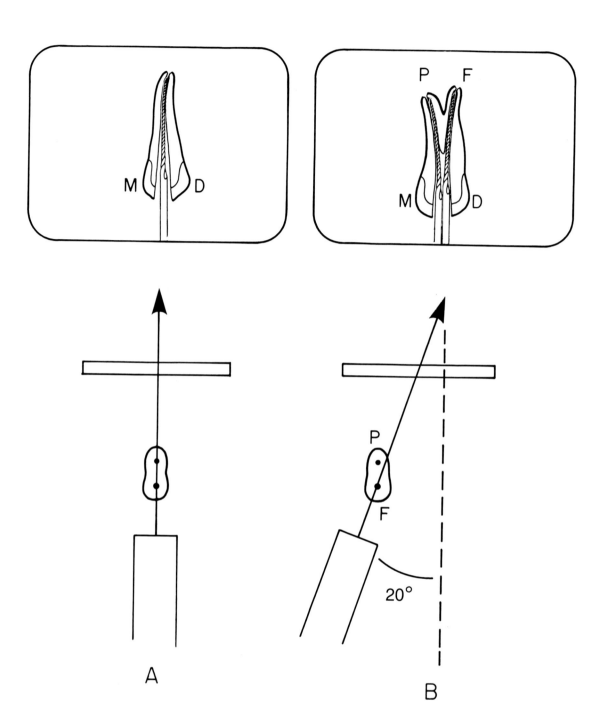

Fig. B—1. *A*, Vertical and horizontal angulation for exposing a periapical radiograph of an upper first premolar. *B*, Radiograph at a 20° horizontal angular change.

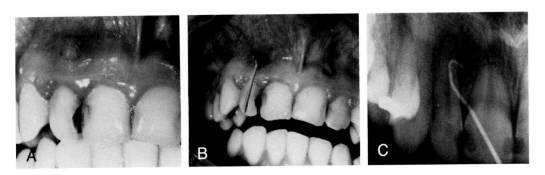

Fig. B–2. *A* to *C*, Radiograph of a sinus tract. *A*, Labial view: sinus tract. *B*, Gutta-percha cone threaded through the sinus tract. *C*, Radiograph of gutta-percha cone tracer in sinus tract.

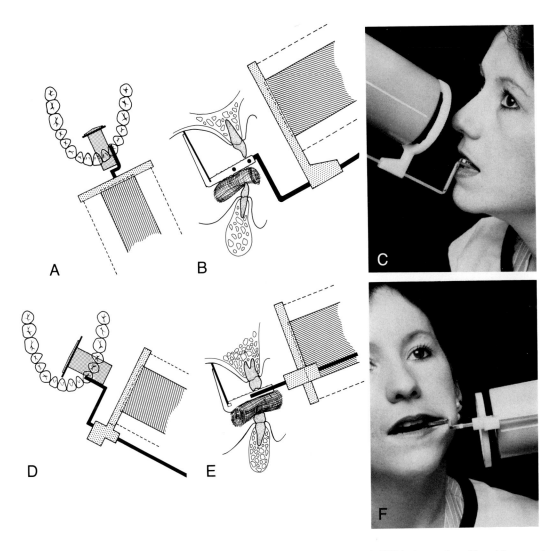

Fig. B–3. *A* to *C*, Paralleling radiographic technique. See text for details. *A* to *C*, XCP instrument positioned for exposing a radiograph of the maxillary lateral incisor. *D* to *F*, XCP instrument positioned for exposing a radiograph of the mandibular premolars.

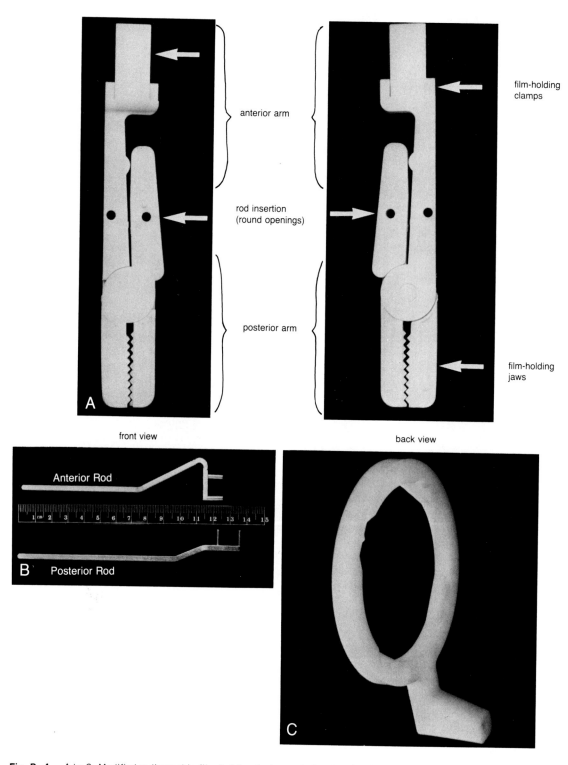

front view

back view

anterior arm

film-holding
clamps

rod insertion
(round openings)

posterior arm

film-holding
jaws

Anterior Rod

Posterior Rod

Fig. B–4. *A* to *C,* Modified radiographic film-holding insrument. See text for details.

bisecting-angle technique because dimensional distortion is less, the image is sharper, and the same angulations are easily reproduced. The paralleling technique may be accomplished with the aid of the Rinn XCP* instrument (Fig. Appendix B–3).

To overcome the difficulties of making radiographs during endodontic procedures, a Rinn Eezee Grip film holding instrument was modified. This modified instrument simplifies the problems of positioning and stabilizing the radiographic film, as well as positioning and angulating the x-ray tube head and cone with the long-cone paralleling technique for endodontic working radiographs (Fig. Appendix B–4).

RADIOGRAPHIC TECHNIQUE FOR ANTERIOR TEETH

1. Assembly of the endodontic film holder
   a. Hold the instrument in the palm of the hand with anterior arm of the instrument up and the label facing away from the operator (Fig. Appendix B–5).
   b. Insert the radiographic film in the anterior arm of the instrument. The front of the film is inserted with the plastic clamps facing the operator (Fig. Appendix B–6).
   c. Holding the instrument in the foregoing position, insert the round prongs of the anterior stainless steel rod into the two small round openings until it is flush with the arms of the instrument (Fig. Appendix B–7).
   d. Slide the beam-alignment ring onto the rod and push it within 2 in. of the film-holding portion of the instrument. Be sure the film is centered in the ring (Fig. Appendix B–8).
2. Taking the radiograph
   a. Remove the rubber-dam frame.
   b. Insert the assembled instrument, and ensure that the tooth is in the center of the film and the film is parallel to the long axis of the tooth (Fig. Appendix B–9). The edge of the film contacting the soft tissues should be about 1.5 to 2.5 cm palatal to the incisal edge of the tooth being radiographed. In the mandibular arch,

this positions the edge of the film away from the muscle attachments and allows the floor of the mouth to flex to accommodate the depth of the film packet.
   c. Instruct the patient to hold the instrument firmly and apply gentle pressure against the incisal third of the teeth in the opposite arch.
   d. Slide the beam-alignment ring along the rod gently, until it lightly contacts the skin.
   e. Align the x-ray tube with the rod and beam-alignment ring to obtain correct vertical and horizontal angulations (Fig. Appendix B–10).
   f. Make the exposure.
   g. Replace the rubber-dam frame.

RADIOGRAPHIC TECHNIQUE FOR POSTERIOR TEETH

1. Assembly of the endodontic film holder
   a. Hold the instrument vertically with the label facing the operator (Fig. Appendix B–11).
   b. Insert the edge of the film with the embossed dot between the jaws of the instrument until it is flush with the bottom edge, close, and lock the jaws (Fig. Appendix B–12).
   c. Holding the instrument with the film-holding jaws toward the patient, insert the round prongs of the posterior rod into the small, round openings. The rod should point to the patient's right for mandibular left or maxillary right radiographs (Fig. Appendix B–13). For mandibular right or maxillary left radiographs, the rod should point to the patient's left (Fig. Appendix B–14). The front of the film should always face in the same direction as the rod.
   d. Slide the beam-alignment ring onto the rod until it is about 2 in. from the film-holding portion of the instrument. Be sure the film is centered in the ring (Fig. Appendix B–15).
2. Taking the radiograph
   a. Remove the rubber-dam frame.
   b. Insert the assembled instrument, and make sure that the tooth is in the center of the film and the film is

---

*Rinn Corp., Elgin, Illinois.

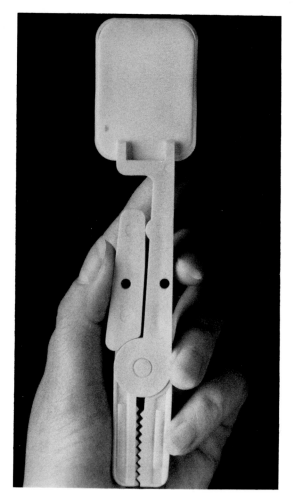

Fig. B—6. Radiographic film correctly inserted in holder.

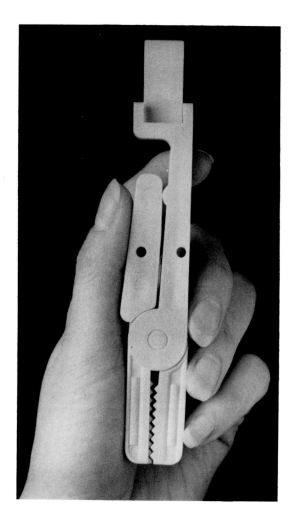

Fig. B—5. Correct method of holding an endodontic film holder for anterior teeth.

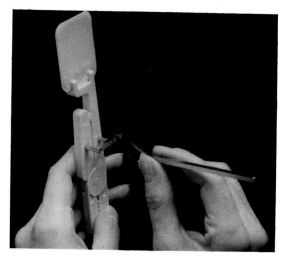

Fig. B—7. Anterior rod inserted in radiographic film holder.

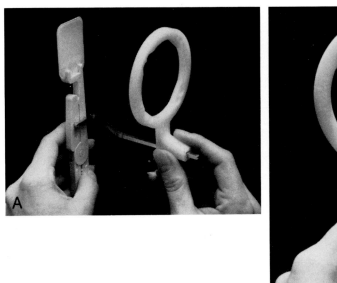

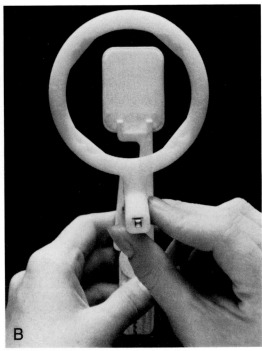

Fig. B–8.   *A* and *B*, Beam-alignment ring in place on an endodontic film holder.

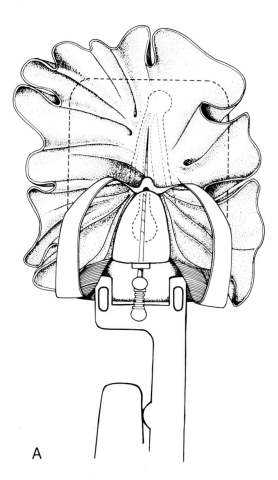

Fig. B–9.   *A* and *B*, Radiographic technique for anterior teeth. See text for details.

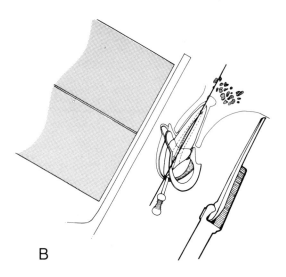

A   B

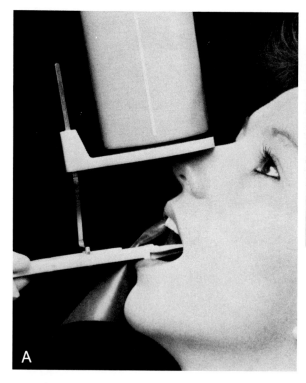

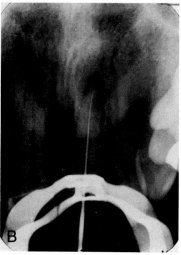

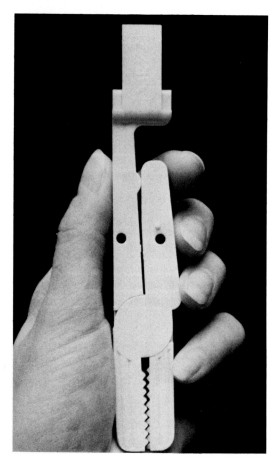

Fig. B–10. *A* and *B*, Alignment for correct radiographic angulation. See text for details.

Fig. B–11. Correct method of holding a film holder for posterior teeth.

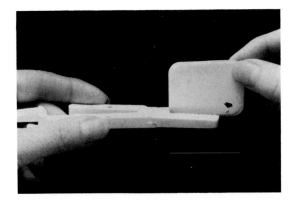

Fig. B–12. Radiographic film correctly inserted in holder, for posterior teeth. The arrow points to the embossed dot on the film.

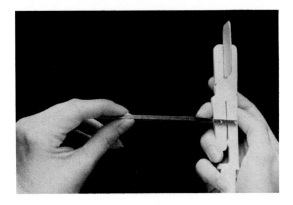

Fig. B–13. Posterior rod inserted in radiographic film holder, for mandibular left or maxillary right radiographs.

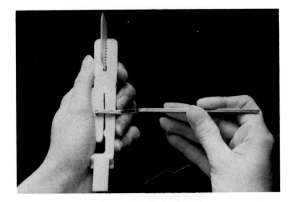

Fig. B–14. Posterior rod inserted in radiographic film holder for mandibular right or maxillary left radiographs.

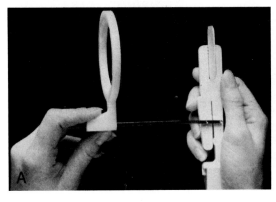
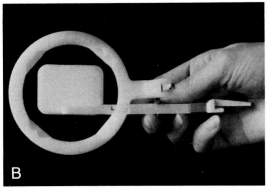

Fig. B–15. A and B, Beam-alignment ring in place for radiographs of posterior teeth. See text for details.

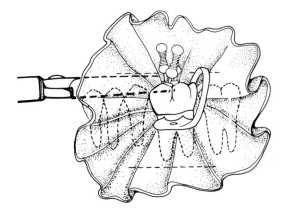

Fig. B—16. Radiographic technique for posterior teeth. See text for details.

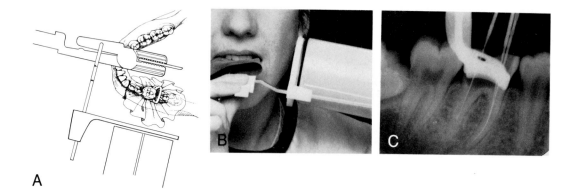

Fig. B—17. *A* to *C*, Radiographic alignment for posterior teeth. See text for details.

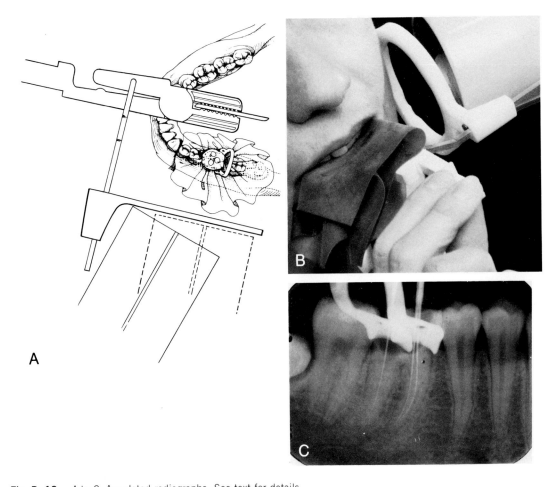

Fig. B–18. *A* to *C,* Angulated radiographs. See text for details.

parallel to the long axis of the tooth (Fig. Appendix B–16).

c. Instruct the patient to hold the instrument firmly in position and apply gentle pressure against the incisal edges of the anterior teeth in the same arch. For mandibular radiographs, position the film between the teeth and the tongue, and make sure that the lower edge of the film does not impinge on the muscle attachments in the floor of the mouth. Care should be taken that the patient does not displace the film by moving the tongue or swallowing when one is making mandibular radiographs.

d. Slide the beam-alignment ring along the rod gently until it lightly contacts the skin.

e. Align the x-ray tube with the rod and beam-alignment ring to obtain correct vertical and horizontal angulations (Fig. Appendix B–17).

f. Make the exposure.

g. Replace the rubber-dam frame.

3. Angulated radiographs

a. Angulated radiographs can be obtained by moving the cone 20° in a mesial or distal horizontal projection (Fig. Appendix B–18).

b. If a change in the vertical projection is needed, it can be accomplished by raising or lowering the cone the desired number of degrees.

BIBLIOGRAPHY

1. Paquette, O.E., Segall, R.O., and del Rio, C.E.: Modified film holder for endodontics. J. Endod., *5*:158, 1979.

Index

Page numbers in *italics* indicate figures; page numbers followed by "t" indicate tables.